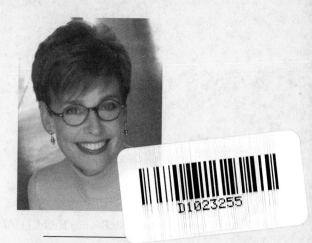

---

*About the Author*

---

JUDITH REICHMAN, M.D., is a gynecologist who practices and teaches at Cedars-Sinai Medical Center and UCLA in Los Angeles. She appears regularly on NBC's *Today* show as a contributor on women's health issues, and she co-wrote and hosted two acclaimed PBS series, *Straight Talk on Menopause* and *More Straight Talk on Menopause*. She is the author of three bestsellers, *I'm Too Young to Get Old; I'm Not in the Mood;* and *Relax, This Won't Hurt*. Dr. Reichman lives in Los Angeles with her husband and is the mother of two daughters.

ALSO BY JUDITH REICHMAN, M.D.

*Relax, This Won't Hurt:*
*Painless Answers to Women's Most Pressing Health Questions*

*I'm Not in the Mood:*
*What Every Woman Should Know About Improving Her Libido*

*I'm Too Young to Get Old:*
*Health Care for Women After Forty*

JUDITH REICHMAN, M.D.

# SLOW YOUR CLOCK DOWN

*A Woman's Complete Guide to a
Younger, Healthier You*

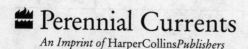
Perennial Currents
*An Imprint of HarperCollinsPublishers*

The Healthy Eating Pyramid on page 138, from *Eat, Drink and Be Healthy: The Harvard Medical School Guide to Healthy Eating* by Dr. Walter C. Willett, copyright © 2001 by President and Fellows of Harvard College, is reprinted with the permission of Simon & Schuster Adult Publishing Group.

A hardcover edition of this book was published in 2004 by William Morrow, an imprint of HarperCollins Publishers.

HarperCollins books may be purchased for educational, business,
or sales promotional use. For information please write:
Special Markets Department, HarperCollins Publishers Inc.,
10 East 53rd Street, New York, NY 10022.

FIRST PERENNIAL CURRENTS EDITION PUBLISHED 2005.

The Library of Congress has catalogued the hardcover edition as follows:

Reichman, Judith.
    Slow your clock down: the complete guide to a healthy, younger you / Judith Reichman.
        p. cm.
    Includes index.
    ISBN 0-06-052727-7
        1. Middle aged women—Health and hygiene.   2. Middle aged women—Diseases.
    3. Menopause.   I. Title.

RA778.R4227 2004
613'.04244—dc22                                          2003066484

ISBN 0-06-052728-5 (pbk.)

05  06  07  08  09  ❖/RRD  10  9  8  7  6  5  4  3  2

*To my mother who has shown me how to savor time*

*To my father who determined I should not waste time*

*To my daughters who have taught me how time flies*

*To my patients who have entrusted me with their time*

*To my husband who has given me the best of times!*

# Contents

# Acknowledgments

Writing this book would have sped my personal clock forward (or, in less prosaic terms, "aged me"), were it not for the invaluable help of some very wise, talented, and dedicated individuals. Dr. Cheryl K. Olson, who holds a doctorate in public health and is the co-director of the Center for Mental Health and Media at Harvard Medical School, helped research, organize, and make sense of the huge number of studies and statistics I used in this book. Her data collection prowess, sense of humor, compassion, and awe-inspiring computer skills were indefatigable and allowed me to "make the case" for the stories, information, and guidelines that I hope will impact the health span of all those who choose to read *Slow Your Clock Down*.

Several medical professionals generously contributed their knowledge: Walter Willet, M.D., of the Harvard School of Public Health, allowed me to use his revised food pyramid. Gene Beresin, M.D., Gary Small, M.D., and Larry Kutner, Ph.D., provided mentally stimulating information on brain health and memory. Alan DeCherney, M.D., my friend and mentor (this will embarrass him) made sure that the section on infertility met his exacting standards. My colleague, Vicken Sahakian, M.D., who directs a large fertility center in Los Angeles, provided much of the economic lowdown on what women need to consider while pursuing their oft-delayed goal of motherhood. Norman Leaf, M.D., a well-known plastic surgeon in Beverly Hills, took the time out of his busy schedule to review the medical and surgical techniques used to slow or reverse the unwanted photoaging and time-aging changes that affect our appearance.

The publishing of any book involves many professionals. I was fortunate to have an extraordinary team behind my efforts. My agent, David Vigliano, encouraged and rallied all of us; Meaghan Dowling, my longtime editor at William Morrow, believed in what the proposed manuscript would become and took on its delivery, together with that of her first child. Toni Sciarra did a phenomenal job of editing; pruning the redundant "book fat" so that the final draft was leaner, meaner, and better (and bore fewer parentheses). Rome Quezada helped guide the final stages of our endeavors. Christine Tanigawa, our production editor, and Sonia Greenbaum, our copy editor, made sure that the manuscript would not cause undue consternation to my former college English professors. Debra Craig did her usual excellent job transcribing portions of the book. Bill Stankey championed this book and has worked diligently to promote it.

The writing of a book in no way guarantees that it will be read. That's where publicists become invaluable, and I am indebted to the efforts of Debbie Stier and Suzanne Balaban at William Morrow, and to my publicists who took on the task of nationally promoting this book because they thought it was important for women: Melody Korenbrot in Los Angeles and Donna Daniels in New York.

I am blessed with friends who were willing to act as editorial springboards and read portions of this book. Thank you, Carole Haber, Lynne Wasserman, Francis Rothschild, and Elena Cates. My staff, especially Deborah Cannon and Judy Casanova, kept our patients and me scheduled and sane despite last-minute phone conferences and deadlines.

The patients' names and the medical histories that are profiled in the book have been changed to protect their anonymity, but all of the stories are based on composites of women whom I have treated during my years of practice in Los Angeles. My patients have bestowed upon me an incredible education in health, disease, human spirit, and "well-gevity." Medical training may be essential in order to translate the research, prescribe the drugs, and perform the surgeries that are inherent to patient care. But how they, the patients, and we, the doctors, care is what makes the practice of medicine so phenomenal. My patients made this book possible, and I hope to slow our collective clocks down, so that we can continue our relationship.

Finally, I want to thank my husband, Gil Cates, who was never ticked off during the times that I was missing in home-action. Your love and encouragement kept me and this book on track. And if I lectured you about what to eat, and not to eat, it's because I want you here forever. . . .

# Timely Thoughts

I love to sleep in. As I lie curled in a fetal position, I embody a revolt against the accumulated demands of medical school and residency, my surgical imperative to get the first time-slot in the OR, the need to see ten patients before lunch, and the pursuit of that New York minute (or thirty) to phone my producers in Manhattan, who have a three-hour time zone advantage. But like most women, when the alarm rings at 6:30 A.M., I rise and—with careful makeup application—create an outward shine. I'm then on the go for the next thirteen hours, until I call it quits or at least break for dinner. The thirteenth hour: just the beginning of the second half of the day. Why call it quitting time? I may crave a later start, but I deplore the notion of ending my day in the middle.

"Middle" is so pejorative, both as an adjective and a noun: *Middle age* connotes a passing from youth, when we were of firm body and sound health, to the middle of our lives (which, by current statistics, occurs in our midforties). Our *middles* become the repositories of bloat, subcutaneous fat, and misbehaving organs. We may be midlife crisising and midcareering. Middle also means compromise, lack of affiliation, or committed direction. I, for one, don't want to settle for half done. I plan to strive to extend the sweetness of my days and years way beyond the halfway point.

This book is both a medical and personal quest to optimize the minutes and hours of our internal and external body clocks, not simply to get more done, but to have time to savor what we've accomplished—and have the good health to do so. Barbra Streisand wrote in a comment for one of my books that "without health, we have nothing." We all fight time because we fear it will take away our health, our well-being. We aspire to look good, but our greatest concern is not feeling good.

The actuaries give us spreadsheets with calculated life spans. As a physician and a member of the woman race, I protest. With medical insight, we should be able to reorganize and redefine our charts in terms of *health spans*. I hope you'll take the time to read on, and let me show you how modern medicine can facilitate your desire to slow your clock down. Sleeping in is an occasional choice. We should also be able to enjoy and luxuriate in the rest of our days and nights.

# Your Reproductive Clock

Our pubic hair—its appearance, what we do with it—is so personal. We can shave it, wax it, depilate it, or just keep it clean. It tentatively makes its appearance as a fine, soft growth, and is often greeted with consternation by its 11-year-old owner. It won't be shamed or tamed, and continues to grow, thicken, curl as the insistent symbol of emerging womanhood.

Pubic hair is created by a marvelously intertwined maturation of centers in our brain, pituitary gland, adrenal glands, and ovaries. It grows after we produce male hormone (testosterone), and is then nourished by our female hormone, estrogen. Its appearance is governed by enzymes in our skin that metabolize testosterone in hair follicles, by genes that determine pigmentation, and by what we eat. And as these factors change with age, so does our pubic hair. It turns gray, becomes sparse and thin, and no longer presents an obstacle to bikini wear, at a time when most of us quit trying to fit into our bikinis.

Celia mourned the passage of her pubic hair. She found (and plucked) her first gray one in her early forties. She ruefully remarked, "It's the only part of my body that's gotten thin! I'm starting to look like my mother down there. God, I hate this aging stuff."

For most of us, diminished fertility, increased PMS, irregular bleeding, rearranged body fat, and the inevitability of menopause all make this pubic hair saga seem trivial by comparison. Yet all of these events occur as a result of the clock that rules our ovaries, and the cellular and molecular changes that occur throughout our bodies.

How can you deal with "this aging stuff"? Can you slow the clock by changing your nutrition or behavior? Can you prevent aging, disability, and mortality with herbs, vitamins, medications, surgery, religion, or inner peace?

Celia wanted her pubic hair back. You probably have different concerns: "Is it too late to have a baby?" "When can I stop worrying about birth control?" "Are 'hot flashes' inevitable?" "Can I put off sagging skin, and keep my figure firm?" "How can I feel good and stay healthy as long as possible—and what should send me running to my doctor?"

Before I get to the "what can be done" part of this book, we'll have to go through the prerequisite "what you should know." Welcome to "Your Hormones and Reproductive Cycle 101." I'll keep it short and sweet.

## THE REPRODUCTIVE CLOCK VS. THE HORMONAL CLOCK

Your body functions to the rhythm of two internal timekeepers—one for reproduction, and one for hormones—and they are not necessarily in sync. Each clock starts, ticks on, pauses, and stops at a different time. In fact, you'll pass through a veritable plethora of pauses: reproductive pause, premenopause, perimenopause, menopause, and postmenopause.

Your reproductive clock began running while *you* were still being "reproduced": as a five-month-old embryo. Your newly formed ovaries teemed with about *five million* pre-eggs, or oocytes. Most of these eggs died of "old age" before you were even born.

At birth, that oocyte number dwindled to a lowly one or two million. As the clock ticked relentlessly, most continued to disintegrate (the medical term for this process is *atresia*), so by the time you began your first period (*menarche*), your oocyte count had plummeted to 400,000.

Over the next twenty-five years, within your ovaries, this cellular loss continues at a fairly steady pace, independent of monthly ovulation. During your reproductive life, each month one plucky oocyte matures inside its follicle and is released as a ripe egg—which, for the next twenty-four hours, is capable of being penetrated by sperm deposited in the neighborhood. Most oocytes never get this chance; less than 0.001 percent of your ovaries' original oocytes are ever sent forth as eggs.

In your late thirties and early forties, the pace of egg death accelerates. As you enter the menopause, just a few thousand aging oocytes populate a shrinking ovarian platform, a tiny remnant of that bountiful original crop. This affects more than your fertility; vigorous oocytes are critical to your hormonal rhythms.

## The Hormonal Clock

The steady ticking of your hormonal clock depends on the monthly march of your oocytes. To help you picture what's happening, here's a quick review of the turn-on and shut-off systems of the glands and organs that coordinate the production of your female hormones and menstrual cycles.

Each month, the development of one dominant follicle (and the failed start of thousands of others) contributes to the estrogen (*estradiol*), progesterone, and intermediary hormones that define your cycle. These attach to receptors in just about every cell—in skin, muscle, fat, brain, bone, and, of course, vagina, uterus, and breasts—and modulate their development, function, and well-being. So when this flow of hormones fluctuates, slows, or stops altogether, the effect is far greater than the mere absence of a period.

Your brain's pituitary gland prompts these follicles into action by producing FSH, or *follicular stimulating hormone,* and LH, or *luteinizing hormone*. This gland, in turn, is under a higher command: an adjacent area of your brain called the hypothalamus, which secretes GnRH, or *gonadotrophic releasing hormone*.

I've often compared the brain, pituitary, and ovarian communication network to a circular control panel, with on and off switches. If levels of the end products—estrogen and progesterone—are high, the network shuts down production of GnRH, FSH, and LH (the ovary says "enough is enough"). But when levels of estrogen and progesterone are low, the system cranks up: GnRH is activated, causing the pituitary to release FSH, then LH, prodding the follicles to develop and release its hormones.

The typical twenty-eight-day cycle (which can vary from twenty-one to thirty-five days) looks like this:

## The End and the Beginning (Period)

This is the lowest point for estrogen and progesterone production, as the remains of the active follicle degenerate. These hormones are necessary for the growth and development of the glands lining the uterus (the *endometrium*). When these endometrial glands lose their hormonal support, they collapse, causing the supplying blood vessels to open and bleed. This hormonal low also triggers the hypothalamus to produce GnRH, which then nudges the pituitary to release FSH (LH comes later). And so, a new follicle gets the go-ahead to mature its egg toward the goal of ovulation.

Unfortunately, pain and cramps tend to come with endometrial shedding. Why? Blame the prostaglandins your uterus produces. These chemical substances cause the uterine muscle to contract, effectively closing off the vessels coursing to your "bruised and bleeding" endometrium. Regrettably, these same prostaglandins are pain mediators; in addition to causing the uterine contractions that are felt as cramps, they can adversely affect your entire body. Some women overproduce or are overly sensitive to prostaglandins, and suffer from nausea, headache, diarrhea, and flulike symptoms; every period leaves them hormonally "down and out."

## The Feel-Good Time of the Month
## (Days 5 to 9: Early Follicular Phase)

The rising FSH stimulates an entire group of follicles. One becomes "the egg of the month" and succeeds in growing faster and better than the others. In order to ensure its superiority, it produces a hormone called *inhibin,* which prevents the other wannabe follicles from maturing. As they die out, the dominant follicle proceeds in its development, producing estrogen along the way. The buildup of this hormone helps repair the wounded endometrial lining, so that once more the glands begin to develop.

This is usually a feel-good time of the month: bloat free, headache free, acne free, and, of course, tampon free.

## Still Feeling Okay (Days 9 to 13: Late Follicular Phase)

That dominant follicle blooms, producing increasing amounts of estrogen. GnRH is still being stimulated, but this time, the pituitary—now aware of all the estrogen on board—responds with production of LH.

The uterine lining, having been fed more estrogen, continues to build up its glands.

That sense of well-being continues, although you may start to develop some breast tenderness as estrogen levels rise.

### "Mittelschmerz" Time: A Pain in the Middle (Day 14: Ovulation)

The surge of LH bursts the bubble of the mature dominant follicle, releasing the egg, which is picked up by the fernlike fimbria on one of the two fallopian tubes. There, it can be fertilized if sperm arrive within the next twenty-four hours. The ruptured follicle is now transformed into a *corpus luteum,* or yellow body (which looks like a minute yellow pea).

As the follicle breaks open, it pulls on the adjacent peritoneum and its generous supply of nerve fibers. Many women know exactly when they ovulate because of this "mittelschmerz," or pain in the middle (of the cycle). The pain can be significant, especially if you've had a previous infection, cyst, or endometriosis that left scar tissue.

### Luteal Phase: LP May Mean PMS (Days 15 to 28)

The corpus luteum produces estrogen and increasing amounts of progesterone. These hormones cause the glands of the endometrium to thicken, and their blood supply increases. This creates a lush, thick bed capable of enveloping and nourishing an embryo. With the rise in progesterone, many women begin to feel bloated, have breast tenderness, mood swings, weight gain, and indeed all the symptoms of PMS (more on that later). Alas, an increase in production of male hormones may also trigger acne.

Fourteen days after ovulation, the corpus luteum and built-up uterine lining are fated to expire—in the absence of a pregnancy. As the corpus luteum dies, the hormonal buttress of its estrogen and progesterone collapses, as does the endometrial lining, and another period arrives.

There you have it: the marvelous ebb and flow that provides us with our extraordinary ability to ovulate, procreate, and "hormonate." Most of us barely notice this hormonal drama, except when our period arrives (to our relief or dismay).

Aside from these monthly hormonal ups and downs, there are variations depending on external and internal stresses, malformations, and, ultimately, the wear and tear (or, more precisely, the using up) of our eggs.

Their number determines when, and how long, we are in the "pre-" or "peri-" of menopause.

## THE REPRODUCTIVE PAUSE

*"He Ran Away with My Sperm!"*

Laura grew up with four brothers in a rural Midwest town, where everyone went to the same general practitioner. He capably wielded his stethoscope but was most reluctant to insert a speculum in young, unmarried women. Laura was in college when she had her first gynecologic exam—at a family planning clinic, where she sought to terminate an unwanted pregnancy. No longer a reproductive novice, she started taking birth control pills, vowing that this would never happen again.

Laura loved the Pill; her periods became light and pain free, and her complexion clear. With her hormonal house now in order, she set her priorities: law school, a job in the right firm, then partnership, marriage to the right man, and yes (eventually), production of progeny. A move to Los Angeles after law school, to join a top entertainment-law firm, knocked the first two goals off her list.

Once I became her doctor, Laura would update me on her career and social life at each annual checkup. By age 35, she'd married an aspiring director (check off goal four) and made partner (goal three).

Medically, Laura got an A. She took her vitamins and calcium, exercised, stayed slim, and ate right. Her meticulous body maintenance and grooming (Armani suit, Prada shoes, exquisite highlights in her hair) hid all public signs of aging; her Pill-regulated cycles gave no hints that her eggs were aging, too.

Through the rest of her thirties, I urged her to start her family. Each year she assured me she was *almost* ready—but couldn't cope with an expanding middle in the middle of this big case, or didn't want to take a maternity leave just when she'd landed a major new client. Meanwhile, her husband had goals of his own, and wanted to wait until he got that hit movie with a salary to match (which would let Laura cut back to forty hours a week).

Ready or not, Laura turned 40. Her client list was one of the best in town. Her husband had embarked on a promising action-and-gore movie for a big studio. At a time when her brothers' kids were having kids,

Laura was just two Pill packs away from allowing her eggs to blossom and conjoin with her husband's obliging sperm . . . and he left her for another woman with twenty-eight-year-old eggs and a body honed at his gym.

Claiming an emotional, legal, and gynecologic emergency, Laura demanded an immediate appointment. As soon as I entered the exam room, she burst into tears: "He ran away with my sperm!"

Laura ticked off her most immediate needs: a private investigator, a divorce attorney, and a sperm bank. And, could we freeze her eggs?

## Did I Wait Too Long? Help!

How long does it take to get pregnant? When it is too late? Unfairly, the older you are, the longer it takes to conceive. Between ages 19 and 26, there's a 50 percent chance of achieving pregnancy in one menstrual cycle (if egg meets good sperm at the right time). This falls to 40 percent for ages 27 to 34, and to 30 percent for women in their late thirties.

What's more, miscarriage rates increase with age: By age 35, the number of spontaneous pregnancies that end in live births is half that of our twenties; by age 45, it's cut by 95 percent. Less than 1 percent of American babies have mothers who spontaneously conceived and delivered them after the age of 40. (This does not include babies born through assisted reproduction.)

Why so low? There are "quality control" issues: Eggs are fewer, of lower quality, and the pituitary hormones that direct their development and release are less coordinated. Damage from infections, fibroids, surgeries, or endometriosis can hamper sperm from reaching the egg, or make it hard for a fertilized egg to get to the uterus and grow. Finally, the risk of chromosomal abnormalities is high; half of midforties pregnancies end in miscarriage.

This doesn't mean all hope is lost. Modern medicine has provided us with some amazing options. But before you start, do all you can to improve your general health and fertility: Give up smoking or using recreational drugs. Have no more than one alcoholic drink a day (quit altogether once you suspect you're pregnant), and cut out caffeine (or have just that one cup of coffee at breakfast).

Try to time your sexual intercourse (not the duration, the occurrence) to promote the chance that your egg will meet his sperm. Fourteen days before your period, an expectant egg is released into your fallopian tube (where fertilization occurs). There are two ways to determine when this is happening. The simplest method is to start counting forward from the day you start your period: this means your target date is day 14 (if you have twenty-eight-day cycles) or day 16 (if you have thirty-day cycles). Because sperm can remain alive and active inside your cervix for up to a week, start trying around day 10, and repeat on days 12, 14, and 16. If you have a long cycle or just want to have fun, keep going on days 18 and 20, etc.

If your usual cycle is twenty-one days, you may ovulate as soon as seven days after your period starts, even if you're still bleeding; in that case, you should start earlier. See a doctor if your cycle is shorter than twenty-one days or longer than thirty-five days, as that suggests you may not be ovulating.

A more scientific method to check for ovulation involves taking your basal body temperature, using a very sensitive basal thermometer you can purchase from your local drugstore. Take your temperature every morning as soon as you open your eyes—so it won't be affected by physical activity or hot coffee. After ovulation, your temperature will go up (under half a degree) due to the production of progesterone from your ovary, and it won't go back down until your period starts. (If you're pregnant, your temp will stay elevated.) You can also use special ovulation kits and computers that test for LH surges in your urine. These will help confirm when and if you ovulate—but I often find that my patients wait patiently for the official confirmation, and then miss the opportunity to have intercourse at the right time. If you are in your late thirties, you can give yourself six months of let's-wait-and-see time. But once you are 40, it's time to stop letting your eggs go one by one (while thousands die) and relying on nature's course of pregnancy action. Acknowledge the fact that you may need medical and even surgical intervention if you want to have that baby.

## What's Wrong? How to Find Out

Initial tests can be ordered by your gynecologist. But as you continue on your reproductive quest, I would suggest that you see a reproductive endocrinologist. First, the quality of your eggs should be checked by testing your FSH level on the second or third day after your period starts. A low level indicates the possibility that your eggs are capable of being fertilized . . . but not the assurance that they can or will.

If your FSH is over 20 mu/ml (milli-international units per milliliter)—and especially if it's over 25 mu/ml for several cycles in a row—you unfortunately cannot conceive using your own eggs. At many fertility clinics, doctors will not even attempt to treat a woman for infertility if her FSH is over 10, or if she's older than 42 or 44, unless she uses donor eggs (see page 17). The cost is just too high, and the odds of success too low, to make it a viable option. (And frankly, centers don't like to lower their outcome statistics with patients who are unlikely to conceive.)

You'll also be checked for medical conditions that can affect ovulation, fertilization, or implantation. If you have had irregular periods, weight gain, acne, and excess hair growth (*hirsutism*) since puberty, you may have a condition called *polycystic ovarian syndrome* (PCOS). This is usually caused by excess production of male hormone and insulin, which prevent the normal monthly development of follicles. The follicles try but fail to produce and "give up" their eggs and instead develop small cysts; hence the name, polycystic ovary. Blood tests often show a high level of LH, testosterone, and insulin. Therapy should be started as soon as the diagnosis is made. Women who do not want to conceive should take birth control pills to stop irregular follicle function and regulate their periods, decrease testosterone levels, and diminish hirsutism and acne. An antimale medication called spironolactone may also help treat these unwanted symptoms. If your insulin levels are high, you should begin therapy with Glucophage, a pill that lowers insulin levels and helps control prediabetes (see page 251). Glucophage alone may also help you establish normal periods and improve your fertility. Once you are actively trying to conceive you may require additional ovarian stimulation (see page 11). Irregular periods can also be due to problems with your pituitary or thyroid glands (detected with a blood test). A cervical infection (checked by culturing material swabbed from your cervix) can prevent sperm from entering the uterine cavity. A pelvic ultrasound should be ordered to see if there are abnormalities such as fibroids, ovarian cysts, or tumors. Hysteroscopy (a procedure using a telescope placed through the cervix) lets your doctor check your uterine lining for any "mechanical" problems (such as a polyp or fibroid) that might interfere with conception or with the progress of a pregnancy.

If your FSH is low, your cycles regular, and a blood test on or about day 21 of your cycle shows adequate production of progesterone, you're probably ovulating. But the sperm need to have access to the egg, which may be blocked if your tubes are scarred by a previous infection or surgery. In the past, your doctor would have ordered an HSG (hysterosalpingography), in which dye is injected through the cervical opening into the uterine cavity at the time that X rays are taken. If this showed blockage, a laparoscopy was often performed "to see what was wrong." Today, however, the experts tend to bypass mechanical tubal issues; instead of attempting surgical repair (tuboplasty), they proceed to in vitro fertilization. (When I reflect on all that time I spent training in order to perform tubal microsurgery, I want to shed a few tears . . . but such is progress in medicine.)

Last but not least: Just because you're older, don't assume the problem with conception is all yours. Infertility is often due to the ominous-sounding "male factor," an insufficient number or poor quality of sperm. For many couples, there is a combination of male/female factors. If you are relying on a partner (as opposed to a sperm bank), the initial infertility workup should include a semen analysis.

## Now What? The Options and Odds

I'm frustrated by the short lifespan of our ovaries. It's not fair that our eggs wither and die while the aging sperm produced by potbellied men wriggle on triumphantly. At this point, you may feel that your biological clock has most unfairly raced ahead, stealing your option to get pregnant when you are, at last, mentally, emotionally, and economically ready to have that baby. The nerve of those eggs! Just when you need them to do their thing. . . .

The fortunate fact (which unfortunately can cost a fortune) is that we now have high-tech options that were not available to previous generations. With the help of assisted reproductive technologies (ART), we can slow our reproductive clock down, or at least speed up and multiply the process of egg development, fertilization, and conception.

### Fixing mechanical problems

Even though ART lets us fertilize an egg outside of the womb, in order to bear your baby, you need a healthy and welcoming uterus to allow the embryo to implant in the lining, receive its nourishment, and grow to term. The uterine lining should not be scarred, or have large polyps or fibroids taking up the room needed by the growing embryo. Large or multiple fibroids in the wall of the uterus are also a concern, since they can instigate premature labor. (The hormones of pregnancy may stimulate these fibroids so that they outgrow their blood supply and, as a result, undergo tissue death or degeneration, which can irritate the surrounding uterus and cause contractions.)

If any of these problems have been diagnosed, you may need a surgical procedure before you proceed with ART. Endometrial polyps and fibroids can be removed with outpatient procedures through a *hysteroscope*. Large fibroids in the wall of the uterus may require removal (*myomectomy*) through an open abdominal incision (a *laparotomy*). Some surgeons feel comfortable performing this procedure through a laparoscope, especially if the fibroids are not deeply embedded in the uterine wall. This involves several small incisions, through which the surgeon inserts telescopic instruments under video screen guidance. The advantage is a smaller scar and faster recovery time.

## Boosting ovulation

*Fertility drugs.* If your eggs are deemed acceptable for use, rather than wait for one egg to be successfully fertilized (at a time when thousands are dying and the chances are slim), your reproductive endocrinologist will push for multiple egg development by prescribing fertility drugs. She or he may begin with an oral medication, called clomiphene. This works by blocking estrogen receptors in your brain, and fooling it into thinking that estrogen levels are low. To correct this perception, the pituitary pumps out large amounts of FSH. In theory, all of this FSH will then stimulate multiple follicles and cause an increased number of ovulations—and chance of conception.

Even if eggs are released, the fertility rates with clomiphene are quite disappointing in "older" women. Most physicians will not waste valuable time persisting in this form of therapy, and proceed to injections of FSH or FSH and LH, followed by hCG (human gonadotropin), which copies the LH surge needed for release of the egg.

These fertility drugs produce better results if we first give your follicles a month of "rest." Your doctor may teach you how to give yourself injections of GnRH analog (Lupron) to block the hypothalamus from producing the GnRH that stimulates your pituitary and thereby your ovaries. After a few weeks of pseudomenopausal inactivity, your follicles are more likely to respond in sync to the FSH and LH that you'll be given to inject in monitored amounts to stimulate ovulation.

The monitoring part is critical. Stimulation of too many follicles can create large ovarian cysts and a medical condition called "hyperstimulation syndrome." This can lead to electrolyte imbalance, abdominal swelling, and—in rare cases—hospitalization and even surgery. And if too many eggs are fertilized, high-order multiple pregnancies (triplets or more) can result (see below). Monitoring includes ultrasound to assess the number and size of developing follicles, along with blood tests for estrogen levels. Too much of a good "follicular thing" will cause the estrogen levels to become sky-high. If this happens the cycle may be cancelled, and the drug that triggers the release of eggs (hCG) not given.

*ART (assisted reproductive technologies).* The drugs and monitoring are expensive, ranging from $2,000 to $3,000 a cycle. So when it's time for fertilization, most specialists will not rely on old-fashioned sex. They'll obtain the sperm, wash it, and put it into a special solution to be "Federal Expressed" via a thin catheter through the cervix into your uterine cavity (intrauterine insemination).

Most likely, you will be encouraged to bypass even this slightly natural course for sperm transport and undergo IVF (in vitro fertilization), GIFT (gamete intrafallopian tube transfer), or ZIFT (zygote intrafallopian tube transfer). All three of these procedures begin with "harvesting" eggs from your ovaries with a needle attached to an ultrasound probe inserted through the vaginal wall, puncturing the ballooning follicular cysts so their fluid can be aspirated. (This can be painful, and is usually done under mild anesthesia.) The eggs are then removed from the fluid under microscopic inspection. The number of eggs harvested (which can be as few as one, or as many as dozens) depends on the amount of fertility drugs used, and your ovaries' response to them.

In IVF, the eggs are then placed together with the sperm in a petri dish (not a test tube) for incubation and fertilization. Three to five days after fertilization, those that successfully develop into embryos (first called *zygotes*, and later *blastocysts*) are implanted via a thin catheter inserted through the cervix into the uterine cavity, where hopefully at least one will "take," grow, and develop.

For women under the age of 37, two to three embryos are usually transferred. Between ages 37 and 40, the number goes up to three or four—and beyond that age, even more may be acceptable, because fewer embryos will go on to develop. This is a balancing act between getting you pregnant or "too pregnant": twins, triplets, or more. Twins might be nice; you've completed your family. But we are very concerned about higher numbers because of the great risk of miscarriage, premature delivery, pregnancy loss, or fetal developmental problems. Many couples decide to decrease the number of developing embryos once they're told about these risks.

In GIFT, the egg and the sperm are introduced to each other during a laparoscopic procedure in which they are inserted into the fallopian tube. In ZIFT, the same technique is used on an already fertilized egg. This requires surgery, and so the majority of infertility clinics have abandoned GIFT and ZIFT in favor of in vitro fertilization. Those clinics that still do them claim that with older eggs, the tubal fluid may be more favorable for fertilization and/or development than the petri dish.

*ICSI (intracytoplasmic sperm injection).* What can technology do for the bestower of the other half of those chromosomes, the sperm? A critical number of active, normal sperm are needed to ensure that one will penetrate the egg and fertilize it, in either a fallopian tube or a petri dish. If your partner's sperm count is low, too many of the sperm appear abnormal, too few embryos develop, or you have failed ART procedures in the past, ICSI is advisable.

Since a single sperm is injected directly into the egg, only a few good sperm are needed to do the job (reminds me of the Marines!). Here's an extreme example of how well this can work: I referred one of my patients, who had a much older husband (in his late seventies) to a reproductive endocrinologist for ICSI and in vitro procedures. The husband had been told that his semen analysis showed absolutely no viable sperm. A few live sperm were obtained through biopsies of his testes, and were injected into several eggs. One of the embryos developed and my patient subsequently delivered a healthy, full-term baby, with her proud husband (holding on to his walker) by her side.

*PGD (preimplantation genetic diagnosis).* Just a few more acronyms. . . . If you've had recurrent failed ART cycles or multiple miscarriages, you may want to consider PGD. This procedure allows the embryologist to identify single gene defects and any chromosomal abnormalities (as well as the gender) before the embryo is implanted. A cell is removed from a three-day-old embryo and scrutinized with gene-detecting technology. Some fertility experts offer PGD to women over 40 in order to lower their chance of miscarriage (only those embryos that pass genetic testing are transferred into the uterus). PGD has also become popular for sex selection. Considering the price (an additional $2,000), this probably should be reserved for couples who have reason to be concerned about genetic disorders.

### Frozen embryos

I noted earlier that there is a need to balance the number of embryos transferred with the risk of multiple pregnancies. When more eggs are stimulated, retrieved, and fertilized than can be used in a single cycle, there will be leftover embryos. These can be frozen for later use, sparing the stress and expense of additional fertility drugs and egg retrieval. The embryos are transferred into the uterus during a future cycle after therapy with estrogen and progesterone have made the lining thick and receptive. You can wait months or even years to do this. Since some embryos do not survive the freezing or thawing process, live birth rates are approximately half of those achieved with fresh embryos.

## Success Rates . . . and How You Rate a Fertility Clinic

Many of the embryos implanted in the uterus don't "take," and miscarriage rates naturally increase with age. The success that counts for the hopeful mother is the live birth rate per cycle. However, many fertility clinics will give you numbers that show *their* success in embryo transfers. This number will always look better.

Statistics compiled in 1999 (reported in 2001) by the Society for Assisted Reproductive Technology (SART), together with the Centers for Disease Control (CDC), showed that overall 30.6 percent of ART cycles led to a pregnancy. Sixteen percent of these pregnancies ended in miscarriage or stillbirth, but this number increased to close to 60 percent in women over the age of 44. Younger women fared much better than those who were older: Women in their late twenties and early thirties had success rates that averaged 38 percent live births per cycle of ART, compared with 18 percent for women aged 38 to 40, 10 percent for women 41 to 42, and less than 5 percent for women over 42. Rates fell to virtually zero after age 46.

These are the overall statistics. Each fertility center has its own figures; those that report to SART have theirs posted on the CDC's website, at www.cdc.gov, under "Infertility." Note that statistics reflect each clinic's

According to the medical journal *The Lancet,* at the start of this century, one in every 100 to 150 babies born in the Western world was conceived through in vitro fertilization (IVF). We've come a long way since 1978 and the birth of Louise Brown, the first baby conceived in a petri dish.

## "Can't I Freeze My Eggs for Later?"

Many of my patients are acutely aware of their biologic clock but haven't found a committed partner, and/or have not reached a financial or professional position that they feel will allow them to start a family. They've all read the "Believe It or Not" stories of successful pregnancies with thawed eggs. (These, by the way, usually involve women under the age of 35 who face loss of ovarian function due to surgery or treatment of disease.) Worldwide, there has been only a handful of births from frozen eggs. Unfortunately, the chance of a frozen egg resulting in a live birth is less than 5 percent. As difficult as it is to preserve the integrity of an embryo during the freezing-and-thawing procedure (almost half don't survive), the egg with its half-number of chromosomes is more fragile.

"Not fair!" we protest. They freeze sperm with such ease; shouldn't our eggs be as freeze-worthy? So far: no. The egg is much larger than a sperm, and its fluid contents are prone to damage by ice crystals during the thawing process. New methods are being developed that may cut down on the freeze-and-thaw "burn."

Don't count on egg freezing as an option to slow your fertility clock. If you must wait (or are faced with imminent loss of your ovaries), and have the sperm of your choice available, consider an in vitro procedure and freezing the embryos to implant later.

patient population. Some clinics refuse to take older patients or more complicated cases so that they'll look better on paper. Choose a clinic based on success rates with women whose stats match your own.

### A Baby, at What Price?

The cost can vary by state and clinic. In California, where I practice, the average cost of an IVF cycle (excluding drugs) is $8,000. The fertility medications needed to stimulate the ovaries can run between $2,000 and $3,000. Several programs have a "risk sharing" plan, requiring a lump sum of nearly $14,000 up front to cover three cycles of IVF. Women under age 34 will get a refund of 90 percent of the cost (excluding medications and anesthesia) if a pregnancy doesn't continue beyond twelve weeks with three attempts. This goes down to 80 percent for women between 34 and 36, and 70 percent for women 37 to 40. (In all cases, the

## ART Fears

*Ovarian cancer.* Some studies have found an increased risk of ovarian cancer among women who took fertility drugs. It's possible, however, that this extra risk was due to incessant ovulation, not to the drugs. We know that women who have never had a full-term pregnancy have an ovarian cancer risk that's 1.5 to 2 times higher than women who've delivered at least one baby. Once a woman who takes fertility drugs has a baby, it seems to cancel out this increased risk.

Ovulating monthly for thirty years or more puts a lot of stress on the ovaries and may result in damaged cells and encourage the action of cancer-causing genes. Suppressing ovulation—via pregnancy, breast-feeding, or oral contraceptives—reduces this risk. If you took fertility drugs to have a baby and succeeded, you don't have to worry. However, if you used these medications for a year or more and did not have a full-term pregnancy, taking birth control pills for a few years will help protect your ovaries.

*Birth defects and low birth weight.* Several studies have shown that infants conceived through IVF and/or ICSI are twice as likely (8.6 percent versus 4.2 percent) as naturally conceived children to have major birth defects. (This applied only to single—not multiple—pregnancies.)

ART-conceived children are also 2.6 times more likely to have low and very low birth weights. This puts them at higher risk for future developmental problems.

But for an infertile couple who would remain childless without ART, the reassuring fact is that if they do become pregnant with one developing embryo, they have a 91 percent chance of having a baby free of major defects, and a 94 percent chance that their "singleton" infant will have a birth weight in the normal range.

woman's FSH level must be below 10.) If you get pregnant on the first try, you get no refunds.

There are insurance plans that will pay for up to three cycles of IVF, depending on your age, but these policies are expensive and employers may exclude them from the coverage they offer. Some states mandate that medical insurers offer IVF coverage for women under a certain age.

Any addition to the "baseline" IVF will drive up the price. For example, ICSI costs between $1,000 and $2,000, and PGD runs over $2,000.

For women using donated eggs (see below), the cost for donor compensation can vary between $3,000 and $50,000! Donors must take fertility drugs to stimulate their ovaries, then undergo egg retrieval. (It's a lot harder than donating sperm.) Agency and legal fees usually add $5,000 to the cost.

Finally, you may choose to use a surrogate if you have viable eggs but are unable to carry a pregnancy due to a hysterectomy, uterine malformation, or a medical condition that makes pregnancy dangerous. Another woman with an intact uterus will carry the pregnancy created through your fertilized egg. The cost is high: $20,000 to $30,000 paid to the surrogate to deliver the baby, and another $20,000 for the agency and legal fees. In some states it is illegal to pay a surrogate mother, so you'd need to find an out-of-state surrogate or a volunteer friend or relative. A fertility clinic can offer advice on agencies that find and screen women willing to donate their eggs or serve as gestational carriers.

## When You Can't Use Your Own Eggs

Despite these marvelous advances, there comes a point when you have to face the fact that your own eggs are not capable of responding. Statistics gathered from established fertility clinics are dismal for a woman over the age of 42. Even if you're younger, once your FSH is over 10, you fall into the "We're not sure we want you as a patient" category, because you may lower their clinics' success rates. Considering the cost and physical rigors, I would advise you to consider using donor eggs. The success rate then depends on the age of the donor, not yours. Eggs from a woman under the age of 30 can result in live birth rates of close to 50 percent per transfer. Women in their early sixties have given birth with donated eggs, but most fertility centers have age limits lower than this.

Even if a woman, with the help of science, succeeds in becoming a single mom in her forties, she faces tremendous societal bias. The gray-haired daddy is applauded for his late-in-life virility, while the older mom doesn't fit in at the Mommy-and-Me classes, birthday parties, and back-to-school nights even if her hairdresser hides her gray. The coup de grace: She simultaneously has to cope with her child's puberty and her own menopause.

It could be argued that as long as a woman is healthy and physically able to handle the stress of pregnancy and delivery, she should be allowed these fertility options. We don't put age limits on men becoming fathers. Having said this, I can't imagine facing the rigors of twenty-plus years of child *rearing* that I know await parents of any newborn, in my fifties or sixties. Maybe it's because I've been there and done that.

This has been a relatively quick overview of the terminology, tests, and therapies in the very specialized field of reproductive endocrinology. I know this section may seem alarming, but an alarm is ringing. "There's a time to sow, and a time to reap," and the sowing should begin before our early forties. We can't change the pace of our reproductive clock, but we can heed the sound of its ticking.

More detailed information is available from Resolve: The National Infertility Association (www.resolve.org, or call 888-623-0744), and from the American Society for Reproductive Medicine (www.asrm.org). I also highly recommend the latest book from Resolve, called *Resolving Infertility: Understanding the Options and Choosing Solutions When You Want to Have a Baby*.

## Laura's Story, Part II

Laura went back to the Midwest to visit her family, for what she thought would be a respite from broken relationships and life in the fast lane. Surrounded by cousins, nieces, and nephews—and their young children—Laura felt out of place. While she loved the kids, being with them was more exhausting than exhilarating. She no longer experienced a void that could only be filled by having a child.

Laura couldn't wait to come home to resume her professional and social activities. She still longed for companionship and love, but the vigilance, energy, and responsibility of child rearing (versus child bearing), especially without a committed mate, were too much to attempt at this time of her life. In her words: "I wanted the pregnancy more than I wanted motherhood."

## THE FLIP SIDE: PREVENTING UNWANTED PREGNANCY

Many women in their forties think that because they are less fertile, or their periods irregular, their eggs are impregnable. This can lead to the ultimate misconception—one that's unwanted. In fact, women in their forties have the second highest rate (after teenagers) of unintended pregnancies!

As you get older, your cycles are less predictable, so the rhythm method (avoiding sex during fertile times of the month) becomes less reliable. Remember, sperm can remain alive and potent inside your cervix for days. Barrier methods (spermicide, diaphragm, condoms) are now good options. If you are in the dating scene and risk exposure to sexually transmitted diseases, condoms may be an especially wise choice; lower estrogen levels mean your vaginal tissue is thinner and more fragile, making it prone to tiny tears that microbes can pass through.

Here are the pros and cons of the birth control options from which you can and should choose.

### The IUD (intrauterine device)

*Pros:* Compared with users of the Pill, IUD users have fewer contraceptive failures, and there's no daily, weekly, or before-intercourse need to remember to use it. You have it inserted and can forget it for ten years if it's the type that's made of copper (the Paragard) or five years if it contains progestin (Mirena).

The copper ions released by the Paragard have a toxic effect on sperm and make the cervical mucus hostile, and the fluid in the fallopian tubes nonconducive, to fertilization.

Mirena, the newest intrauterine system (IUS) on the block, works by releasing minute amounts of progestin to alter the lining of the endometrium and the cervical mucus, dissuading sperm from swimming up. It also affects ovulation and inhibits active egg release. Because progestin "calms" the uterine lining, preventing heavy buildup and decreasing blood loss and cramps (which sometimes increase with other IUDs), Mirena may be an excellent choice for women with a history of heavy periods or fibroids. It is also used "off label" by doctors to protect the lining of the uterus in women who are taking estrogen replacement therapy.

Once inserted, this IUS is good for five years at a cost of about $550, or less than $10 a month—a relative bargain. And it's over 99 percent effective! One Mirena change may be all you need in your last decade of contraceptive use. If you happen to become menopausal while it's in there, you also have the option of starting estrogen therapy without adding a progestin.

*Cons:* The IUD will not stop ovarian cycles and won't provide the ovarian cancer protection you get with the Pill. If you have never given birth, it can be somewhat difficult to insert. The copper IUD can cause spotting or heavy periods, provoking concern for women in their forties (and their doctors).

Does an IUD or IUS increase your risk of uterine and tubal infections, or pelvic inflammatory disease (PID)? For years the media brouhaha over infections caused by the Dalkon Shield virtually eliminated the use of all IUDs. We now know that the infections and subsequent scarring were due to the Dalkon Shield's multifilament tail, which wicked bacteria from the vagina into the uterine cavity.

All subsequent and current IUDs have monofilament tails that are essentially inert. Recent studies have shown that PID is associated with the presence of antibodies to *Chlamydia* (a sexually transmitted bacterium), not IUD use, even in women who've never had children. But tradition and underlying "let's play it safe" recommendations prevail (and appear in the physician and patient information inserts). I, like most doctors, don't insert IUDs in women who have a significant risk of exposure to sexually transmitted diseases.

### Depo-Provera and Lunelle (the Shot)

*Pros:* Depo-Provera has been an old standby for the treatment of heavy periods as well as providing "hands off" contraception for three months at a shot. It stops periods in half of the women who use it, and may also reduce the risk of developing uterine cancer. Depo-Provera contains progestin only, while the newer monthly shot, Lunelle, contained both estrogen and progestin (giving a monthly period). In 2002, this latter injection was found to have inconsistent dose concentrations and was withdrawn from the market by its manufacturer.

*Cons:* PMS, weight gain (two to four pounds a year), acne, spotting, and headaches can occur with Depo-Provera therapy. Once given, it may take months for these annoying symptoms to stop.

### What About Implants?

The Norplant, progestin-bearing matchstick-sized rods that were inserted under the skin of the arm, turned out to be difficult to remove—and the product was removed from the market in mid-2002 due to concerns about effectiveness (which turned out to be unfounded), dissatisfaction with side effects such as bleeding, and the problem with extraction. An updated version with fewer rods, called Implanon, awaits FDA approval.

## Ortho Evra (the Patch)

*Pros:* This new birth control patch basically has all the pluses of birth control pills. It can be placed on your lower abdomen, your rear, or your upper arm. The amount of hormone absorbed through the skin is equivalent to what your body receives from a low-dose birth control pill. The patch offers "I don't have to remember to take a pill every day" convenience; but you do have to remember to change it once a week (three weeks on, one week off—creating a period). It costs about $30 a month.

Because the route of hormone delivery is through the skin and not the gastrointestinal tract, the patch avoids "first bypass" through the liver. Whether this makes it any "safer" has not been established.

*Cons:* If you have contraindications to using oral contraception, they are just as pertinent for the patch (e.g., a history of clots, stroke, heart attack, or liver problems—or cigarette smoking). Also, while it's designed to withstand showering and swimming, the patch can occasionally fall off. If it won't stick back on easily, don't use a Band-Aid to keep it there. The hormone is in the adhesive, so you should apply a new patch within twenty-four hours for the Ortho Evra to continue to be effective as a contraceptive. A small percentage of women stop using the patch due to skin irritation. There are also warnings that in heavy women (over 198 pounds) the contraceptive failure rate increases.

## NuvaRing

*Pros:* Like the patch, this new form of contraception offers levels of estrogen and progestin equivalent to those of a low-dose birth control pill. But these hormones are absorbed through the vaginal lining, which (like skin) is good at releasing the medication in a slow, steady fashion.

The ring looks like a thin hollow diaphragm and should not be felt once inserted, nor should your partner feel it during intercourse. Unlike the diaphragm, it does not seem to increase urinary tract infections (UTIs). You have to keep it in for three weeks and then take it out for a week, at which time you'll get your period. Its hormone release is not affected by condoms and/or spermicide. If you take it out or if for some reason it falls out (it only comes in one size), you can simply reinsert it and it will continue to work over its three-week lifespan. It, too, costs about $30 a month.

*Cons:* The same contraindications as for the Pill.

## Tubal ligation (sterilization)

This is the most common form of contraception for American women who are 35 or older. Tubal ligation blocks the fallopian tubes so that sperm can't reach an egg. "Ligation" means tying (the tube), but in most procedures a portion of the tube is cauterized or electrically destroyed, or stapled with special clips through a laparoscope.

A newer method, called Essure, involves using a scope inserted through the cervix, through which a little metal coil is placed into each fallopian tube. This can be done on an outpatient basis without general anesthesia. It takes up to three months for the coils to cause the scarring that blocks the tubes; a special X ray should then be taken to ensure that this has been accomplished.

*Pros:* Tubal ligation is the most fail-safe method of contraception available; among all women who have tubal ligation, two out of one hundred will get pregnant within ten years. It also decreases your future risk of ovarian cancer by one-third. We're not sure why—perhaps by preventing cancer-causing contaminants such as talcum powder from traveling to the ovaries through the vagina, uterine cavity, and tubes. Similarly, blocking your tubes may also keep out microbes and decrease your risk of pelvic inflammatory disease.

*Cons:* The cost ranges between $1,000 and $3,000; so check to be sure your medical insurance will cover it. There are also the small but real risks associated with any surgical procedure (e.g., problems with anesthesia or infection).

Finally, some women experience regrets after sterilization. If you've already had tubal ligation and changed your mind, you may be a candidate for in vitro fertilization.

## Reasons to Consider the Pill in Your Thirties and Forties

Here are some of the valid reasons to consider the Pill at any age, but especially if you're in your thirties or forties and have any of the health concerns below:

*Fibroids.* At least one-third of women over 35 develop these noncancerous tumors. Made of smooth muscle fibers, they can appear inside the wall of your uterus (intramural), project into the lining (submucosal), or grow on the outer surface (subserosal). They constitute a problem if they become very large (the size of a four-month-plus pregnancy) or cause abnormal or heavy bleeding, pain, or pressure. (For more on submucosal fibroids and bleeding, see page 32.)

Fibroids are more likely to grow during our late thirties and early forties, due to unopposed surges of estrogen and lack of balancing progesterone. Combined birth control pills contain both estrogen and progestin, and so may prevent this exuberance of growth. The Pill also thins the endometrium and may decrease excessive bleeding caused by the fibroids.

In the past we were taught that the Pill made fibroids grow, but a literature review spanning thirty years found that fewer than ten cases were reported that showed that fibroids enlarged in response to an estrogen-progestin pill. If you have sizable fibroids (as large as or larger than a three-month pregnancy), you should be checked at least annually to make sure they remain stable in size.

*Ovarian cysts.* If too much fluid accumulates in the developing follicle or corpus luteum, a cyst develops. This type of "functional" cyst (so called because it occurs as a result of our ovarian "functioning") can quickly reach walnut or even lemon size and, when it ruptures, cause considerable pain.

The Pill, because it stops ovulation, prevents this fluid buildup. Monophasic pills, which have an unchanging dose throughout the cycle, may have superior cyst-cessation ability than triphasic pills, which contain increasing amounts of progestin over the three "active" weeks of the pill pack. Smokers have a twofold-increased risk of developing functional ovarian cysts compared with nonsmoking women. If they continue to smoke past age 35, they shouldn't take the Pill (at risk of dire health consequences), and so forfeit this medical option to "decyst"—unless they stop smoking.

*Endometriosis.* This insidious disease is a common cause of severe menstrual cramps, pelvic pain, and infertility, affecting at least 10 percent of women. Endometrial cells (the ones that grow in response to your cyclical production of hormones) grow in the wrong places: on the surface of the uterus, ovaries, fallopian tubes, or anywhere in the abdominal cavity.

How do these cells get "lost"? Possibly through retrograde menstruation; that is, instead of exiting the uterine cavity via the vagina, the cells go the wrong way, up through the fallopian tubes, seeding onto neighboring organs. Or they may wander to the wrong place through blood or lymph vessels. Multipotential cells may also be present almost anywhere in the pelvis or abdomen, and convert to hormonally stimulated endometrial-like cells.

These out-of-place cells should be destroyed by the immune system. But if this control fails, they take root and respond to your hormones, causing local reactions such as scarring and blood-filled cysts (*endometriomas*).

The Pill decreases buildup of the endometrium, so there are fewer cells to wander in a retrograde fashion. It also prevents some of the cyclical hormonal "feed" of these stray cells, and reduces prostaglandin production, which participates in the formation of scars and adhesions.

*Endometrial cancer and ovarian cancer.* Unopposed estrogen increases the risk of endometrial cancer (cancer of the uterine lining; see page 279). The Pill's daily dose of counterbalancing progestin reduces that risk by as much as 80 percent after eight years of use. And when it comes to ovarian cancer, aside from surgery the Pill is currently our *only* recourse for prevention. Because the Pill inhibits ovulation and "quiets down" ovarian activity, it seems to muffle the production and replication of the abnormal cells that could turn into cancer. Just three to six months of Pill use (while our ovaries are functioning) can reduce future risk of ovarian cancer by 40 percent. And studies show that the longer you take it, the lower the risk: after seven-plus years on the Pill, there is an 80 percent reduction in risk.

*Osteoporosis.* We need estrogen in order to build bone until age 30, and to maintain bone in the decades after. Low estrogen levels—which can occur in anorectic or very thin, athletic women whose periods are irregular or totally absent—cause bone loss and are a major factor in premature development of osteoporosis. The Pill provides the missing estrogen and protects bone health throughout the reproductive and perimenopausal years. You don't have to be *amenorrheic* (without periods) for your bones to benefit; the Pill prevents the fluctuations in our estrogen levels that can confuse bone-building cells, especially in our late thirties and forties.

*Acne and skin.* Acne is not just a problem for teenage girls. It can raise its ugly head(s) at any age. As long as we produce androgens, or male hormones, in our adrenal glands and ovaries, we are in the oil-production business. Male hormones promote oil secretion (sebum) in the skin. When this oil meets bacteria, the result is pimples. In preventing ovulation, the Pill decreases ovarian production of testosterone. Additionally, the estrogen in the Pill encourages the liver to make a protein that deactivates male hormones so they can no longer blight our skin with blemishes.

However, not all Pills are created equally skin-friendly. Most of the progestins used in older brands of the Pill are chemically similar to testosterone. So despite the Pill's estrogen component, these don't always clear—and indeed sometimes cause—acne in pimple-prone women. The newer progestins (norgestimate and desogestrel) have a lower androgenic activity. Ortho Tri-Cyclen and Alesse have been specifically approved by the FDA to treat acne. The latest Pill on the block, Yasmin, has a progestin that actually has *anti*-androgenic activity, potentially making it the best oral contraceptive acne blocker.

*Lumpy breasts.* If you tend to have lumpy breasts, taking a low-dose Pill may reduce fibrocystic changes in your breasts. It can take three months before you notice the difference, but ultimately your breasts should feel less tender and cystic.

## The Cons: When You Shouldn't Take the Pill

At one time, we were told that women over the age of 35 should not take birth control pills. This admonition has persisted, as many old wives' (or young to middle-aged women's) tales do. Ample studies have shown, however, that unless you smoke, there are no age restrictions on the use of birth control pills. You can stay on them until you're menopausal—which, for some of us, means our midfifties.

There are, of course, the usual warnings against use with certain medical conditions that apply at any age. These include pregnancy, liver disease, history of venous clots or pulmonary embolism (lung clots), heart attack, active liver disease, or uncontrolled hypertension. Don't take the Pill if you have, or have had, breast cancer. However, new studies have shown that there appears to be *no* connection between use of birth control pills and future risk of developing breast cancer.

I would like to add another, newly identified contraindication: the inherited abnormal clotting factors called *factor V Leiden* and *prothrombin mutation,* which increase a woman's lifetime odds of developing venous clots. These are present in about 2 percent of women. When this condition is combined with birth control pills, the risk of clots may increase thirtyfold.

How do you know if you have abnormal clotting factors? If you or several close relatives (parents, siblings, children) have had any problems with blood clots, such as deep-vein clots or a pulmonary embolism, talk to your doctor about having diagnostic blood tests.

### Can the Pill Help Me Look and Feel Younger?

I'm going to couch this answer in a lot of medical terminology, but my over-all conclusion is—yes. The Pill helps prevent all those perimenopausal symp-toms that can leave you drained, irritable, and depressed (if you don't have those symptoms, ignore this last sentence). It's good for your bones and pre-vents diseases—and if anything will age you, it's certainly disease. Estrogen has been found to increase collagen, water content, and elasticity of skin, and that translates into fewer wrinkles.

On the subject of skin, I have to add the warning that estrogen can in-crease pigmentation or dark areas on the face around the upper checks and lip (*cloasma*) after sun exposure. But if you want to prevent skin aging, it's im-portant to use lots of sunblock and stay out of the sun, anyway!

## When Can I Stop Using Birth Control?

I have a patient who had her IUD removed at 47 because her periods were getting heavy and she felt she no longer needed contraception. Six weeks later she felt nauseated, tired, and cranky: "Is this hormonal?" Yes, but not the hormones she expected. . . . To her amazement and dismay, her pregnancy test was positive!

The average age of menopause is 51.7 years (more on this later). The official word, according to the medical societies, is that we should con-tinue to use contraception for six months to a year after our periods stop. Not all my patients follow this recommendation, and I've yet to see a pregnancy in a woman over 52 with menopausal FSH levels. If you want to know whether you're menopausal, stop the Pill for two weeks and have a blood test to measure your level of FSH. If it's over 30, welcome to menopause. If it's lower, and you feel fine, you can go back on the Pill. Studies show that staying on the Pill beyond the actual date the ovaries quit working causes no harm.

## Annette's Story

Annette loved the Pill; she had regular periods, great skin, no PMS, and none of the hormone problems her friends in their early fifties were suf-fering through. She was more than willing to stay on them forever.

When she turned 52, I called a "time out." I pointed out that the estrogen in the Pill was nearly five times more potent than the estrogen in hormone replacement therapy (HRT)—and that the Pill had masked her probable entry into the world of lost ovarian hormone production. Annette had avoided the clinical symptoms of perimenopause, and even though she had not paused in her periods, she was probably menopausal.

Reluctantly, she went off her Pill for two weeks. I then tested her FSH—it was 18. She happily restarted her Pills, stating, "I told you I wasn't there!"

A year later, we repeated the off-Pill blood test. This time, Annette's FSH was 35. Continuing without the Pill "to see what menopause felt like," she developed hot flashes and night sweats . . . and decided to start a course of HRT.

## PERIMENOPAUSE

### "So What Am I, Pre- or Perimenopausal— or Has an Alien Taken Over My Body?"

Although the "alien" part is generally ignored in our medical literature, this question of definition has confused both doctors and patients. One near-frantic patient told me she wasn't sure if she needed a gynecologist, a psychiatrist, or an expert on extraterrestrials!

After numerous committee meetings, various professional societies have agreed: the only difference between pre- and perimenopause is that "peri-" includes the year beyond your last menstrual period. But to individual women, definitions matter far less than predicting and understanding symptoms—and what can be done about them.

### Premenopause

We are always "pre" something, and as someone who is always late, I consider it a positive term. Premenopause begins when your cycles vary two to seven days from your personal norm (they are often closer together and last longer, so you may feel like you're bleeding all the time).

Premenopause represents an era of accelerated depletion of the follicles in your ovaries. Each month, a dominant follicle may or may not develop. Its production of estrogen and ability to form a working corpus luteum become hit-and-miss. The pituitary doesn't receive its usual signals of ovarian well-being, so it puts out more FSH, trying to right an ovarian wrong.

Often a patient will ask to be "tested" for premenopause: "Does the late period mean my ovaries are failing? Is it just stress? Could I be pregnant [an entirely different stress]? Is something else wrong with me? Does this mean I'll reach menopause next month, next year?"

The best but not infallible guide is a blood test that shows an elevated FSH at day 2 or 3 of the cycle, when FSH should be at its lowest level. We once thought that as our ovaries aged, their estrogen output gradually dwindled, but "going, going, gone" does not describe our premenopausal state. There are days, or even months, when the remaining follicles respond to elevated levels of FSH and burst forth with surges of estrogen that can be as high as those produced in pregnancy. If we test FSH during this revived-follicle time, it will be low. This rapid firing is, however, short-lived, and the next generation of follicles may be unimpressed and unresponsive. Estrogen levels then plummet, and FSH ascends.

This hormonal roller coaster explains the symptoms of premenopause—irregular or missed periods and bouts of menopausal symptoms (especially before and during a period), which include hot flashes, sleep disturbances, memory and concentration problems, and mood swings. Indeed, because estrogen drops from superhigh levels, these symptoms may be worse than those we experience postmenopause, when the levels remain consistently low.

Add to this the breast tenderness, bloat, and weight gain that some women experience during high estrogen output (reminders of how we felt during pregnancy), and the severe headaches that can be triggered when high estrogen levels drop . . . and our sense of "this isn't me" can be explained by the fact that our hormonal clock has entered a state of disequilibrium. Even when the follicles behave and our cycles are fairly regular, albeit longer, there tends to be an inequity in the production of estrogen and progesterone, so PMS may get worse and last longer.

During the final peri- year, there are very few oocytes left in your ovaries. FSH's valiant efforts to coerce them to become functioning follicles will soon be of no avail. For the rest of your life, you will continue to have high levels of FSH. Even if you decide to use hormone replacement therapy, FSH will not go down to premenopausal levels, so routine testing of FSH ("to see what your hormones are doing") is unnecessary and expensive and, although ordered by many physicians, does not determine appropriate dosing of estrogen replacement (see page 65).

## Physical and Emotional Symptoms of Perimenopause: What Can I Expect?

> "I go from PMS to hot flashes. I don't know when my period is coming, and when it shows up, it's heavy and painful. When will this be over?"—JEAN, AGE 45

I'm not a speculum-bearing soothsayer, so I can't tell Jean exactly when these symptoms will abate and menopause (and *its* symptoms) will begin. Indeed, they may slowly merge, as menopause starts with a whimper, not a bang.

One study suggested that the average woman may have symptoms for nine years. I've had patients who have had perimenopausal symptoms that make them feel run-down and prematurely old from their early or midthirties.

While the average age at which a woman has her last menstrual period (menopause) is 51.7, it's considered "normal" for it to occur between the ages of 47 and 55. Smokers tend to reach menopause at an earlier age; those cigarette chemicals seek and destroy vulnerable follicles. Most women have a tendency to copy their mother's reproductive pattern. Jean might get a better sense of when "this will be over" from her mom rather than from me, her doctor.

A lucky 10 percent of women have few or no symptoms, and wake up one day to realize that they haven't had a period in months. Voilà! They're menopausal.

## Treating Jean's Perimenopausal Symptoms

Philosophically, it could be argued that Jean (quoted above) is going through a natural transition that should be left to take its course. Note that a hundred years ago, the "natural course" of many women's lives was to die in their late forties. This makes it difficult to look to our ancestors for examples or advice.

## Common "Menopausal" Symptoms Before, During, and After Menopause

*Hot flashes.* As with labor, you'll know when they occur.... You may sense their coming and start to feel anxious. Suddenly, you're hot and can feel your face turning red. Your heartbeat quickens, and you begin to sweat. Perhaps you feel a surge of irritation, edged with panic. Unless you've left an air-conditioned environment and ventured into a tropical climate, you're having a hot flash.

As you get older, your brain's inner thermostat becomes acutely sensitive. This, combined with a decline in estrogen levels, can leave it utterly confused. Just before the hot flash, it raises your core body temperature, and your nervous system is then presented with the task of doing something to cool you down. Temperature physics take over: Your heart beats rapidly to rush blood to the surface of your skin, where small blood vessels dilate (hence the flushing), and heat is dispersed outward (your skin feels hot to the touch) with the help of evaporation (you perspire). Your inner core temperature now comes down, leading to an overreaction to this temperature-control "oops." Your body attempts to bring back some of its lost heat by contracting small muscles (you shiver), and closing surface blood vessels (you turn pale). An exhausting process—which can occur a few times a day or hourly.

Any event that incites a temperature rise can trigger a hot flash: exercise, warm rooms, body heat under your blanket at night, hot beverages, spicy foods, alcohol (especially wine), or ubiquitous stress.

There are a lot of hot-flash jokes, but they are nothing to laugh about. They interrupt our activities and our rest, and undermine our composure at work. We may avoid close encounters of an intimate kind.

*Night sweats.* Hot flashes may awaken you several times a night, leaving you drenched with sweat, throwing off blankets, opening windows, or setting air-conditioning to "maximum freeze."

*Insomnia.* Hot flashes can occur throughout the night without actually waking you. Whether they rouse you or not, they disrupt the REM (dreaming) stage of sleep, leaving you feeling exhausted, irritable, and depressed. I refer to this as "menopausal jet lag" (without the reward of arriving at a vacation spot). Lack of estrogen also increases risk of *apnea:* breathing pauses (often accompanied by snoring) that leave you oxygen deprived at night and fatigued during the day. This may occur with diminished estrogen at any age: before a menstrual period (when your estrogen level drops), during perimenopause, and throughout menopause.

*Mood changes.* Twenty percent of us will experience a serious clinical depression at some point in our lives. While this number does not increase at menopause, that transition may trigger a recurrence if you have a history of clinical depression. Not all "I'm feeling down" symptoms represent true depression. Sleep disturbances alone could account for the fatigue, low energy, irritability, and nervousness of perimenopause and menopause.

However (and there's always a "however" in medicine), there is another explanation for menopausal mood changes: Estrogen can affect serotonin levels. Women produce roughly half as much serotonin as men, which could partially explain why we're twice as likely to experience depression. If the level of this "feel good" neurotransmitter drops as estrogen decreases, its absence may be felt. From an artistic point of view, this might be considered our "Blue Period."

*Vaginal dryness.* The vagina seems to be more sensitive to estrogen fluctuations than any other organ in our bodies. Normally, during arousal, blood vessels in the vagina become engorged and fluid is pushed out. Any drop in estrogen level (even before your period) can affect lubrication, making intercourse uncomfortable (*dyspareunia*). Long term, lack of estrogen makes the vaginal lining thinner, less elastic, and pale. (I can often assess a woman's estrogen levels by looking at the vaginal mucosa during a speculum exam.) This condition is disturbingly but accurately described as "vaginal atrophy." Ultimately, this causes changes in the normally acid vaginal pH, affecting the ecosystem of bacteria. Abnormal bacteria can grow, causing bladder infections and irritating vaginal discharge.

*Less interest in sex* (decreased libido). Remember when sex was a consuming passion (though we may have been less laser-focused on it than men)? Now you may feel less interested or even disinterested. Libido is governed by so many factors—a sense of well-being, body image, the attractiveness of your partner, communication, and finding time to make love, not work—but it's also ruled by your hormones, both female (estrogen and progesterone) and male (testosterone).

While your female hormones may fluctuate like crazy in the years before menopause, your male hormones are consistently lower: 50 percent lower than when you're in your twenties. Many women in their forties are just not in the mood, although they may enjoy sex once they get started and, with some work, go on to achieve orgasm.

*(continued)*

If this lack of interest is global (in a personal, not geographic, sense—no person or fantasy turns you on), it may be due to a low level of testosterone. It's not the total testosterone that counts, just the small percentage that's "unbound" by proteins, called "free testosterone."

How can you tell whether it's hormones or him? A blood test can determine if you have a low level of free testosterone and a high level of the protein that binds testosterone (SHBG, or sex hormone binding globulin). Testosterone therapy may help, and I'll address this in the next chapter.

Perimenopause presents us with a therapeutic dilemma: Birth control pills used to treat its symptoms can increase levels of SHBG. As a result, you may feel better, have smoother cycles—but also feel less lusty. There's no free lunch (or date).

*Short-term memory loss... I almost forgot.* Are you forgetting familiar phone numbers, whether you took your vitamins this morning, or the name of the person you're supposed to meet for lunch? Is it harder to concentrate? As estrogen levels decline, there can be changes in the production, utilization, and breakdown of neurotransmitters in those areas of the brain that deal with short-term memory.

Estrogen loss at the beginning of menopause may be a factor in the development of Alzheimer's disease later in life (see chapter 8). But the good news is that long-term memory, as well as our ultimate intelligence, seems to be unrelated to estrogen level.

The need for treatment depends on the severity of symptoms and whether these symptoms are merely annoying or are warning us of present or future diseases.

If your symptoms are like Jean's, here's what you should know:

### Treating heavy periods

These can be due to Jean's hormonal changes, which may cause an inconsistent buildup of the endometrial lining, or uneven (and prolonged) shedding, or both. A trial of therapy with birth control pills would be helpful. If the bleeding lightens up, this lights the way to diagnosis.

Fibroids (see page 22) are another possible cause for her heavy periods. Those that project into the lining (submucosal) are the worst offenders. A saline ultrasound exam (using sterile fluid to separate the walls of the uterus for a better view) would help establish whether this type of fibroid is contributing to perimenopausal blood loss. Submucosal fibroids can also be detected through a hysteroscope inserted through the cervix. If the Pill or a progestin intrauterine system (IUS) doesn't control the heavy bleeding, it may be necessary to remove (resect) the fibroid. This is an outpatient procedure requiring general or epidural anesthesia.

Other types of fibroids can also cause heavy bleeding. The abundant and abnormal blood supply that develops to feed them also feeds the endometrial lining. Fibroids don't contract, and these tumors can prevent the uterine muscle contractions that constrict and close bleeding vessels. Once more, the Pill or the progestin IUS may help. If not, a surgical procedure may be needed. Obviously, if the fibroids are very large they, or the uterus, can be removed. Submucosal fibroids can be removed or resected through a hysteroscope. In addition, the endometrial lining can be *ablated* (destroyed) with cautery, laser, ultrasound, or heat.

Another, less surgically invasive treatment is also available. A catheter is inserted through the large artery in the upper thigh and threaded up into the vessels that supply blood to the uterus and fibroid. Tiny synthetic particles are then injected. These block the vessels (*embolization*) and deprive the offending tissue of its blood supply, so that it undergoes tissue death (*necrosis*). There can be post-op pain, ranging from minimal (take some Tylenol) to so severe that hospitalization is necessary. In the best-case scenario, fibroids shrink by 60 percent, decreasing bleeding and other fibroid symptoms.

Of the 600,000 hysterectomies done annually on American women, 30 percent are performed for excessive bleeding. The average age of women undergoing hysterectomy is 42.7 years. Between the Pill, the Mirena IUS, ablative techniques, and embolization, Jean and at least two-thirds of women like her could control their bleeding and forgo this major surgery.

Bleeding, spotting, and pelvic pain can also signal other serious problems. For example, actress Fran Drescher saw several doctors for heavy and irregular bleeding before she received a diagnosis of endometrial cancer. If Jean, or any other woman in her forties (or even thirties), cannot control her bleeding with the Pill, an ultrasound should be done to check if the endometrial lining is unusually thick. If so, an endometrial sampling (suctioning or scraping cells from the uterine cavity for microscopic diagnosis) should *always* be done prior to ablative or embolization procedures.

### Treating menstrual cramps (dysmenorrhea)

These clutching pains near your pelvis—which can radiate forward, back, and downward to the legs—are due to uterine contractions, triggered by prostaglandins released when your uterine lining sheds. Medications that prevent this prostaglandin production can be very effective. Some, such as ibuprofen (Advil, Motrin) and naproxen (Aleve), are over-the-counter. They work if they are started before the cramps are strong. As long as you don't have gastrointestinal problems, you can try up to three 200-mg tablets of ibuprofen every six hours, or two Aleve every eight to twelve hours, for a day or two—but make sure to take them with food.

If these don't do the job, stronger anti-inflammatory meds (NSAIDs), such as prescription-strength naproxen (Naprosyn, Anaprox), or a new type of COX-2 inhibitor (Bextra) may help.

Once more, use of birth control pills will lessen the pain and heavy bleeding by limiting endometrial buildup and prostaglandin production.

### Treating PMS (premenstrual syndrome)

It's more than a coincidence that the same initials, PMS, stand for pre-menstrual syndrome and perimenopausal syndrome. The symptoms—bloating, weight gain, mood changes, depression, food cravings, sleep problems, and overall feelings of mild to moderate woe—recur monthly, and may last for days or weeks between the midcycle and day 3 or 4 of menstrual bleeding. As we get older and our cycles change, PMS symptoms can intensify and last longer.

For up to 8 percent of women, the symptoms seriously interfere with daily routines, work, or relationships, and are given an official medical title: PMDD, or *premenstrual dysphoric disorder*. In the past, both PMS and PMDD were dismissed as "all in our heads" phenomena. But once accepted by the gynecologic and psychiatric communities, these disorders became a battleground over causes and cures, argued with religious fervor.

The "progesterone supporters" proclaim that most PMS (and peri-menopausal symptoms) arise from lack of an appropriate rise in proges-terone. They promote "progesterone predominance" as a way to cure/treat the symptoms. Modes of natural progesterone therapy will be covered more completely in chapter 2.

Others—I guess we can call them the "estrogen blamers"—feel that the trouble lies in too much estrogen, not too little progesterone. Studies in Sweden have shown that high levels of estrogen produced after ovulation are associated with increased PMS symptoms. The fact that PMS worsens as we age may be due to elevations or swings in estrogen production. Estrogen sensitizes progesterone receptors in parts of the brain that create our emotions. So when the progesterone hits, it does so with a vengeance!

PMS encompasses the effects of these hormones not only on the brain but also on our adrenals, kidneys, and blood vessels. Fluid leaves the vessels and accumulates in our tissues; we bloat and gain weight.

It would make sense that preventing the midcycle rise of these two hormones would cancel these effects. In other words, the Pill should cure PMS.

Going back to Jean's story: There are now two reasons for me to suggest that she try the Pill: her heavy bleeding and her PMS. Remember that much of what Jean is experiencing is due to her hormonal ups and downs. The Pill provides the ultimate corporate takeover for her erratically responding ovarian follicles. By providing even doses of estrogen and progestin, it turns off the hypothalamus and pituitary so that GnRH, FSH, and LH are not secreted as get-going messengers to the ovary.

With over forty brand name and generic birth control pills on the market, what's best for perimenopausal PMS? Over the past thirty years, the amount of hormones in combined pills (containing both estrogen and progestin) has decreased; today's low-dose birth control pills contain 35 mcg (micrograms) or less of the estrogen component (ethinyl estradiol) and some form of progestin. The hormone combination in a low-dose pill should work for Jean, without making her feel over- or underhormoned.

For most women, the two important differences between the various birth control pills are the type of progestin they contain, and whether the amount of progestin is the same in each pill throughout the month (*monophasic*) or gradually increases during the three-week pill pack (*triphasic*) to help prevent breakthrough bleeding. The triphasic pills contain an estrogen dose of 25 mcg (Cyclessa, Ortho Tri-Cyclen Lo) or 30 to 35 mcg (Triphasil, Ortho Tri-Cyclen).

Women who find that their PMS mood changes actually become worse on the Pill may be sensitive to its synthetic progestin. A new progestin, drospirenone, could resolve this problem. It not only mimics our natural progesterone but also has an anticorticosteroid effect—meaning it works like a mild diuretic and prevents fluid accumulation and bloat. The birth control pill Yasmin contains this progestin. This is probably what I would initially prescribe for Jean's PMS.

For some women, the estrogen content is the important factor for their Pill well-being. The lowest dose of 20 mcg of ethinyl estradiol is available as Alesse, Loestrin ½₀, and Mircette. Estrogen-sensitive women who develop breast tenderness, or bloating, or just feel "out of sorts" on regular low-dose pills (or just like the idea of using the very lowest dose available) may prefer these. Asian women tend to be slow metabolizers of estrogen, and should start at the lowest estrogen dose. Women using these very low-dose pills may experience more breakthrough bleeding, especially if they don't take them at the same time every day.

Finally, if getting a period makes you miserable because of heavy bleeding, cramping, fatigue, headache, hot flashes, or a general sense of "letdown," try using the Pill to extend your cycle so you bleed less frequently. This can be done with *any* monophasic birth control pill; just continue the active pills (the first three weeks of the pill pack) month after month and omit the placebo pills. I suggest you do this until you start to spot or have breakthrough bleeding, at which time you can stop the active pills and take the placebo (or nothing) for one week. (When I took birth control pills I would do this for two to three months at a time, until it was "convenient" for me to bleed.) One birth control pill has been packaged and marketed for this bleed-just-four-times-a-year purpose. It's called Seasonale. It is a triple-tiered pill pack that contains eighty-four days of active pills followed by seven days of placebo pills. Initially, there may be some breakthrough bleeding (during the pharmaceutical trials this occurred in more than 60 percent of the women), but this should decrease with ongoing use.

As your clock advances, life events may reduce your contraceptive concerns. Perhaps you've had a tubal ligation or use an IUD; your partner had a vasectomy or uses condoms; or you are not sexually active. Realize that at least one-third of women taking the Pill use it for noncontraceptive reasons; fear of unwanted pregnancy is not a necessary prerequisite to starting the Pill.

## Other Therapies for Symptoms of Perimenopause

Now that I've sung my paean to birth control pills for controlling perimenopausal symptoms, let me go over other therapies: pharmaceutical, behavioral, and alternatives in between.

### Pharmaceutical category

*Progestins.* Heavy bleeding and irregular periods can be treated with progestins alone. An old standby has been the synthetic progestin called medroxyprogesterone acetate (MPA), also known as Provera. It thickens the lining of the uterus, and will limit bleeding due to irregular shedding of the endometrium. It's usually prescribed for ten to fourteen days, and then stopped; the sudden withdrawal of progestin support leads to collapse of the built-up lining and a "cleansing" period. This can be repeated monthly to control cycles, or every other month to see what happens without medication during the month.

This is not my favorite therapy. MPA can induce PMS-like symptoms, as well as headaches in women prone to menstrual migraines. I prefer micronized natural progesterone (usually Prometrium) for endometrial stability, because it's more like the hormones produced in our ovaries. "Micronized" means the progesterone is broken down into minuscule pieces to improve absorption and to prevent deactivation in the gastrointestinal tract. Versions of natural progesterone can also be made by compounding pharmacies (see chapter 2 for more on those).

Progesterone therapy is an option for women with abnormal bleeding who are smokers, and therefore can't take birth control pills.

One caveat: Progestin won't work without some estrogen on board. If bleeding does not occur after a course of MPA or progesterone, it's usually a sign that menopause has occurred and estrogen is no longer being produced by the ovaries. Some doctors use a trial course of progestin therapy to test for menopause; it's cheaper than a blood test.

*Drugs that treat depression, anxiety—and PMS.* Antidepressants have been found to be very effective in reducing the mood changes associated with PMS. The earliest PMS studies were done with Prozac. And in fact, Prozac (which is now available in less expensive, generic form) is now marketed under the name Sarafem for the express purpose of treating PMS. Antidepressants are usually prescribed daily, but because these drugs may lower libido, some women prefer to take them only during the one or two weeks a month in which their PMS symptoms occur. Studies support this intermittent therapy: Taking antidepressants on a timed "need to treat" basis for PMS can be effective.

The anti-anxiety medications Xanax and BuSpar are often effective for women whose chief PMS symptoms include a heightened sense of irritability and anxiety. Again, they should be used on a need-to-take basis, when you know PMS will ruin your day (or night).

The following medications can help control life-stressing PMS mood changes:

| *Antidepressants* | *Dosing* |
|---|---|
| fluoxetine (Prozac) | 20–60 mg per day (daily or during luteal phase)* |
| sertraline (Zoloft) | 50–100 mg per day (daily or luteal phase) |
| citalopram (Celexa) | 20–40 mg per day (daily or luteal phase) |
| paroxetine (Paxil) | 10–30 mg per day (daily or luteal phase) |
| venlafaxine (Effexor) | 50–200 mg per day (divided doses, twice daily) |
| clomipramine (Anafranil) | 25–75 mg per day (daily or luteal phase) |
| escitalopram (Lexapro) | 10 mg per day (daily or luteal phase) |

| *Anti-anxiety agents* | |
|---|---|
| alprazolam (Xanax) | 0.25–0.5 mg, 2 or 3 times a day (luteal phase) |
| buspirone (BuSpar) | 7.5–15 mg twice a day (luteal phase) |

*Note: The luteal phase is the last two weeks of your cycle before your period.

These brain-chemistry-altering drugs do have side effects (see chapter 8), and it may be easier (and cheaper) to initially try an appropriate birth control pill for PMS—if there are no contraindications—before working up to these medications.

*Estrogen.* Before we close this drug story, there's one more pharmaceutical option to treat the symptoms of perimenopause: HRT (hormone replacement therapy). While birth control pills even out the ups and downs of our ovaries' own hormone production, hormone replacement therapy (HRT) delivers an add-on, helping the lows but possibly making the highs too high. Some physicians prescribe HRT and report that patients have a good response, especially if their chief complaint is hot flashes.

Transdermal estrogen (the patch) may work the way your ovaries used to, providing even levels of estrogen slowly absorbed through the skin. Doses can range from mini-amounts (0.025 mg) to complete replacement amounts (0.1 mg). As with all HRT, progestin should be used for twelve days every one to three months in order to protect the endometrium.

There is a product called FemHRT that combines the same estrogen and progestin in birth control pills, but at much lower doses, and this may be an option for women during this transition. It won't work as a contraceptive, nor will it override natural cycles.

I've often found that giving any type of HRT at this stage may leave a woman feeling overdosed so that she develops bloating and breast tenderness. My concern is that she'll give up on HRT forever—for the wrong reasons. We'll revisit HRT for menopause in chapter 2.

There is one form of HRT that I frequently prescribe for perimenopausal women who suffer from *menstrual migraines:* the estrogen patch. In this case, the patch is applied only for that low-estrogen week just before or during a period. Adding estrogen helps prevent the premenstrual hormone drop that instigates the inflammatory and vascular changes triggering migraines in susceptible women.

If a patient is on the Pill, I instruct her to put the patch on the day before she stops her last "active" Pill and to keep it on during her week on "placebo" pills (the last row in the pack). She should take the patch off when she starts her new pill pack. If a patient is not on the Pill and knows when her period is going to start, she anticipates this event with a patch.

### Behavioral treatments for perimenopause symptoms

*Quit smoking.* Practically every time I mention behavioral therapy in this book, I'll start with this injunction: Don't smoke! Smoking hastens the onset of perimenopause. It worsens estrogen loss; speeds skin wrinkling, bone crumbling, and vaginal thinning; *and* prevents your doctor from prescribing birth control pills that could treat many of these symptoms.

This book is about what we can do to slow down the aging process. If, however, you want to *accelerate* aging, keep on smoking. . . .

Beyond that, adding exercise, changing your diet, and learning controlled breathing techniques can help alleviate your perimenopausal symptoms. See chapter 2 for these techniques, as well as some alternative therapies.


Has this all been a dress rehearsal for the final show: menopause? Not necessarily. The hormonal changes in our late thirties and forties cause unique symptoms and health problems and should be treated as a distinct category.

Once your ovarian follicles are depleted, you enter a whole new time zone. Read on to see what this means and whether you should do something about it.

# 2

## *When Your Hormonal Clock Stops*

**TWO TALES OF MENOPAUSE**

Dana phoned me in a state of considerable apprehension. She hadn't had a period for several months and wanted to find out if she was menopausal. When I questioned her about her symptoms, she said, "I can't discuss this with you. I'll come in for the tests. When you get the results, please call my psychiatrist. He'll tell me."

Dana's FSH was 50 ml, and her *estradiol* (estrogen level) was less than 10. These results, combined with her lack of periods and her age (50½), made it obvious that she was indeed menopausal.

I phoned her psychiatrist: "I'm calling at Dana's request; I know this is unusual."

"No, I was expecting your call." Once I'd explained the test results, there was a pause, followed by a deep sigh. Then he said, "Well, I guess we're going to have some major work ahead."

Dana called back several weeks later, crying. "This is the beginning of the end. I started antidepressants. Dr. Smith also suggested I talk to you about hormone therapy."

Sally came in for her annual checkup with a smile and announced, "I haven't had a period for almost a year. I have a few hot flashes; they're not too bad. I guess this is it: I'm finally menopausal. Can we do a blood test and make it official?"

When told her FSH was high, Sally's response was, "Thank God, I'm done! No more contraception. Let's talk about what I should and shouldn't do. . . ."

## MENOPAUSE: AM I THERE YET?

Officially, menopause occurs with your final menstrual period. If you've had twelve consecutive months of no periods, with no other obvious cause, you've passed menopause. After that last period, you are considered postmenopausal whether your menopause happened naturally or was caused by surgery (removing both ovaries), chemotherapy, or radiation.

"Postmenopausal" is a clinical, distressing term that I (like most women) dislike, because of all it implies: post-having fun, post-being able to have a baby, post-having the attributes conferred by our natural hormones. Medically, the adjective "postmenopausal" is not meant to convey a judgment; it simply denotes "the rest of your life after your menstrual period."

Assuming this occurs naturally, when can you expect it? The average age of menopause is 51.7. Most women will reach it between the ages of 47 and 55. As with other life events, we don't all fit the norm; indeed, 1 percent of women become prematurely menopausal before age 40.

### Premature and early menopause

This is most frequently caused by destruction of the ovarian follicles by chemo or radiation therapy used to treat cancer in childhood or early adulthood. Rarely, follicles are destroyed by a woman's own antibodies; this may become a multiglandular attack, with early "failure" of the thyroid and pancreas.

Heredity and behavior also play a role. If your mother or older sister had very early menopause, you may as well. Inherited abnormal genes on the X chromosome may fail to promote the development of sufficient numbers of follicles to last for thirty years, and once they're used up the ovaries cease to function at some point between puberty and the "normal" age of menopause. If you have short menstrual cycles, or never experienced pregnancy, you may also use up your oocytes more rapidly than other women and become menopausal in your midforties.

Smoking can hasten the onset of ovarian failure by two years. Oddly, living at high altitudes (above ten thousand feet) also contributes to early menopause. (I would hasten to add that smoking at high altitudes becomes a hormonal blitz.)

**Late menopause**
Again, look to your mother's experience. If she was a late finisher, you will probably follow in her hormonal footsteps. The good news is, you won't need to deal with the dilemma of taking HRT in your early fifties. The bad news is, the later you go through menopause, the longer your breasts are exposed to your own estrogen production, and this may minimally increase your risk for breast cancer.

## How Long Will These [expletive deleted] Symptoms Last?

Up to 20 percent of women continue to have symptoms of menopause for more than fifteen years. For the other 80 percent of women, symptoms do fade over time. If you decide to go off HRT, will your symptoms recur?

Consider a recent study of over 2,700 women between 55 and 88 (average age 67) who had not taken HRT for at least three months. Their hot flash occurrence rate was:

47 percent between ages 55 and 59
37 percent between ages 60 and 64
almost 20 percent between ages 70 and 74

Also, over a quarter of these women complained of vaginal dryness, and 10 percent of vulvar irritation. Sleep problems were perhaps the most life-disrupting symptom—affecting 55 percent of these women.

## IS MENOPAUSE A DISEASE?
## WILL "TREATING" IT SLOW
## DOWN THE CLOCK?

I saw a new brouhaha about menopause intensifying, and my own feelings of uneasiness and dismay increased. . . . There seemed to be a suspicious coincidence of the demographic emergence of this incredible market—fifty million women hitting menopausal age—with the revived definition of menopause as disease. . . .

If we didn't define menopause, which is undeniably the end of youth and reproductive function, as a disease, why would we try to cure it?—BETTY FRIEDAN, *THE FOUNTAIN OF AGE*

All women over 35 experience declining estrogen levels and, eventually, menopause. They and their families continue to struggle with the impact of menopause on their physical and psychological well-being, many having to deal with severe and extreme symptoms. . . . [We] encourage the advancement of private and public research for the treatment and management of menopause, and to facilitate the approval of remedies designed to alleviate the symptoms of menopause.—AMERICAN MENOPAUSE FOUNDATION

Disease: A condition of the body or one of its parts that impairs normal functioning.—*WEBSTER'S DICTIONARY*

I would defend menopause against the accusation of "disease." We don't attribute that label to puberty—though I must admit that when I mothered pubertal daughters, I considered all possible remedies (medical and behavioral) to ensure our survival! Menopause is a *transition:* one with clear implications for our cells, tissues, and systems. Just as each segment in our lifespan has its specific health-related problems, we can't deny the special concerns of postmenopause just because it's "natural."

As a gynecologist, I was taught to look at women's bodies through the lens of their reproductive organs—but have always felt that a speculum limits one's view. We're more than our mammary glands, uterus, and ovaries. Yet there's no question that our reproductive hormones and organs put us in a gender-specific medical situation; our physiology, diseases, and responses to medications very different from those of men. (When asked what kind of doctor I am, I now say I specialize in "female medicine" rather than "just" gynecology.)

The rush to medicate menopause has been widely criticized. On the other hand, a similar, more recent scuttle to proselytize and market so-called natural supplements and herbs has become more socially acceptable. Those who are cynical might say that the marketing of both approaches is driven by women's willingness to spend money to allay their fears of aging. We, the women, are dazed by the onslaught of information: conflicting medical reports ("This will save your life/kill you"), drug commercials ("This product will keep you young, dry, energetic, and strong"), cosmetic ads ("You'll look like this model if only you . . ."), and proclamations by "naturalists" that we should ignore all of the above and gracefully accept whatever happens to our bodies.

New studies about menopause or hormones elicit frantic calls from patients: "Should I stop taking this? Should I do what my friend is doing? Why can't you doctors get your story straight?"

I empathize with their frustration. Unfortunately, there are no simple, one-size-fits-all answers. The "ifs, buts, and therefores" are not just medical-legal hemming and hawing; they reflect the tremendous diversity of human beings. A given study may pertain to medical conditions, genetic variations, gender, species, lifestyles, or environments that do not reflect your individual situation. Each study is a building block, not a completed structure, and it is almost never the final word.

So the explanations and advice I offer here will be qualified, but within those limits I promise to be as up-to-date as possible. Each woman has to consider her personal physical and mental health, social situation, family history of disease, past and present risky behaviors, and fears of what will happen to her body in the future if she takes (or does not take) a certain course of action. None of us can really know how fast our clock is ticking. All we can do is inform ourselves about the options that might slow it down, and make the best decisions we can as we move ahead with our lives.

# DISEASES THAT MAY
# BE LINKED TO POSTMENOPAUSAL
# ESTROGEN LOSS

## Osteoporosis

Don't think of your bones in the context of those inert white skeletons displayed in biology class. Bones are living tissue, undergoing constant breakdown and reconstruction. Cells called *osteoclasts* eat away like Pac-Men, creating tiny holes that are filled with new bone by cells called *osteoblasts*. When the filling is greater than the drilling, we build bone. When the drilling (the medical term is *resorption*) dominates, the bones become more porous, and may go from a state of *osteopenia* (low bone density) to *osteoporosis* (weakened, fracture-prone bones). Estrogen increases the number of bone-building osteoblasts and their ability to fill in those holes.

We create 30 to 60 percent of our adult bone mass during the growth spurt at puberty. Once the ovaries produce enough estrogen to initiate menstrual periods, the emphasis shifts from building longer bones to building stronger (more dense) bones. Because girls have an earlier and briefer growth spurt than boys, the average woman ends up shorter and has smaller, less dense bones than the typical man.

With proper nutrition and regular periods, women slowly build bone density until the age of 30. Once that peak density is reached, women as well as men begin to lose bone density at an average rate of 0.5 percent a year. But since we start with a lower bone mass, it takes less time for us than for men to reach the critical bone density level that defines osteoporosis. Loss of estrogen at menopause accelerates this descent: The osteoclasts are unleashed, and the osteoblasts become less competent. Bone mass can decrease by 2 to 3 percent per year during the first eight to ten years of menopause, totaling as much as 30 percent by our sixties.

## Tooth Loss

In our jawbones, loss of density leads to tooth loss. Falling estrogen levels also have been linked to gingival inflammation (diseased gums), which causes teeth to loosen, decay, and require extraction, or just fall out.

## Coronary Heart Disease

The average age for the onset of coronary vascular disease in women is seven to ten years later than that in men. This cardiac superiority has been attributed to our estrogen production prior to menopause. Once we enter our perimenopausal years, our risk of heart attack begins to rise. By age 70, we are just as likely as men to have heart attacks; in fact, beyond this age we outnumber men in the occurrence of and death from heart attacks.

The earlier we go through menopause, the more likely we are to develop coronary heart disease. The Harvard Nurses' Health Study, which was begun over twenty-five years ago with approximately 120,000 nurses, found that women who had an early surgical menopause (i.e., their ovaries were removed) were more than twice as likely to develop coronary artery disease as women of the same age who did not become menopausal. If women were given hormone replacement after this surgery, their risk of disease was no greater than that of their nonmenopausal peers.

Estrogen replacement therapy was thought to protect our hearts as well as our own estrogen does. Combined results from three decades of research (over forty observational studies) have shown that post-menopausal women who took estrogen had a 30 to 50 percent lower risk of coronary heart disease than women who did not take estrogen. These results seem to make sense when we look at the biological effects of estrogen on our cardiovascular system.

Estrogen helps keep the "good" cholesterol (HDL) up, and the "bad" cholesterol (LDL) down. It also helps prevent the oxidation of LDL, which is known to contribute to atherosclerotic plaque formation. Estrogen improves the resiliency of blood vessels and the health of their linings (*endothelium*). It increases substances that keep blood vessels open (such as nitric acid), and limits production of substances that cause blood vessel constriction (such as renin and angiotensin).

Estrogen also improves insulin sensitivity and helps prevent the rising insulin levels found with prediabetic conditions that are linked to atherosclerosis. Finally, it lowers levels of homocysteine, a "bad" amino acid that also promotes plaque.

But—and here's where we get to the heart of the controversy—oral estrogen therapy (ERT) may increase levels of substances that have been linked to a higher risk of coronary vascular disease (biomarkers). These include certain clotting factors, triglycerides (fats), as well as markers of inflammation such as C-reactive protein. (Note: We now recognize that atherosclerosis results from more than fats accumulating in blood vessels. It also involves inflammation or irritation of the blood vessel lining.)

The argument has been made that many of the women taking estrogen in past studies were healthier to begin with, or developed healthier lifestyles as the study continued, than those women who did not take estrogen. Estrogen users were more likely to comply with medical advice: not only to take their pills, but also to exercise, eat right, and maintain a healthy weight.

That's why there have been such high expectations for randomized, prospective studies that could assess what happens to equally healthy (or unhealthy) women if they take estrogen replacement therapy (ERT), estrogen plus progestin (HRT), or a placebo—with neither patients nor doctors knowing who's taking what. Results for some of these studies are now in (more on this later in this book).

## Colon Cancer

Estrogen is probably good for our guts (at least, our large bowel and rectum) and may decrease the risk of colon and rectal cancer, probably due to the fact that estrogen lowers the production of irritating bile acids and their secretion into the bowel. It also decreases the production of insulin-like growth factor I (which can promote cancer cell growth) and has a calming effect on the colorectal epithelium (cells lining the colon).

## Alzheimer's Disease

Is estrogen brain food? Biologically, our brains are different (I'm not saying better) from those of men. They are chock-full of estrogen receptors, especially in areas related to the sound and structure of language, including verbal and visual memory. Estrogen affects important neurotransmitters such as acetylcholine (which facilitates our memory and thought processes), as well as the mood-improving serotonin and dopamine. Estrogen also appears to make neurons more sensitive to nerve growth factor, promoting growth of neurons and their connecting fiber networks.

Estrogen helps protect brain cells from free radicals, potentially damaging molecules produced as a by-product of oxygen metabolism. Estrogen also appears to help prevent abnormal protein plaque (*amyloid*) from accumulating in the brain and killing cells, a key factor in Alzheimer's disease (AD). Estrogen may also favorably alter apolipoprotein E, which injures neurons; indeed, a gene that increases production of this lipoprotein is linked to early onset of AD.

Before I forget . . . there is a correlation between severe hot flashes and decreased blood flow and glucose transport to the hippocampus, a memory-storing area of the brain. This means that hot flashes may be a warning or symptom of neuronal damage from low levels of estrogen.

Taken together, it appears that loss of estrogen can be detrimental to our brains. In one study, women who experienced surgical menopause (leading to severe, abrupt estrogen loss and disabling hot flashes) were more likely than women experiencing natural menopause to show memory impairment five years after menopause. Thirty-five years after surgery, more of the first group had developed Alzheimer's disease. We also see AD more often in women who have other conditions associated with low estrogen levels, such as osteoporosis, hot flashes, and low body mass (the fewer fat cells we have, the lower the conversion of adrenal hormones to estrogen).

## Mental and Mood Disorders

Freud suggested that at menopause, women were destined to sink into a morass of melancholy. Already burdened with penis envy, once we suffered the indignity of lost reproductive capability, we were doomed to a life of sad resignation. In fact, men need estrogen for *their* brains' well-being; that's where testosterone is converted to estrogen. I wonder if Freud's well-documented smoking and drug use affected his brain estrogen, and his theories on women!

Estrogen appears to influence the brain's production of—and sensitivity to—neurotransmitters such as serotonin, dopamine, and norepinephrine, but clinical depression does not seem to be more prevalent at menopause. There are three exceptions: women who experience a sudden change in estrogen levels (as in surgical menopause, which deprives women of both estrogen and testosterone), women who have a prolonged perimenopause, and women with a previous history of psychiatric illness. The *change* in estrogen, not its lack per se, seems to be responsible.

## Eye Disease and Blindness

Women with early-age menopause have been found to have a 90 percent increased risk of developing macular degeneration later in life, compared with women who have a later menopause. (Macular degeneration is responsible for 25 to 60 percent of all new cases of legal blindness in the

United States.) We don't have sufficient studies to know whether estrogen replacement will prevent this. We do have evidence that HRT may protect against cataracts.

## ESTROGEN AND HRT:
## TO TAKE, NOT TO TAKE, OR STOP?

This question has been extraordinarily divisive for all of us who are involved in women's health. Some physicians feel that menopause is a state of hormone deficiency, akin to thyroid deficiency or diabetes, and should be treated indefinitely with the missing hormones. Others adamantly state that hormones are being rashly prescribed for women who don't need them—and who indeed may be harmed by them—violating the sacred rules of evidence-based medicine.

Evidence-based medicine is the Holy Grail of health care: The benefits of any treatment must be shown to outweigh the risks, based on very large, long-term prospective double-blind trials. This means waiting almost a lifetime (or what seems like one) to see if years of treatment help or hurt. Few medications, especially when prescribed to women, have undergone this rigorous analysis. Our personal clocks can't always wait for all pertinent data to come in. We often have to take our chances and choose therapies based on the best currently available evidence.

Let's review the largest, most publicized trial of hormone replacement therapy, which was expected to provide some of the evidence we seek. (See the box on page 50.)

When the results of this study hit the airwaves, I was vacationing in Cape Cod, far away from my practice—and briefly considered hiding out there until the brouhaha passed. It didn't, and I came home to return frantic calls from my patients, then went to New York to explain the study for the *Today* show viewers. Was the "I've got to get off my hormones immediately!" panic justified?

The numbers suggested a personal risk for an individual woman taking the HRT Prempro as less than one-tenth of 1 percent per year. But this study raised public health concerns for the more than forty million menopausal women, one-third of whom had been taking some form of hormone replacement therapy (and almost half of those were taking Prempro). Taken together, the individual risks for these women became significant.

# The Women's Health Initiative (WHI) and What It Means for You

This ongoing study, sponsored by the National Institutes of Health (NIH), was designed to follow more than 160,000 postmenopausal women and determine if medical, nutritional, and/or behavioral therapies could reduce death and disability from heart disease, osteoporosis, and breast and colorectal cancer. One branch of the study looked at the effects of hormone replacement therapy (HRT); it included over sixteen thousand healthy women ages 50 to 79 (average age: 63) who had not had hysterectomies.

Half of these women took Prempro (0.625 mg of Premarin, an estrogen made from pregnant mare urine, combined with 2.5 mg of Provera, a synthetic progestin). The other half did not take HRT. Another branch of the WHI looked at the effects of Premarin taken alone.

The WHI was the first truly large study that followed women prospectively (forward in time) in which neither doctors nor patients knew who was getting hormones and who was getting look-alike placebos (a double-blind trial). Results were eagerly awaited. Would the women taking HRT develop fewer diseases than those women who took placebos—without increasing other risks to their health?

The Prempro study was planned to continue for 8.5 years but was unexpectedly stopped after 5.2 years; based on the interim results, the study's safety committee felt that the benefits of this therapy were not sufficient to offset its risks. Translated into practical terms, here were their calculations:

## Negative outcomes

Over the course of a year, if ten thousand women taking Prempro were compared with another ten thousand not taking HRT:

- 8 more women on Prempro would develop invasive breast cancer.
- 7 more women would have a heart attack.
- 8 more women would have a stroke.
- 8 more women would have blood clots in the lungs.

Complicating the picture: The increased breast cancer risk did not appear in the first four years of hormone use. Risk for blood clots was greatest during the first two years of HRT use.

**Positive outcomes**
- 5 fewer women on Prempro would have hip fractures.
- 6 fewer women would develop colorectal cancer.

This reduced risk for colorectal cancer was seen after three years.

## Understanding relative risk

Another way of looking at the WHI results and Prempro's risks and benefits involves the concept of "relative risk": the rate of the disease or condition among those receiving a treatment, divided by the rate among those not receiving it. Given a large enough study (like the WHI), the farther the relative risk number is from 1 (equal risk), the more meaningful it is.

An example: Studies show that a smoker's relative risk of lung cancer is between 10 and 25; put simply, smokers are *at least* ten times more likely to get lung cancer than nonsmokers (a 1,000 percent higher risk). By comparison, the relative risk of heart attack, cancer, and blood clots for HRT users in the WHI study was about 1.3 (30 percent higher), and the relative risk of osteoporosis and colon cancer among HRT users was about 0.67 (33 percent lower). If the WHI had continued long enough, sad as it sounds, for more women to get sick or die, we might have learned much more.

## Questions not answered by the WHI study

The medical community had hoped that WHI would answer the question of whether giving HRT at the beginning of menopause made a difference for women later in life. Unfortunately, the majority of the women who joined the study had been postmenopausal for years (their average age was 63), so arguably this question was not adequately addressed. The typical HRT user that I and most doctors see is in her fifties.

It's possible that some of the negative outcomes in the study were due to Provera (the "pro" part of Prempro), which may partially block estrogen's cardiac benefits and might, when added to estrogen, increase the risk of breast cancer. The risks that were the cause for concern might not occur with the use of Premarin by itself. Indeed the women in the WHI study who used this estrogen alone have continued to do so, and will until 2005. (We can also expect results in 2005, from other branches of the WHI, on the effects of eating habits, dietary supplements, and lifestyle.)

Finally, the WHI did not adequately address the value of HRT in treating hot flashes, sleep disturbances, and mood and memory problems at the *onset* of menopause. Women with severe menopausal symptoms were less likely to enroll in a study in which they knew they might be given a placebo. (Less than 12 percent reported significant menopausal symptoms when they entered the study.) Previous research has found that women who suffered from hot flashes felt their mental health was improved with HRT, whereas women who did not flush or flash felt no better and even complained of some decline in their sense of well-being.

### Are all HRTs created equal?

Do the findings of the WHI study apply to all hormone replacement therapies, or just to Prempro? I, and many of my colleagues, feel that there are some very important differences in the clinical effects of various modes and delivery methods of HRT (see below) and that the WHI should not be used as a blanket condemnation of all of them.

However, the FDA has decided, in its watchdog role, to add a "black box warning" to all HRT products. A black box is meant to draw attention to potentially serious side effects or newly discovered adverse reactions, and is found on the labels of many prescription remedies. The new warning describes the WHI findings, and recommends that if any form of HRT is prescribed, the smallest amount should be used for the shortest duration in order to reach treatment goals. The debate over what these treatment goals should be will keep medical journals busy for years to come. Most experts agree that the treatment of severe menopausal symptoms is a legitimate goal.

## Reasons to Start Hormone Replacement Therapy

### How do you feel . . . and look?

Here's what I tell my patients: The most important factor in deciding whether to begin HRT is how you feel at the onset of menopause. If you suffer from severe hot flashes, night sweats, insomnia, vaginal dryness, fatigue, mood swings, loss of short-term memory, or other "I feel so below par" symptoms, you should consider HRT, especially for the short term. Nothing can treat all of these symptoms as well as estrogen therapy, and you should notice a difference within a few weeks.

Less important, but not insignificant, are estrogen's effects on your looks. Estrogen helps keep the skin thicker, more supple, and better supplied with collagen and moisture. A study of nearly four thousand post-menopausal women found 30 percent less wrinkling among those who had ever used HRT, even after adjusting for sun exposure and smoking. A much smaller study, but one that I found fascinating, was done on sixty menopausal Canadian nuns. Half took estrogen for a year; the other half didn't. By the end of one year, the nuns who took estrogen had a 30 percent increase in their dermal thickness (as documented by skin biopsies); the other nuns saw no improvement (despite their habits). (For more on skin, see chapter 7.)

## Aside from Treating Symptoms, Can HRT Prevent or Treat Disease?

### Estrogen replacement and osteoporosis

They call osteoporosis "the silent epidemic." But there's nothing silent about the pain associated with fracture of bones so porous that they cannot support your head, your chest, or your body weight. The crippling effects of osteoporosis—being unable to stand up straight, move without pain, expand your lungs, have room for your heart to beat, or walk or even get out of bed—are the absolute, horrific antithesis of our anti-aging goal (see page 285).

Much of our later-life bone loss is attributed to estrogen loss, and more than fifty randomized, placebo-controlled clinical trials corroborate that use of estrogen (and estrogen-progestin therapy) prevents much of the typical thinning.

Estrogen therapy also was found to *increase* bone mineral density in spines by 4 to 6 percent, and in hips by 2 to 3 percent, within three years of starting treatment. In some studies, women still had thicker bones five to fifteen years after treatment. Even the newer low-dose estrogen therapies increased density 3.5 to 5.2 percent in older postmenopausal women who had low bone mass. (A few-percent gain may sound small, but remember most women are *losing* bone during that time. This small increase can make the difference between a broken bone and one that holds up.) We still don't know the optimal duration of estrogen therapy for osteoporosis, but it probably works best if started within five years of menopause and is used for ten-plus years.

The goal of prevention and treatment is not simply to "pass" your bone mineral density test (more on this in chapter 6). What really counts is whether your bones will break. Unfortunately, most of the studies used bone density as their measure of success (it's easier and cheaper to run imaging tests than to wait for a large group of women to break their bones). Right now, the medical literature talks about a 24 to 34 percent reduction in risk of hip fracture and other nonvertebral fractures in postmenopausal women who ever used ERT or HRT. The WHI study using Prempro showed that treated women had modestly fewer hip fractures than those not treated: a decrease of five per ten thousand women (remember, however, that the study did not follow these women long enough to monitor their bones into old age).

Until there are more randomized prospective trials, the Food and Drug Administration (FDA) has instructed drug companies not to promote estrogen for osteoporosis treatment, but only for osteoporosis prevention. They also recommend that HRT not be prescribed solely for this purpose. I look at it as one factor among many in the estrogen-prescribing decision process I go through with my patients.

### Estrogen replacement and heart disease

Prior to the WHI study, there was a veritable alphabet soup of studies looking at ERT/HRT and its effect on women's hearts. They looked at signs and symptoms such as angina (heart pain), arterial blockage, and heart attack, as well as deaths due to heart disease.

Here is a quick summary of some of the latest randomized, controlled studies whose acronyms are being bandied about with abandon:

*HERS I study* (Heart and Estrogen/Progestin Replacement Study). This involved 2,763 women (average age 67) with established coronary disease, treated with Premarin (estrogen) plus Provera (progestin), or a placebo, followed for 4.1 years.

*Results:* Overall, there was no difference in heart attack or coronary heart disease–related death (defined as heart "events") between the groups—but there were more events in the first year in the hormone-treated group, and fewer during the last two years. Because cholesterol (lipid) levels improved, it was thought that perhaps the study had ended prematurely and that with time, these healthier lipid levels would prevent further events in the HRT-treated women. So, on to the sequel . . .

*HERS II study.* This study included 93 percent of the women who survived HERS I, so they were four years older.

*Results:* There were no significant decreases in heart events among women in the hormone group, compared with those taking a placebo.

*Note: These were older women who already had significant heart disease and then were given a form of HRT that might not have been ideal for this condition. The progestin (see PEPI study below) may have blocked any heart-improving effects of estrogen.*

*ERA trial* (Estrogen Replacement and Atherosclerosis in Older Women). Three hundred and nine postmenopausal women (average age 66) whose angiograms were abnormal (i.e., they had arteries clogged with plaque, a condition called *atherosclerosis*) were followed for a little over three years. They received Premarin, Premarin plus Provera, or a placebo.

*Results:* None of the hormones slowed the progression of atherosclerosis in these women with established disease.

Based on all these studies, cardiologists advise that women with known heart disease not be started on HRT. The question now remains: What about those of us who don't have heart disease, yet want to prevent it?

*PEPI trial* (Postmenopausal Estrogen/Progestin Interventions). This included 875 *healthy* postmenopausal women (ages 45 to 64) who received (1) Premarin with Provera for twelve days a month, (2) Premarin with Provera daily, (3) Premarin with micronized progesterone for twelve days a month, or (4) a placebo. They were followed for three years, and their lipids tested.

*Results:* When Provera was added, the heart-healthy effects of estrogen on total cholesterol, HDL, and LDL were partially blocked. Micronized oral progesterone caused the fewest problems.

The American Heart Association states that HRT does not provide a benefit, in either preventing heart disease from the get-go (primary prevention) or preventing its getting worse if you have it (secondary prevention).

Before you assume that you'll put your heart at risk if you decide to take some form of estrogen, let me give you some reassurance. Certain women do have a genetic risk for abnormal clotting and inflammation, which can be aggravated by initial use of HRT. Few women in the above studies were screened for this. In the very near future, we may routinely assess this risk, with blood tests for markers such as C-reactive protein

(CRP), interleukin 6, lipoprotein (a), factor V Leiden, protein S, and pro-thrombin gene mutations (to name a few).

There's some evidence that having abnormal or elevated baseline levels of these markers may be more important for predicting your risk of CHD (coronary heart disease) than use or nonuse of HRT. Future studies might well show that women with healthy hearts and normal levels of these markers not only will be unharmed by HRT but may attain cardiac benefit.

One final heartfelt (sorry!) comment: Estrogens and progestins other than Premarin and Provera, derived from other sources and delivered through a different route (e.g., through the skin or vagina), may have very different effects on our coronary blood vessels. We just don't have WHI-type studies to demonstrate this. Currently, the FDA, in its infinite caution, warns that we cannot assume this difference is present.

### Estrogen replacement and colorectal cancer

Colorectal cancer is the third leading cause of cancer death in women (after lung and breast). So anything we can do to reduce this risk certainly has major implications for our longevity.

A review of eighteen studies found a 20 percent reduction in risk for women who had ever used HRT, compared with those who never used it. Moreover, women who were still taking hormones had a 34 percent decrease in risk; the Nurses' Health Study showed similar results. Finally, the WHI study seems to confirm this benefit. This is still not considered "conclusive evidence," or sufficient reason by itself, for prescribing HRT.

### Estrogen replacement and Alzheimer's

As we tick on to age 85 and beyond, roughly 40 percent of us may be afflicted by Alzheimer's disease. Diagnosing Alzheimer's is still very difficult, making prevention studies hard to perform and harder to interpret. So, much of the estrogen pro-brain data focuses on known symptoms such as changes in problem-solving ability, verbal and visual memory, and attention span. (For more information, see page 358.)

A variety of studies have found as much as a 50 percent reduction in risk of developing symptoms of Alzheimer's among women who have *ever* used estrogen. Some researchers speculate that short-term estrogen therapy to treat hot flashes—which may correlate with or cause reduced flow of blood and glucose to critical areas in the brain—could be key in preventing or delaying AD. Unfortunately, studies have not shown that once Alzheimer's is diagnosed, its progression can be altered by giving estrogen. And if we wait ten to fifteen years after menopause starts, estrogen doesn't seem to help, as was demonstrated by a study with the delightful name of WHIMS: the Women's Health Initiative Memory Study.

WHIMS compared the effect of Prempro and placebo on women who were 65 or older. After four years, more women (40 out of 2,229) on this HRT were diagnosed with dementia (mostly Alzheimer's disease) than those taking placebo (21 out of 2,303). In the real world, this would be equivalent to an extra twenty-three cases of dementia per year among every ten thousand Prempro users. The study also found small *gains* in all of the women's brain function test scores (a Modified Mini-Mental State Examination; see chapter 8 for a description), perhaps because they were getting used to taking the test . . . practice makes perfect. But those on Prempro did slightly better.

This highlights the possibility that years of estrogen "loss" may result in a loss of estrogen receptors in the brain. We can't expect estrogen to repair a damaged neuron, but if it's given at the onset of menopause, it may help protect the neuron's future.

### Estrogen replacement and mood disorders

During bouts of clinical depression, levels of neurotransmitters (norepinephrine, dopamine, serotonin) as well as opioids (natural antipain substances) decrease. When estrogen reaches the brain, guess what happens? All of the neurotransmitter levels increase. Many psychologists and psychiatrists feel that if a postmenopausal woman is seen for treatment of depression, estrogen should be prescribed before or in conjunction with antidepressants.

### Estrogen replacement and insomnia

Lack of sleep speeds up our clock and ages us. Although there are many causes for insomnia, and estrogen is not a panacea, it will prevent interruption of REM (dreaming) sleep and may improve the quality of your rest. Natural progesterone also enhances sleep. So I encourage use of this combination for some of my sleepless-in-L.A. patients prior to resorting to other, habit-forming sleep aids. For more on ways to sleep better, see chapter 8.

## SIDE EFFECTS OF ERT/HRT:
## REAL VS. FEARED

I've been helping patients make decisions about HRT for more than twenty years. Concerns and fears have come and gone, influenced by media reports, friends' experiences, word-of-mouth horror stories, direct-to-consumer advertising—and, oh yes, what the doctor said. Some are valid; some are based on innuendo instead of data; and some are completely unfounded. Let's look at these one by one.

### Concerns We Can Do Something About

#### Vaginal bleeding

Jeanine had been on hormone replacement therapy for over a year. She cleaned out her bathroom closet, giving all of her pads and tampons to her daughter. Then suddenly, she started to bleed. She immediately called me: "I thought I was done menstruating. And now I've ruined two pairs of pants!" Then she voiced her real fear: "Do I have cancer?" And she stopped her HRT.

Bleeding is one of the key reasons that women quit HRT. Adding progestin to estrogen can instigate a "period." In theory, if HRT is given continuously (a daily dose of estrogen and progestin or progesterone), the glands of the uterine lining are suppressed (the progestin "opposes" the estrogen); the endometrium is not built up and shouldn't shed. But between theory and reality, there's a lot of soiled underwear. Absorption, metabolism, and the levels of hormones can vary as a result of antibiotics, steroids, stress, gastrointestinal upset—or just forgetting to take them. When this happens, remnants of the lining break off, and bleeding results.

Some of my patients prefer to bleed every month; it makes them feel that they're not really menopausal. One woman recently told me, "I just love getting my period; it's such a cleansing experience." (There is no evidence, by the way, that monthly bleeding keeps you younger or cleaner.) For these patients, I prescribe cyclical hormones: estrogen daily, and progesterone (or progestin) twelve days a month. Some women have trouble tolerating any progestin product, I then suggest they take it for twelve days every two to three months and watch over their endometrium with yearly ultrasound exams.

While taking cyclic HRT, a woman should bleed when she stops the progesterone. But often, especially if the hormone doses are low, nothing happens. *Lack* of bleeding is never a problem. The only time I become concerned is if bleeding occurs at the wrong time, or is heavy or prolonged. In most cases, abnormal bleeding means something went wrong with the way the hormones worked. If so, we can fix it by increasing the progestin for a while, decreasing the estrogen, or adjusting the timing and/or delivery of the hormones (patch or Pill).

But one must never make medical assumptions, and I advise all women with abnormal bleeding on HRT to have a pelvic ultrasound to measure the thickness of the endometrium. If it's greater than five millimeters, it could indicate a precancerous condition (*atypical hyperplasia*) or even endometrial cancer. To rule these out, I perform an endometrial sampling, inserting a very small suction catheter into the uterus to scrape off some superficial cells.

In sum, if you have unexplained bleeding, don't panic—but do seek medical advice. Your doctor can make sure you don't have cancer, diagnose the cause of the bleeding, and adjust the hormone dose or method of therapy. Remember this comforting statistic: Women who take some form of combined estrogen/progestin therapy are less likely to develop uterine cancer than women who do not.

**Weight gain**
A major fear for most of my patients is weight gain (I practice in Los Angeles, where tummies are flat and often bared, with ring-adorned navels!). As we get older, fat is deposited in an apple pattern around our waists— and, yes, we gain weight. (See the chapters on eating and exercise.)

Studies have shown that postmenopausal women who take hormones gain *less* weight than women who do not. HRT has actually been found to limit abdominal obesity.

Having said this, I do have a few patients who believe their appetites increase when they take HRT (maybe because they feel better). Others claim that when they go off hormones, they lose weight. A few say they fare better on transdermal estrogen (the patch), or a natural progesterone. I'm willing to let them try all of these and come to their own conclusions.

There are some data indicating that estrogen combined with testosterone may increase lean body (muscle) mass, but I don't think the evidence is sufficient to prescribe this routinely for all women on HRT. (I reserve it for those with low libido; see next section.)

## Libido

Does HRT improve sex? Hormones are only part of the issue. The absence of a desirable partner or at least a fantasized one, depression, chronic fatigue, or an unsexy body image may be more damaging than lack of estrogen.

Then there's *dyspareunia,* that sandpapery, "it hurts like the dickens" feeling during intercourse. There's nothing like anticipated pain to make the act unappealing. Estrogen therapy helps improve sexual response by improving vaginal health; it not only stops pain but also promotes arousal: increased blood flow to the vaginal wall, along with lubrication.

Note I haven't used the word "libido" yet, and that's because there is an estrogen dichotomy: Its replacement is good for the vagina but can dampen desire. Oral estrogen increases liver production of the protein that binds up testosterone (sex hormone binding globulin, or SHBG) and renders it "impotent." Bound testosterone is of no benefit in maintaining fantasies, desire for sex, and orgasmic response. Only free, unbound testosterone (think Samson with his unshorn hair), which attaches to receptors in our brains, genital tissue, and all the other cells in our bodies, has this libidinous effect.

So I'm not surprised when a patient tells me she thought oral HRT would help her libido, but the opposite occurred. The estrogen may be counteracting the small but critical amounts of testosterone she's making in her adrenal glands and her ovaries, so I'll suggest that she switch to a transdermal patch or vaginal ring. The estrogen absorbed through the skin or vagina does not initially pass through the liver—where it can increase levels of SHBG. If this doesn't help, she may be a candidate for testosterone supplementation (see below).

### *Well-Founded Fears About HRT*

#### Cardiovascular diseases (clotting, heart disease, and stroke)

Harking back to those acronym-laden studies, we found that women with heart disease may do worse on HRT, and HRT may not prevent heart disease (or stroke) in still-healthy women. Does that mean you should be worried that taking HRT will give you a clot, a heart attack, or a stroke? There's no simple answer. It depends on your personal risk factors. I would definitely advise you *not* to take estrogen if:

- You've had a *previous heart attack* or have coronary vascular disease.
- You have a *history of blood clots* in the deep veins of your legs (*throm-*

*bophlebitis*) or of pulmonary embolism (clots that traveled to your lungs). HRT seems to double the risk of deep-vein thromboses (leg clots), with the greatest danger seen in the first year of treatment. This suggests that certain women are more susceptible—and if they are going to develop clots, they'll do so fairly early in their course of therapy. They may have underlying clotting or inflammatory abnormalities, such as an increased Leiden factor V, a prothrombin gene mutation, or an elevated C-reactive protein, that place them at risk—made even higher by estrogen.

- You have a *history of stroke* or "ministrokes" (transient ischemic attacks). These, too, may have been due to small clots or vessel obstruction, and constitute a risk for new clots.

If you are at risk for or have *diabetes,* HRT poses a dilemma. Estrogen has been shown to increase insulin sensitivity and delay the onset of diabetes. In the past, doctors have prescribed estrogen for diabetic women without compromising their diabetic control. However, since many diabetics have underlying coronary vascular disease, there's the issue of heart protection. Tests to assess coronary arteries (see page 233) may help you and your doctor decide whether HRT is right for you.

### Breast cancer

For many of my patients, the predominant HRT fear is: "Oh my God, will I get breast cancer if I take estrogen?"

Despite fifty years of hormone use, and almost as many studies, this question has not been definitively answered. Some very well regarded, large studies found no increase in risk; others found a slight increase, especially with longer use. Here is an overview of the best-known studies.

The Harvard Nurses' Health Study found a slow increase in risk of breast cancer each year, up to about 30 percent, among women who took estrogen (most used Premarin) for more than five years. Adding progesterone (again, Provera) seemed to slightly increase this risk to 40 percent. The WHI found that what the statisticians stated was a "barely significant" increased cancer risk of 27 percent after five years among women using Prempro.

The Iowa Women's Health Study (comprised of more than 37,000 women) found that only 5 percent of cancers were correlated with estrogen use, and these were of a highly treatable type; in other words, 95 percent of breast tumors were not estrogen linked. What about breast cancer mortality rates? A huge study by the American Cancer Society that followed more than 400,000 women over ten years found that those who ever took estrogen had a 16 percent *decrease* in risk of *dying* from breast cancer. Combined with the Iowa study results, this may mean that hormone replacement contributes to a slight increase in risk of developing estrogen-receptor-positive tumors. However, such tumors respond to therapy, and are less likely to spread or to be fatal than estrogen-receptor-negative tumors.

It may turn out that progestin is the greater culprit, as was concluded by a recent NIH-sponsored five-city study involving over 3,800 post-menopausal women, comparing those with a history of breast cancer and those without. The women who took combined continuous HRT (daily estrogen and progestin) for five years or more had a risk of breast cancer that was approximately 50 percent higher than that of the women who did not take HRT. But six months after they quit this hormone regimen, this extra risk disappeared.

Perhaps more intriguing was the finding that estrogen replacement alone did not increase cancer risk. A 2003 study in the *Journal of the American Medical Association* looked back at the hormone-taking history of 975 "older" women (between the ages of 65 and 79) who were diagnosed with breast cancer. Estrogen-only therapy did not appreciably raise their risk of breast cancer—even if they took it for over twenty-five years! But women who took progestin either continuously or cyclically together with the estrogen increased their chance of developing a type of breast tumor that had estrogen and progesterone receptors. (These types of tumors are considered less aggressive than those without these hormone receptors.) This risk increased with years of use, becoming 2.6 times greater after fifteen years.

Additional breast-concerning results from the WHI were reported at the same time. In the five years of that study, there were 245 cases of breast cancer in women who were assigned to take HRT (not all took it) versus 185 in women who were assigned to take a placebo. But compared with those in other studies, the cancers in the HRT group were found when they were larger and more advanced. The women on HRT were also more likely to have abnormal (harder to read) mammograms, even one year after starting HRT. This could have hindered early pickup of small cancers.

Shortly after the WHI breast findings were announced, the Million Women Study was published in *The Lancet*. Between 1996 and 2001, nearly 1.1 million women aged 50 to 64 enrolled in a British government–sponsored breast cancer screening program. The study was designed to look at the effects of HRT on breast cancer incidence and deaths. About half of the women reported past or current use of HRT. These women received mammograms just *once* every three years (annual mammograms are recommended by the American Cancer Society).

For current HRT users, an increase in breast cancer risk was seen within a year or two of starting HRT. Those who took estrogen alone (pills or patches) had a mild increase in their rate of breast cancer, compared with the women who were not currently taking hormones. Translated to a thousand women, five years of ERT use would be expected to cause 1.5 "excess" cases of breast cancer, and ten years of continued use would cause five extra cases. Women using combined estrogen and progestin (Provera or other synthetic progestin pills) on either a continuous or sequential schedule faced a higher risk: an additional six cases per thousand after five years of HRT, and nineteen cases after ten years. In other words, when calculated for thousands of women, the cancer risk became significant, but for an individual woman (absolute risk), it was small. Breast cancer mortality in the women on long-term HRT had a far smaller increase, and this statistic was considered to have "borderline significance." Finally, past users of HRT had little or no overall increase in their breast cancer rates; whatever risk was present wore off within five years of cessation of their HRT use.

It's not clear how we can explain the combined findings of these studies. It may be that adding progestin to estrogen can promote abnormal breast cell division and growth by stimulating both estrogen and progesterone receptors. Rather than triggering new cancers, HRT may make existing cancer cells grow, develop, and come to diagnostic attention more quickly. Women on HRT may also develop denser, more glandular breasts, making initial diagnosis through mammograms more difficult.

However, before you clutch your breasts in despair, remember most of these studies were done on "traditional" doses of estrogen and synthetic progestin. The risk may be lower when other forms of progesterone are used, or when we limit the systemic (breast) effect of this hormone with lower or "local" endometrial progesterone therapy (see next section); we can create an "almost" estrogen-only effect that may be less breast-worrisome, at least for short-term use.

### Endometrial cancer

It's well established that taking estrogen unaccompanied by progestin or progesterone stimulates the uterine lining (endometrium). Studies have shown that this creates a five- to eight-times-greater risk of developing endometrial cancer. Fortunately, adding even small amounts of progestational hormone will cancel this risk. That's why, unless you no longer have a uterus, HRT (not plain ERT) is the standard for hormonal care.

### Gallstones

One final concern is that estrogen concentrates and diverts cholesterol from your liver into bile, promoting formation of irritating cholesterol stones (gallstones). Estrogen therapy has been shown to double the risk of gallbladder disease.

### *What to Do?*

Yes, this is complicated. What's more, there are many types of hormones available, and their benefits and risks may differ. In the next section, I'll review your options—and as usual, I'll conclude with the phrase "Discuss this with your doctor."

## THE MANY FACES OF HRT: WHAT YOU AND YOUR DOCTOR NEED TO CONSIDER

> A hormone remake of the old Paul Simon song would feature
> this refrain: "There must be fifty ways to prescribe HRT."

In these days of managed care, doctors often lack the time to go over all our options carefully. That may be why one-third of women who are given an HRT prescription don't fill it. They don't know why it's prescribed, what it can or cannot do, or what to expect once they've started it. Armed with the information below, you'll know the buzzwords, be able to ask better questions, and feel more comfortable with your choices, whatever they may be.

### *Natural vs. Synthetic*

The way to sell anything today is to label it either "natural" or "designer." The word "synthetic" has acquired a negative aura in this so-called New Age.

When endocrinologists say "natural," they are not referring to where the hormone came from, but to whether—once inside your body—it's treated like the "homemade" estrogen (*estradiol*) produced by your ovaries. To them, natural means naturally metabolized like estradiol and broken down into less potent estrogens, called *estrone* and *estriol*. These estrogens enter your body cells, attach to receptors, and do their thing. Most of the estrogens in oral ERT are extensively processed and metabolized in a woman's liver, whereas the "synthetic" estrogen (ethinyl estradiol) in birth control pills is not. Because of this, even though the Pill is now "low dose," it's five times more potent than naturally processed estrogen, which is why it can block ovarian hormone production and stop ovulation.

Many of the estrogens in ERT originate from plants: soy and wild yams. If you consider animal products natural, the estrogen in Premarin is, too, since it comes from the urine of pregnant mares. (Animal activists and vegetarians can fight this one out.) Once the hormone is extracted, from whatever source, it is isolated, enhanced, purified, and condensed in a lab to become hormone therapy. It's a mistake to think that someone is out in a field, gathering plants, crushing them with a pestle, and packaging them from their farm as pure estrogen. Whatever combination of animal, vegetable, and laboratory was involved in the production of the following ERTs, it matters more to the marketers designing labels and slogans than it does to your estrogen receptors.

## Estrogen Options

Here are the types of estrogen used for ERT that are approved by the FDA and available by prescription from your pharmacy. (Note: This information also applies to generic versions.)

Is one better than another? Who gives the "Good Body-keeping Seal" of approval? Alas, we don't have prospective, long-term studies for forms of HRT other than Premarin and Prempro. Appropriate doses of all these estrogens "cure" acute menopausal symptoms.

### ERT pills

*Conjugated equine estrogen (Premarin).* The first estrogen therapy, introduced over half a century ago, this was the estrogen used in most American studies of ERT, including the WHI, HERS, ERA, and PEPI studies. This product is made up of many types of estrogen, including equine (horse) estrogens. Premarin is prescribed in doses ranging from 0.3 mg to 1.25 mg.

*Micronized estradiol (Estrace).* Made from plants, this type of estrogen is identical to that which we produce in our ovaries, and is a favorite in Europe. "Micronized" means that the estrogen is granulated into minute pieces, so it's more stable and easily absorbed.

*Other plant-derived oral estrogens.* These include Menest and Cenestin. The chief component of Menest (estrone sulfate) is one of the forms of estrogen produced in our bodies after we metabolize estradiol. Cenestin, a more slowly released, conjugated estrogen, may keep blood levels of estrogen more constant—a plus for women who develop hot flashes eighteen hours after taking some shorter-acting pills.

*Estropipate (Ogen, Ortho-Est).* This estrogen is made in the lab from purified crystalline estrogen. It behaves in the body like the estradiol metabolite estrone and, dose for dose, is slightly less active than Premarin or Estrace.

### ERT patches

*17 (beta) estradiol (Alora, Climara, Esclim, Estraderm, Vivelle).* These contain plant-derived estradiol that is processed so it can be absorbed through the skin from the adhesive in a patch. This mode of ERT delivers a very steady dose of hormone, which most closely mimics your ovarian estrogen production prior to menopause.

I find that the patch's even dosing is especially helpful for women with a history of menstrual or menopausal migraines. Even the tiny variation in estrogen that can occur with the time delay between doses, or between absorption of oral estrogen and its action in the bloodstream, can instigate headaches, hot flashes, or night sweats.

These patches differ in their adhesive, color, size, and duration of use. Climara needs to be changed only once a week; the others require twice-weekly changes. The patches come in many doses, from the very low 0.025 mg to 0.1 mg. And in between, they vary from 0.0375 mg, 0.05 mg, 0.06 mg (Climara), and 0.075 mg. The 0.05-mg dose is roughly equivalent in its final effect to 0.625 mg of Premarin or Cenestin, and 1 mg of Estrace. So, if you switch from an oral ERT to the patch, your dose can be matched, or you can gradually lower it.

### Low-dose ERT

Lower may be better—and may become the norm in the future—when it comes to minimizing side effects, or at least allaying fears about them. Low-dose estrogen formulations (0.3 mg Premarin, Menest, and Cenestin;

0.05 mg Estrace; or 0.025 mg Climara, Vivelle, or Esclim) are currently available. This amount may relieve many symptoms of menopause, especially if not severe. Low-dose ERT is also a good option if breakthrough bleeding is a problem on higher doses, if you're a petite woman or an Asian (with slower estrogen breakdown), or if you've been taking estrogen for many years and decide to continue. Studies show that we "need" less estrogen as we get older. Even though endometrial buildup may be less with low-dose ERT, the majority of doctors will also prescribe a progestin to protect against endometrial cancer (see below).

These doses have been found to preserve bone in most women if taken with 1,500 mg of calcium (although this amount of estrogen may be too low to increase bone density to the extent that higher doses can).

## Pill vs. Patch: Making a Choice

The chief difference between pill and patch is in the way the estrogen is initially metabolized, and the consistency of its level once it's introduced in your body. When you take a pill, the hormone is absorbed through the gastrointestinal tract and passes directly to the liver, where it is metabolized. This is called "first bypass." The pill contains higher doses of estrogen in order to get past the liver barrier breakdown and go on to reach physiologic levels of estrogen in your body. Estrogen from a patch is absorbed directly into the bloodstream without this initial bypass and deactivation. The initial dose is therefore lower. While oral estrogen stimulates the liver to produce higher levels of "good" HDL and lower amounts of "bad" LDL, it also increases triglycerides, a type of fat found to be an important predictor of heart disease risk.

The estrogen from a patch eventually enters the liver, but it takes longer to affect HDL and LDL, the effect is weaker, and triglycerides are not increased. The patch does not cause an increase in the inflammatory marker CRP (C-reactive protein), also implicated in our cardiac disease risk.

Other advantages: Bypassing the liver means less production of a substance called *renin,* which can elevate blood pressure. Estrogen absorbed through the patch has actually been shown to lower blood pressure in hypertensive women.

## Consider the patch if:

- You have high triglycerides or high levels of C-reactive protein (CRP).
- You are hypertensive (have high blood pressure).
- You have poor absorption of oral medications (when you take oral estrogen, you continue to have symptoms, and blood tests show low estradiol levels).
- You have a history of menstrual headaches, or headaches when taking oral estrogen.
- You smoke. Smoking affects absorption and breakdown of oral estrogen—and nicotine, combined with oral estrogen, may increase your risk of abnormal clotting. (This becomes so complicated . . . just quit smoking!)
- Your hot flashes return eighteen hours after taking oral estrogen (when blood and tissue levels may diminish).
- You feel nauseated after you take oral estrogen.
- You gain weight and think it's due to oral ERT.
- You have a low libido.

## Estrogen in pill form may be preferable if:

- You develop unacceptable redness or itching in the area of the patch (this occurs in less than 2 percent of women).
- You don't want even a private display of menopausal therapy (i.e., you don't want your lover to see your patch).
- You perspire profusely or take lots of hot baths, and the patch keeps falling off.
- You prefer to take a pill once a day with your vitamins and get ERT over with.

### Vaginal estrogen

*Estrogen creams (Premarin, Estrace, Ogen).* These can be used alone to treat vaginal dryness. Inserted into the vagina with a plastic applicator (generally twice weekly), creams help maintain the vaginal blood supply, moisture, elasticity, pH—and the general health and comfort of this previously-taken-for-granted lining. Because estrogen absorption with these products is low, you don't have to worry about potential total-body side effects, nor do you need progestin to protect the lining of your uterus.

*Tablets (Vagifem).* These are usually prescribed daily for two weeks (if you're first beginning therapy and already have symptoms of vaginal atrophy), after which a tablet twice weekly should suffice. These are placed into the vagina with a special applicator. Many of my patients like tablets because they dissolve quickly with little mess, while others prefer the extra moisture and soothing sensation of a cream.

*Estring.* This is a hollow ring that looks like the rim of a diaphragm. It contains 2 mg of estradiol (a typical two-day dose for oral estrogen), which is slowly released over three months, producing a negligible rise in blood estrogen levels. It may be the product of choice if you want the least possible estrogen without compromising vaginal health. I prescribe it for patients who have had breast cancer, and it's made a huge difference in their ability to have intercourse and to ward off vaginal and bladder infections.

The only problem: It comes in one size, which doesn't fit all. The Estring may be too big for women who never gave birth, had surgery that narrowed or shortened the vagina, or have severe narrowing due to atrophy—and too small for those who had several vaginal deliveries or have vaginal prolapse. ("Prolapse" means a loss of vaginal support, so that the cervix, uterus, and/or bladder protrude down or out from the vaginal cavity.)

*ERT by ring (FemRing).* The latest ring on the block that can provide full estrogen replacement therapy (as opposed to just locally treating the vaginal mucosa) is FemRing. It provides 0.05 mg of estradiol a day. It was FDA-approved in 2003 for HRT.

Like the Estring, it comes in only one size. And, as with the patch or any other form of ERT, if you have not had a hysterectomy, you need to add some form of progesterone to protect the uterine lining.

### Skin creams and gels

Estradiol gels and creams are not yet sold by pharmaceutical companies in the United States, but are widely used in Europe. There, many women rub estrogen gel on their arms, shoulders, or abdomen. A low-dose estrogen cream can also be used for local skin therapy on your face or hands, and may indeed help combat collagen loss and wrinkles.

Several companies are working to obtain FDA approval for these products. In the meantime, with a doctor's prescription, you can obtain estrogen cream from compounding pharmacies; they take the raw ingredients and make it up in small individual batches. Dosage control can be more difficult with cream than with pills or patches. For more on this skin secret, see chapter 7.

## Compounding Pharmacies: Another Option

These pharmacies make up capsules, creams, and gels according to a physician's very clearly specified prescription. Such pharmacies state that their products are "natural," meaning plant derived. They often mix various types of estrogen and estrogen metabolites: estriol, estrone, and estradiol (the latter is the most potent).

Unlike prescription pharmaceuticals, these products are not reviewed by the FDA; while the FDA can provide guidance to the compounding industry, it does not have the power of law for enforcement. On the plus side, there is a professional association of compounding pharmacists that provides some oversight.

Occasionally, at a patient's request, I will write a prescription for an estrogen made by a compounding pharmacy. But I feel far more comfortable prescribing FDA-approved medications: I know what's in them, their dose and quality are consistent, and their makers must answer to higher standards than those imposed on compounding pharmacies. Most medical associations and editors of peer-reviewed journals take the same position. And many insurers will not pay for a specially compounded drug.

Note: In a 2002 FDA survey of prescriptions filled by compounding pharmacies, ten of twenty-nine prescriptions failed assays. Of the ten, nine were below the potency prescribed (this included oral progesterone) and one had a high level of a toxic substance. The survey included the twelve biggest compounding pharmacies in the country.

## What About the "H" in HRT? (The Progestins)

By the time we reach our fifties, two-thirds of us still have a uterus. Fifty years ago, when postmenopausal estrogen supplementation was introduced with "Here, this will keep you young forever," doctors didn't know that without adding progesterone, as nature does in the reproductive years, women could end up with uterine cancer. Over time, researchers garnered sufficient evidence to show that the risk for endometrial cancer was five to eight times greater in women who took unopposed estrogen. Because natural progesterone was poorly absorbed and unstable, chemists created synthetic compounds called *progestins*. These continue to be widely used.

Most synthetic progestins are actually derived from testosterone. The flagship product has always been *medroxyprogesterone acetate* (MPA), sold under the brand names Provera and Cycrin. MPA is also the "pro" of Prempro and the "phase" of Premphase. Another progestin, *norethindrone acetate,* is sold as Aygestin. Its chemical cousin, *norethindrone* (NET), is sold as Micronor.

Since they are derived from testosterone, they may possess some male hormone (*androgenic*) activity and may also have an effect similar to that of adrenal hormone (causing fluid retention or bloat). MPA seems to be the most androgenic, and NET the least. Unfortunately, these progestins' success at endometrium protection has not always been matched by comfort promotion. The more androgenic the progestin, the more women complain of bloating, breast tenderness, headaches, irritability, sleeplessness, and general PMS-like feelings that we thought would end with menopause. Another concern is that adding some of these progestins to estrogen might diminish the latter's beneficial coronary effects. The PEPI study showed that MPA tended to undermine estrogen's good effects on the cholesterol profile. The WHI study found that this translated into an increased risk of heart attack and stroke.

If you prefer a "natural" option that may cause fewer PMS-like effects, there are several:

*Micronized natural progesterone capsules.* Natural progesterone (found in Prometrium) is similar to that produced by our ovaries, and doesn't oppose the positive effects of estrogen on cholesterol and perhaps heart disease. The PEPI study showed that this could be as effective as MPA in protecting the endometrium. It should be taken at night because it can make you sleepy.

*Vaginal progesterone gel.* Since for some patients, even oral natural progesterone can cause dizziness, drowsiness, and headaches, I sometimes prescribe an alternative route for this product—through the vagina or directly into the uterus. Natural progesterone supplied in a 4 percent vaginal gel has been shown to protect the endometrial lining from estrogen effects. But this product was FDA-approved only for *secondary amenorrhea* (lack of periods) in women of reproductive age.

The original 4 percent gel, Crinone, is not currently available, but marketing rights have been acquired by another company, which markets it under the name Prochieve. (They also make an 8 percent gel, used to treat infertility caused by progesterone deficiency—hence the name.)

One prefilled applicator is inserted vaginally every other night for twelve nights, and can be used as infrequently as every other month. Some of my patients have vaginal bleeding when they finish this course of progesterone, as they would with other cyclic HRT (see page 73). Since this is not officially approved, I monitor these patients with yearly pelvic ultrasound exams to ensure that their endometrial lining remains thin and is sufficiently protected by this form of progesterone.

*Transdermal progestin.* Currently, a progesterone or progestin-only patch is not available. There are two FDA-approved patches that contain progestin combined with estradiol. The first one to be marketed was CombiPatch, which comes in two doses of the progestin norethindrone acetate and one dose of estradiol (0.05 mg). It is changed twice weekly. Climara Pro received its FDA approval at the end of 2003. This patch contains slightly less estradiol (0.045 mg) and one of two doses of the progestin levonogestrel (LNG), which has been extensively used in birth control pills and has less male-hormone-like activity than many other progestins. This patch makes transdermal HRT very simple; just change it once a week. It may be more physiologic and steady-state to get our progestin through the skin, vagina, or even the uterine lining (see below). This, together with estrogen, most mimics what our ovaries did when they were young and active.

*Drospirenone.* The first in a new class of progestins, *drospirenone* has effects closer to those of natural progesterone, and holds promise for women sensitive to progestins. Its antimale-hormone qualities (meaning less acne) and mild blood-pressure-lowering and diuretic action (less bloat and breast tenderness) have made the birth control pill Yasmin very popular. Drospirenone is available in Europe; it is undergoing testing to allow it to be marketed in the United States together with estrogen therapy.

*Intrauterine progestin.* The Mirena IUS, placed directly into the uterus, slowly secretes minute amounts of progestin over five years. The amount absorbed is negligible, and so are the side effects, but being in the right spot at the right time helps prevent endometrial buildup. This, too, awaits FDA approval for HRT use.

One alternative form of progesterone treatment that I do not recommend is 4 percent progesterone skin cream. The best-known version is marketed under the name of Progest. An article in the prominent medical journal *The Lancet* concluded that Progest does not raise blood progesterone levels sufficiently to protect the uterus during estrogen therapy. Moreover, there is little evidence that progesterone cream by itself builds bone or prevents or cures hot flashes. I've had two patients who took estrogen and prior to seeing me had used Progest cream for endometrial protection—and despite this, went on to develop endometrial cancer.

## Modes of HRT

There are all sorts of inventive ways to add progestin to estrogen, affecting if and when you bleed.

### Cyclical schedule

Don't throw away those tampons! This form of HRT mimics the cycles of the reproductive years. You get your estrogen (any type) either daily or on days 1 through 25, and add a progestin or progesterone for twelve days. Your HRT calendar will look like this:

| Hormones | Days on | Days off | Days of possible bleeding |
|---|---|---|---|
| Estrogen | 1–25 | 26–30 or 31 | |
| Progestin | 14–25 | rest of month | 26–31 |
| *or* | | | |
| Estrogen | every day | never | |
| Progestin | 1–12 | rest of month | 13–17 |

(Note that bleeding occurs when you stop the progestin, and usually lasts three to five days.) If you hate your "progestin-ated days," some doctors let you take higher doses every two or three months for fourteen days, and remain progestin free in the intervening months. The advantage of cycling is that you know when you should bleed. The disadvantage is that you *will* probably bleed. Premarin and MPA are packaged together as cyclical hormones in the form of Premphase: Premarin 0.625 mg is taken daily, with 5 mg of MPA added for the last two weeks of your cycle. If you take natural progesterone, the cyclical dose is usually 200 mg. I prescribe less for patients on very-low-dose estrogen.

### Continuous schedule

If you want to do away with "periods" or feel better keeping your hormone levels consistent throughout the month, you can take estrogen and progestin (or natural progesterone, 100 mg) daily. Estrogen has been combined with various progestins in a pill or patch to help ease this rite of continual hormonal passage:

| Hormone | Days on | Days off | Days of "planned" bleeding |
|---------|---------|----------|----------------------------|
| Estrogen | all | none | none |
| Progestin | all | none | none |

Brands that combine estrogen and progestin include:

- Prempro (0.65 mg Premarin, 2.5 mg MPA)
- Low-dose Prempro (0.45 mg Premarin, 1.5 mg MPA)
- Activella (1 mg estradiol, 0.5 mg norethindrone acetate)
- FemHRT (0.05 mg ethinyl estradiol and 1 mg norethindrone acetate)
- Climara Pro (0.045 mg estradiol and 0.03 or 0.04 mg levonorgestrol)
- CombiPatch (0.05 mg estradiol and 0.14 or 0.25 mg norethindrone acetate).

If you take a separate estrogen and add natural progesterone, the dose of the latter is usually 100 mcg nightly.

**Alternating schedule**
Finally, there is a continuous-dose therapy called Ortho-Prefest, which alternates three days of tablets containing 1 mg of estradiol with three days of tablets containing estradiol plus a low-dose progestin (0.09 mg norgestimate). It should act like the abovementioned continuous dose products to protect the uterine lining. The "on and off" progestin is supposed to help reset progesterone receptors so they don't become overburdened by progestin stimulation. For some women, this may reduce breakthrough bleeding.

## Should Hormone Replacement Therapy Include Testosterone?

> Why can't a woman be more like a man?
> —HENRY HIGGINS, IN MY FAIR LADY

Your hormonal clock undergoes other pauses that don't grab the titles of perimenopause and menopause. A gradual decrease in male hormone levels (*androgens*) can affect how your bones, skin, muscle, vagina, and hair age, as well as how you feel. Since puberty, your ovaries and adrenals have been making male hormones. Adrenal glands produce DHEA and *androstendione,* prehormones converted into testosterone in other parts of the body.

As testosterone circulates through the bloodstream, most of it will be bound to protein made in your liver (SHBG). Only that portion which is "free" can penetrate a cell, where once more it's converted so it can attach to receptors and do its androgen thing. When it comes to hormonal loss, the adrenals predate (or preage) your ovaries by far. From your twenties to your forties, the amount of DHEA they produce decreases by as much as 50 percent.

During these reproductive years, the rest of your male hormones are produced by the follicles in your ovaries. As you deplete these, you experience an even greater male hormone loss. But know that your androgen loss is not complete. Ovarian tissue surrounding the now-defunct follicles continues to produce premale hormone, which can be converted to more potent androgens in peripheral tissue.

How efficiently tissues convert and use even small amounts of male hormone precursors may be more important than a critical "normal" level. Even though all of us eventually notice we're missing our periods, we may not notice that we're missing our male hormones. Less estrogen means less liver production of SHBG, so the testosterone we do have is allowed to enter cells and work. Maybe this is the hormonal reason that some women experience a "menopausal zest."

### The woes of missing androgen

Our medical understanding of symptoms linked to low testosterone levels comes from studying premenopausal women who are abruptly deprived of this hormone (together with estrogen) due to surgical removal of their ovaries. Even when estrogen is prescribed to restore presurgery levels, many women experience mood swings, lack of motivation, and fatigue, as well as decreased libido, sexual fantasies, and sexual pleasure—and they continue to have hot flashes. They may also suffer accelerated bone loss, decreased muscle strength, increased body fat, and changes in memory. If testosterone is added to their hormone replacement regimen, many of these symptoms improve.

So, how do you know if you are testosterone-deficient? At the risk of sounding like the comedian Jeff Foxworthy (author of *You Might Be a Redneck If . . .* ):

You might be testosterone-deficient if:

1. You had your ovaries removed before menopause.
2. Your libido was always great, nothing has changed in your life except perimenopause or menopause—and now it's gone.
3. You are taking oral estrogen and your libido has become non-existent.
4. You are taking steroid medication (which prevents your adrenals from producing DHEA).
5. Your menopausal symptoms, especially hot flashes, do not improve with estrogen.

You'd think that if we can measure estrogen levels, we could do the same for male hormones, but total testosterone levels don't mean much; we need to know what portion is "free." Right now, this can only be done by measuring SHBG and making calculations to estimate the level of free testosterone. If this is low, and you have the "right" symptoms, then you could benefit from androgen therapy.

### Types of male hormones for women: "Will this give me a beard and a deep voice?"

When it comes to androgens, there is no doubt that too much of even a good thing can be a disaster. Testosterone can cause oily skin, acne, excess hair growth, male pattern hair loss—and very high doses of it can result in deepening of the voice and enlargement of the clitoris. It can also decrease production of good cholesterol in the liver (although it does lower total cholesterol, LDL, and triglycerides) and contribute to fluid retention.

A woman's dose of male hormones should provide physiologic levels that mimic those produced during her reproductive years. If you decide to use androgens to boost your sex drive, I have to pronounce the required medical disclaimer: There are no FDA-approved androgen therapies for female sexual dysfunction, and any use of them is considered "off label." (Once a drug is approved by the FDA to treat a particular condition, physicians can choose to prescribe it for other uses.) Studies have shown that when testosterone is given to menopausal women with low levels of free testosterone (or to younger women who've had their ovaries removed), it can increase libido, sexual fantasies, orgasmic response, and energy levels. It also can help build bone and muscle, thicken skin, and may increase lean body mass.

*Testosterone pills.* The only FDA-regulated testosterone pill comes combined with estrogen, in two strengths: *Estratest* and *Estratest HS* (for half-strength). The testosterone used (methyl testosterone) has been chemically altered so that it will be absorbed and won't be broken down or converted to estrogen. (Note: "Pure" testosterone is quickly metabolized and can become estrogen.) It was approved to aid estrogen in combating resistant hot flashes.

The full strength is probably too much for most women, and I prefer the half-strength form (equivalent to a mid-dose estrogen, such as Estrace 1 mg, and the normal production of testosterone in a 30-year-old woman, 1.25 mg). Even so, some of my patients develop acne, so I have them alternate estrogen-only and Estratest HS every other day. Since blood levels of methyl testosterone cannot be measured (the lab can only test for non-methylated testosterone), we have to rely on how you feel, as well as any side effects such as acne or hair growth, to fine-tune the final dose.

To avoid deactivation during first bypass through the liver, there are testosterone formulations that can be absorbed under the tongue or through the skin. These can be obtained with a prescription, but only through compounding pharmacies. They include:

*Topical testosterone.* A 2 percent testosterone proprionate ointment, applied nightly to the genital area. Some doctors prescribe a 2 to 4 percent cream rubbed on the inner thighs. (Their application can be a sexual experience in itself!) When I talked about this form of male hormone therapy on the *Oprah* show, she created a run on testosterone by turning to the cameras and proclaiming, "Show me this cream!"

*Methyl testosterone drops or troches (lozenges).* These are placed under the tongue; usual doses range from 0.5 to 1.5 mg.

*Testosterone patch.* These are currently available for men; "weaker" ones for women are being developed.

There is one other gentle male (somewhat of an oxymoron) hormone being used off label to improve energy, sense of well-being, and libido in women: DHEA. Since it is a prehormone, and to some extent undergoes conversion to more effective androgens in our cells, theoretically it should be effective. So far, studies on this are few, small, and short term. This product is unregulated in the United States (but is tightly regulated in Canada and Europe) and can be bought over the counter—I've even seen it at airports next to *People* magazine. For more detail on the intriguing DHEA story, see chapter 5.

## Making sure that male hormones cause no harm

A woman's sexuality requires a healthy cardiovascular system and nervous system, genital health, a good body image, and reasonable self-esteem. The latter includes feeling worthy of sex as we get older and our bodies change. Unlike European women, American women often have a sense that after 40, they're not entitled to feel sexy. Good sex also requires a healthy relationship and a low level of stress. While men sometimes use sex to destress, this doesn't seem to work for us.

Even if testosterone deficiency is at the root of your decreased sexuality, you won't feel better with supersized male hormone doses—but you may get sick with liver problems, high cholesterol, and even heart disease. The lowest effective dose should be used, and you should be monitored with blood tests for abnormal liver function and cholesterol, and have exams for hypertension and heart disease. If acne and hair loss occur, report these to your doctor and decrease the dose.

Hormone bells chime at various frequencies and intensities throughout our first six decades of life. These rhythms vary in each of us. All chiming does not cease in our fifties. And there are things we can do to keep up a comfortable internal rhythm, with or without hormone therapy.

Will hormones keep us young? Perhaps, given their effects on bones, skin, and brain. Can they make us feel better? Most likely, yes. Can they cause harm? For some, yes. Do we *need* to use hormones to live longer? No. It's an option, not a medical requirement. Below are other options.

### About SERMs (Selective Estrogen Receptor Modulators)

These "designer estrogen" compounds actually oppose the effects of estrogen on some areas of the body—but promote estrogenlike effects in selected cells. *Tamoxifen* (see page 270) decreases breast cell activity and proliferation. Hence, it has the ability to decrease recurrence in women who've had breast cancer, and lower the risk of the disease in women who—because of family history, previous biopsies that showed "overactive" cells, or BRCA2 genetic mutation—are known to be high risk. This SERM's antiestrogen effects also extend to menopausal symptoms, so it does not help (and indeed may worsen) hot flashes and vaginal dryness.

A second SERM that is used to combat osteoporosis is *Evista* (raloxifene). It has most recently been studied in the MORE (Multiple Outcomes of Raloxifene Evaluation) trial. Researchers followed 7,700 postmenopausal women who had osteoporosis (average age 67) for four years. Women who took the 60-mg dose had a roughly 50 percent lower risk of having a *first* vertebral fracture, or a 30 percent reduced risk of suffering a *new* vertebral fracture (if they showed evidence of broken bones before the study began).

When raloxifene also was found to lower by 84 percent the risk of estrogen-receptor-positive breast cancer in the treated women, the finding was heralded by the media and the manufacturer. The researchers involved with this study warned, however, that while the result looked promising, it applied only to women with osteoporosis who in general are at low risk for breast cancer. Further studies are needed before we can officially recommend this drug for cancer prevention.

For the entire group of raloxifene users, no significant effect was seen on the risk of heart attack or stroke. But when the statisticians separately analyzed the data for women judged to be at cardiovascular risk (they smoked, or had diabetes, high cholesterol, or a previous heart attack or stroke), they found that women who took raloxifene had a 40 percent reduction in their risk of heart attack and a 62 percent decrease in strokes at the four-year mark, compared with those who did not take the drug.

Like estrogen, SERMs increase the risk of clots; however, they do not increase the proinflammatory factor C-reactive protein, and hence may stabilize plaque and prevent the shearing off of pieces that lead to heart attacks and strokes (see page 231). However, once more the authors of the study were quick to point out that only 13 percent of the women in the study fell into that cardiovascular risk group. Until larger studies can confirm these good results, it's too soon to prescribe Evista to reduce cardiovascular events.

Also, Evista does not act like an estrogen on our inner thermostat control. It does not reduce hot flashes (indeed, it may worsen them) or improve mood swings, short-term memory, or vaginal dryness. I prescribe the SERMs for very specific reasons: tamoxifen to lower breast cancer risk in patients at high risk, and raloxifene to treat osteoporosis (and perhaps give an added edge if they are at risk for coronary vascular disease).

## When You Still Need a Prescription: Nonhormone Options for Hot Flashes

Nonhormone drugs found to diminish hot flashes include:

*Bellergal.* This is FDA-approved to treat hot flashes, and was the past standard nonhormonal medical therapy for hot flashes, night sweats, insomnia, and restlessness. It contains belladonna, which may make your pupils dark and mysterious, but also causes dry mouth and dizziness. It also includes an ergot compound, which constricts blood vessels and helps prevent the flush, and phenobarbital, which sedates and may help regulate the brain's temperature control system. Unfortunately, this last substance is also addictive. Not my favorite combination, nor—after months of use—does it seem to be effective.

*Catapres (clonidine).* This is usually prescribed for high blood pressure. Given as a patch or a pill, it reduces blood vessel sensitivity and the dilation of vessels in the skin that occurs during a flush. But it often causes side effects such as drowsiness, constipation, and dry mouth.

*Antidepressants.* Drugs targeting our neurotransmitters (particularly feel-good serotonin) have become the newest "use instead of ERT" therapy to combat hot flashes. In a 2003 study, 165 women over age 34 who had gone through either natural or surgical menopause were given either Paxil (paroxetine) or a placebo. These (nondepressed) women were coping with at least two or three bothersome hot flashes a day. After six weeks, the daily flash count was reduced by over 60 percent; a low dose of controlled-release Paxil (12.5 mg a day) worked as well as a 25-mg dose, with fewer side effects. This study, published in the *Journal of the American Medical Association,* is the first of what is likely to be a series of randomized double-blind trials of SSRI (selective serotonin reuptake inhibitor) antidepressants—such as Prozac, Celexa, Zoloft, and Lexapro—for treating menopausal symptoms. I've prescribed many of these SSRIs for my symptomatic patients who can't or won't take estrogen (many of whom are also depressed—not always a coincidence), and so far have not seen outstanding hot-flash results.

A different type of antidepressant, Effexor (venlafaxine), was tested as a hot-flash suppressor in 191 women with a history of breast cancer. Three doses were tested against a placebo for just four weeks. The most appropriate dose was 75 mg daily—this reduced hot-flash scores after two weeks by 61 percent (compared with a 27 percent reduction with placebo pills).

I suggest starting with a lower dose of 37.5 mg, because side effects of mouth dryness, decreased appetite, nausea, and constipation increase with higher doses. If this doesn't work within two to three weeks, it's reasonable to increase it to 75 mg. This dose of Effexor can favorably affect serotonin levels, but at higher doses it also prevents reuptake of the neurotransmitter norepinephrine—which can *cause* hot flashes. (See chapter 8 for more on antidepressants.)

Finally, there's some data suggesting that Neurontin (gabapentin) can reduce hot flashes. This drug is typically prescribed for epileptic seizures or nerve-related pain, and can cause significant side effects. Most of my patients who have tried it complained more about drug-related drowsiness and dizziness than about their original hot flashes.

## Can an Alternative Method (or Two) a Day Keep Hormones Away?

> When I heard about that WHI study, I stopped my hormones. Find me a gentler, kinder way to feel good and stay young!
>
> —SANDRA, AGE 57, WHO QUIT HRT AFTER USING IT FOR FIVE YEARS

In our world of instant gratification, many of us would rather take a broccoli pill than eat the vegetable. The same could be said for managing menopausal symptoms: Why can't we *take* something (an herb or vitamin) rather than *do* something? Alas, the "taking" has a low success rate; lifestyle and nutritional changes may be far more successful alternatives.

### Foods, herbs, and flashes

*Eat right, flush less.* Avoiding certain foods can help prevent hot flashes. Here are the usual stay-away-from substances: caffeine, alcohol, spicy foods, foods that contain nitrites or sulfites, hot drinks, and sugar. Big, heavy meals are more likely to cause hot flashes than small, frequent ones. And what should you *add* to your diet? Lots of plants that provide phytoestrogens (I'll explain what these are in chapter 5) and fiber.

In health food stores and on the Web you'll see all kinds of claims for herbal medicines. And do those "flash and flush not" supplements work? The National Center for Complementary and Alternative Medicine, part of the NIH, is supporting research on herbs that could have some potential to lessen the symptoms of menopause, including black cohosh, red clover, dong quai, flaxseed, and dietary soy. These studies are looking at safety and effectiveness, as well as trying to understand if and why they work. For an overview of these herbal remedies, turn to chapter 5.

*Vitamins.* One randomized trial found that a daily dose of 800 units of vitamin E had a small beneficial effect on hot flashes (see page 174).

*Wild yam cream.* Many prescription estrogen therapies are produced from wild yams. Going back to "nature's source," some enterprising individuals have marketed creams made with wild yam extract. This, unfortunately, is a yam scam; wild yam cream is no more than an expensive moisturizer. The progesterone in wild yams cannot be absorbed through the skin; it needs to be extracted in a lab. So don't expect it to relieve the symptoms of hot flashes. Some of these creams have been found to contain no yam at all; others are spiked with progesterone.

## Keep moving and think cool

*Exercise.* A Scandinavian study showed that women who took fitness classes three or more hours per week had fewer hot flashes than those who were physically inactive. Exercise increases natural opioids, known as endorphins, in the brain. Filling that opioid void may help quell hot flashes.

Exercise also increases general well-being; reduces muscle tension, anxiety, and insomnia; and helps our hearts, bones, and weight management. If you exercise an hour a day, you'll get your gold star from the Institute of Medicine. While you'll sweat during your workout, you may feel dryer for the rest of the day—and certainly more virtuous.

*Deep controlled breathing techniques (paced respiration).* Every morning and evening, find a quiet place with minimal distractions. While sitting, slowly breathe in (count five seconds), then breathe out (count five seconds). Do this for fifteen minutes.

It works best if you breathe deeply, from your diaphragm (instead of high, shallow breaths from your chest). Once it becomes routine, use paced respiration when you feel a hot flash coming on. In small studies, this technique reduced hot-flash frequency by an average of 50 to 60 percent.

*Meditation techniques.* At the onset of a hot flash, go to a cool place in your mind (snowy mountains with icy streams). Picture heat escaping from your hands and feet. (If you're a ski fan, remember how cold these extremities get when you've been on the mountain for a while.)

## Environment Management

With forethought, you can reduce your exposure to hot-flash triggers and hasten flash relief. Keep rooms cool, especially your bedroom. When you feel a flash coming on, try putting ice on your forehead or the back of your neck. Dress in layers that you can shed quickly when your temperature spikes. Employ that ever-reliable fan.

While managing your outer environment, remember your inner one. *Stop smoking!* Nicotine constricts blood vessels and can make hot flashes worse.

## Acupuncture

Acupuncture has been shown to raise both our central brain endorphins as well as those within the nerve fibers elsewhere in our bodies. There is good evidence that it can control nausea and some types of pain. Some women feel a sense of well-being along with a decrease in the frequency of their hot flashes with acupuncture therapy. Once more, the studies are small, with varied results, and it's difficult to completely rule out a placebo effect.

As our hormonal clock winds down, some of us hear nothing. Others sense a change in the tone of the bells that ring out the hour . . . or they fear a dreadful silence.

My intent is not to sound an alarm. I hope my discussion of perimenopause and menopause has, however, been a gentle wake-up call to what's happening to your body, giving you a sense of what you can do to enhance the privilege of getting older, as you outlive your ovaries.

We've gone through so many hormonal start-ups and slowdowns. It's time to start the count on all the other events, behaviors, and medical discoveries that can maintain the steady ticking and amazing cadence of our bodies in the years to come.

# 3

## *Minuets and Other Exercises to Slow Down Aging*

### SHAME ON US

"The weather's awful today." "I hate to get sweaty." "I despise gyms." "It's too boring." "I don't have time." Excuses, excuses. . . .

Up to 70 percent of American women are sedentary or only irregularly active. Our bodies were shaped by evolution to plant fields, gather firewood, carry water, and walk (or run when chased) for miles. Oh, the motions past generations went through! Walking, not driving; climbing stairs instead of taking elevators; farming rather than shuffling paper. Most of us can remember (or at least saw in movies) when women did things by hand: washing clothes, whipping cake batter, pushing the lawn mower, and manually opening the garage door. Our electrical contraptions have made these manual tasks, and so many others, mostly obsolete.

While physical prowess is no longer necessary to care for, feed, and protect ourselves and our families, physical activity is critical to our health. It's not enough that we listen to the music. We'd better start dancing—be it the slow, stately minuet (or the walking equivalent), or the jumping, bumping, and bobbing of hip-hop and its corollary, rigorous aerobic exercise.

Unless you make exercise one of your top four priorities on a given day, you won't get to it. And if you don't fit in exercise, there are a lot of other things that, ultimately, you'll *never* get to do. Aside from antibiotics for a life-threatening infection, *there's no medicine I, or any physician, can prescribe that can have the effect on the quality and length of your life that you will get with regular exercise.*

The dance of death, as expressed by the dying swan, is a beautiful adieu in *Swan Lake*. The more piteous finale for most women is expressed not through the movement of dance but through the absence of movement.

> "I'm eating the same. How can I weigh this much?"
> —DORLA, AGE 45

Dorla is married, has two preteen daughters, and a full-time career as an executive at a television production company. She refers to her "pre-baby weight" (118 pounds) as her "normal" weight, and bemoans the increase she's experienced over the years. During her visit to my office last year, she ultimately had to slide that heavy weight to the "150" slot so the smaller one could be shoved along to balance the scale, at 152 pounds.

"I haven't changed a thing in my diet!" she insisted. "You'd better check my thyroid . . . or maybe it's my hormones."

No, she didn't exercise. There was no time, between the kids, the job, and the fact that her hair frizzed when she perspired. But this was her first over-150 experience, and it scared her. If it wasn't the food (well, yes, maybe she could change that a bit) and it wasn't underactive glands, then maybe she would break down and tone up.

She already had the requisite L.A. treadmill at home—until now a convenient place to drape discarded clothes—but she was tired of buying ever-larger clothes, and eager to regain her smaller body. I suggested she spend thirty minutes daily on the machine, either in the morning before she went to work, or in the evening watching the nightly news. If the only TV she turned on was in the room with the treadmill, since her work as a producer made some viewing a necessity, she'd be forced to combine both priorities.

Every night as she went to sleep, Dorla mentally scheduled her next day's workout. If she had a dinner engagement, or evening plans with her family, she'd get up thirty minutes earlier and get on the treadmill in the morning. If not, she'd sleep in and tread to decompress before she tackled dinner. She left weekends "exercise optional," but since she still wanted to watch the news, she often ended up walking while viewing the day's disaster summaries.

Six months later, she gleefully returned and slid the large weight back to the "100" spot and the smaller one to "42." She had not bought a new wardrobe, but she bulged less in her current one. She felt better, slept better, and was contemplating renewing a gym membership which she'd let expire many times in the past.

## THE HIGH COST OF WEIGHT GAIN

Researchers in the Netherlands have found that women who are overweight at age 40 lose an average of three years from their lifespan; obese women lose *over seven years*. (To put this in context: A five-foot-five woman who weighs at least 150 is overweight; at 180-plus pounds, she's obese. See chapter 4 for more.) For smokers the news is worse; the typical obese smoker can expect to die 13.3 years earlier than a normal-weight nonsmoker.

### Exercise and the Well-Rounded Woman

You don't have to be slim to get a big payback from exercise. A recent review of studies found that regular physical activity partially offsets the health risks of extra pounds: heart disease, diabetes, and early death. Believe it or not, an active 180-pound woman is likely to be healthier and to live longer than a 120-pound couch potato. Inactivity and poor cardiorespiratory fitness are killers of women of all sizes.

### Action! The directorial order for long life
L.A. is full of actors, writers, and waiters who just want to direct. Each scene starts with the command "Action!" and continues until the shout of "Cut!" Individually, we direct something more important than a "movie of the week": our health. As long as we heed the "action" part, we lessen the risk of "cutting" the duration and quality of our lives.

Physical inactivity accounts for at least 25 percent of deaths from chronic disease.

Nearly every aspect of our appearance and well-being is improved by exercise. *Exercise is the ultimate anti-aging prescription.* If the above stats don't convince you, I hope the following will:

*Pound away the pounds of life.* Without exercise, we're destined to gain weight as we go through:

- Pregnancies, and an average 3-pound weight gain with the birth of each child.
- Years of caloric excess. We're fed more, cook larger quantities, cook for more people (and our kids love calorie-dense high-sugar foods), eat out more, snack more, and expect more food for our money.
- A 4 to 5 percent decrease in metabolic rate per decade. As we age, there's a gradual decline in our high-energy-using muscle cells, which make up our lean body weight—so it takes less food to maintain our weight. We also tend to move around less with age.

The average American woman gains "just" 0.8 pound a year. But "weight" (okay—wait): that's 20 pounds between the ages of 25 and 50. This partially explains Dorla's dilemma: She's eating the same but gaining weight. She's probably burning 100 fewer calories per day than she did ten years ago; 100 calories over thirty-five days equals 3,500, which equals one extra pound. In a year, that's more than 10 pounds. And if Dorla unthinkingly adds one additional 100-calorie cookie a day ("How bad can it be? It's low fat"), this may turn into twenty pounds. Exercise builds muscle mass, and muscle metabolizes calories more efficiently than fat tissue—burning that accumulation of stored calories.

*Reduce abdominal fat.* Age, not menopause, receives the scientific blame for the growing circumference of our waists. This midabdominal or visceral fat is present under the abdominal wall. It's this type of fat that leads to changes in how we process glucose—resulting in insulin resistance (see chapter 4), type 2 diabetes, high blood pressure, and heart disease.

The Physical Activity for Total Health Study recruited 173 overweight postmenopausal women to find out if moderate, regular exercise could fight this vicious visceral fat. These well-educated but sedentary women were randomly assigned to exercise or just stretch—and asked not to

## Exercise: How It Adds Up

Here is what it takes to burn 150 calories, if you weigh 150 pounds:

| Activity | Duration (minutes) |
| --- | --- |
| Playing volleyball | 43 |
| Moderate walking (3 mph) | 37 |
| Brisk walking (4 mph) | 32 |
| Table tennis (Ping-Pong) | 32 |
| Leaf raking | 32 |
| Social dancing | 29 |
| Lawn mowing (powered push mower) | 29 |
| Jogging (5 mph) | 18 |
| Field hockey | 16 |
| Running (6 mph) | 13 |

(Source: *Physical Activity and Health: A Report of the Surgeon General.*)

change their usual diet. The first group aimed for forty-five minutes of moderate-intensity exercise five days a week—mostly treadmill walking and stationary bicycling. After one year, those who exercised at least 3.25 hours a week showed remarkable changes compared with the stretch-only control group, losing an average of 3 pounds (the controls gained a bit), along with 4.2 percent of their overall body fat and nearly 7 percent around the waist, as measured with a body scan. Aside from being more svelte from the inside out, they also had measurable improvements in cardiorespiratory fitness.

*Prevent heart disease.* The Iowa Women's Health Study of forty thousand women found that those who engaged in moderate exercise four times a week or vigorous activity twice a week had a 30 percent lower risk of death from all causes than women active only a few times a month. A different, Harvard-based Women's Health Study, involving nearly forty thousand health professionals aged 45 plus, found that while vigorous exercise cut risk, so did walking—and that the *amount of time* spent walking was more important than the walking pace. Women who walked just sixty to ninety minutes a week had *half* the risk of coronary heart disease (the leading cause of death for American women) compared with those who did not walk regularly.

Other research has found that regular activity is linked to lower levels of C-reactive protein, a marker of inflammation that may be an even better predictor of heart disease than your cholesterol level (see chapter 6). So, for your heart's sake, just get out and move!

*Prevent diabetes.* Exercise lowers insulin levels and increases your body's ability to recognize and use insulin (insulin sensitivity) so that you don't overproduce insulin in response to consumed sugar. High insulin levels encourage the deposit of fatty plaque in coronary vessels, and heart disease. Thus begins a vicious cycle: The insulin increases visceral fat, which increases insulin resistance, which increases heart disease . . . you get it.

The Nurses' Health Study found an inverse relationship between regular exercise (including walking) and developing diabetes: the more exercise, the lower the risk. Interestingly, the pace of walking affected diabetes risk (independent of hours walked); "brisk or striding" walkers had just 41 percent of the risk of "easy" walkers. A related study found that too much sitting—especially in front of the TV—increases your risk of diabetes and obesity. Just standing up or walking around the house makes a significant difference.

Even if you are already diabetic, get out and walk: The nurses' study shows it can significantly cut your risk of heart disease and stroke.

*Reduce cancer risk.* Exercise decreases the incidence of cancer. There's overwhelming evidence that physical activity reduces the odds of developing colon cancer by as much as 50 percent. One reason is that exercise helps move food (and potential carcinogens) through your G.I. system more rapidly (food that sits there is not good for your bowel or your body).

*Improve sleep.* One study published in the *Journal of the American Medical Association* looked at adults over 50 with "moderate" sleep problems (taking at least twenty-five minutes to fall asleep, and getting only about six hours of sleep a night). Half the group began a sixteen-week aerobic exercise program, working up to about forty minutes four days a week of low-impact aerobics, brisk walking, and/or stationary cycling. There was little difference after eight weeks, but after sixteen weeks the exercise group reported significant improvements: They fell asleep faster, slept better, and awoke feeling more rested. Note that exercising within four hours of your bedtime may interfere with sleep (sexual activity is not included in this warning).

*Prevent osteoporosis and fractures.* Weight-bearing exercise—walking, running, jogging, stair climbing—stresses your bones, making them stronger. Menopausal women who exercise for an hour three times a week can increase their bone mass by 5.2 percent, while their couch-potato peers will lose 1.2 percent of their bone mass every year. Among those oft-mentioned nurses, the regular walkers (at least four hours a week) cut their risk of hip fracture by 41 percent. So, stand up for stronger hips: More time on your feet, even standing still, reduces fracture risk.

*Improve balance and reduce risk of falling.* When an older woman falls, weak muscles and poor balance are often to blame. A fall can be dead serious, especially if you have osteoporosis. (Twenty percent of women who fracture a hip will die within a year; many more will be disabled.) Can exercise help?

In a New Zealand study, elderly women prone to falls were asked to do thirty minutes of simple exercises three times a week. These included leg exercise with light ankle weights, stretching and rotations, heel-toe walking, and walking backward, as well as moves that mimicked everyday activities (climbing stairs, bending and picking up things, stepping over things). They were also encouraged to walk around a bit. At the end of a year, these women had roughly half as many falls as did women in a control group. In another study, older women assigned to learn tai chi experienced similar protection from multiple falls.

*Prevent disability and pain.* A decades-long study of over 1,700 university alumni found that regular exercise (combined with not smoking and keeping a moderate weight) helps prevent arthritis and back pain, as well as heart disease and stroke. These healthy habits delayed the onset of disability by an average of five years and reduced levels of disability at all ages.

Vigorous exercise helps even more. A study that followed members of a "50+" running club for thirteen years found that runners postponed serious disability by almost nine years (versus nonrunning controls), and the women benefited even more than the men.

*Improve mental alertness.* Exercise increases blood flow to the brain. Tests show that it improves mental agility and the ability to react quickly—meaning that for all practical purposes, exercise makes you smarter.

*Lift mood.* Exercise raises brain endorphin levels, causing a feeling of well-being. Evidence is mounting that regular exercise reduces depression and anxiety; a Duke University study found major benefits, especially in combating mild depression. (If you walk with friends or visit a gym, the social contact helps, too.)

*Strengthen your immune system.* Getting physical may mean getting fewer colds. Moderate exercise boosts the functioning of killer cells, T- and B-lymphocytes, and other immune system stalwarts, helping your body fight off infections.

*Slow your clock down* (the reason you're reading this book!). Exercise is truly an anti-aging panacea. You'll not only live longer—you'll look, act, and feel younger. You'll have greater strength and energy, a more confident stride, and a trimmer body.

## Vary Your Exercise for Longer Life

Exercise of all types offers important benefits:

1. *Endurance (aerobic) exercises.* These strengthen your heart and lungs, helping you plow through everyday activities with more energy and less fatigue. Aerobic exercise is your disease prevention (or at least delaying) mainstay—against heart disease, diabetes, and some cancers. Many aerobic activities are also weight bearing (e.g., jogging, walking, stair climbing), protecting bones and reducing fractures. Last but not least, they help you lose (or maintain) your weight and convert fat to lean tissue.
2. *Strength exercises.* Beginning in our thirties or forties, most of us start to lose muscle and gain fat. Lifting weights and other objects can stop or reverse this process. Maintaining your muscle tissue helps your body better use insulin to clear excess sugar from your blood, reducing your risk of diabetes. Strength training also increases bone mineral density (see chapter 6). Stronger muscles can mean less strain on your back, knees, and hips. And if you stick with it, working with weights will significantly improve your shape (more on this on page 101).
3. *Flexibility exercises.* Regular stretching not only feels good; it keeps you limber and active. Physical therapists sometimes recommend these to prevent injuries or speed recovery.
4. *Balance exercises.* These are easy to do, help you move more gracefully, and serve as insurance against falls.

While you should include some activities from each category, your choices may vary depending on your personal health risks and goals. Do you want to lug that computer briefcase through the airport without strain and pain? Does heart disease run in your family? Do you want less body fat and a svelte figure? Are you at high risk of osteoporosis? Do you want more energy and better sleep?

There are also practical considerations, such as how to work exercise into your schedule and budget, and integrate it with competing priorities. Continue reading to learn about ways to gradually move exercise from "I'll get to it someday" into what you do today . . . and tomorrow.

## I Did It—So Can You

I empathize with any woman who has to borrow time to sleep and can't "for the life of her" figure out when she can possibly exercise. For years I made sporadic attempts to get physical. I tried going to Jane Fonda's workouts but usually showed up late and was not admitted to the classes. I had an aerobics instructor come to my house, and worked out with my colleague before we went to the office. That lasted until we realized that our surgery schedule was going kaput.

I tried jazzercise, then jogging—and indeed was running five miles a day until I fell and had some nasty contusions, which left scars on both knees. (My rationale for quitting was, "This is a dangerous sport!") I did learn to ski in my thirties (thankfully, no injuries there) and to scuba dive in my forties. But these are vacation sports; I can't rely on them for my daily caloric output.

In my forties, I wised up and joined a gym near my hospital. I hired a trainer and scheduled appointments three times a week. He was my nightmare exercise drill sergeant, exhorting me to go faster on that treadmill, increase weights on the machines, and break into a hair-frizzing sweat. But I learned the routine, and after about two years (I was a slow learner) realized that, yes, I could mount that treadmill, climb that Stairmaster, and pedal that elliptical runner (my favorite) *by myself*. I could also count to 15 reps twice on the machines or while doing free weights. And I would pick those weights up on my own.

Dismissing the trainer was a declaration of self-determination. He was one more appointment that I had to make, break, be late for, and pay for even if I didn't show up. I proudly graduated to "I can be responsible for my own exercise" status.

I bought a treadmill; it's in my den, near the TV, and is clear of junk. If I can't get to a gym, I use it mornings to watch the *Today* show or—if I have surgery or early meetings—evenings before dinner. I rapid-walk at a 4-mph pace for thirty minutes. Three times a week, I spend twenty minutes lifting free weights and doing floor exercises. On weekends, if I'm not on a plane, I hike or bike for at least an hour. When I travel, as soon as I check into a hotel, I scurry to the gym for a thirty-minute treadmill walk; if it's nice out, I take a fast walk in the park.

As I penned this personal ode to exercise, I was caught in New York City in the worst blizzard they'd had in years. It was also a holiday, and the hotel gym was closed. To ease my guilt, restlessness, and sour mood, I ran in place for thirty minutes while I watched the news about closed roads and cancelled flights. I then took the two huge phone books (the white and yellow pages were about the same size) and used them as weights for arm lifts. Finally, I plopped on the floor to do sit-ups and push-ups, and used the edge of the bed for back-arm extensions. A nice hot bath, and I was ready to venture out into the two feet of snow to find something to eat. I find that working out before dinner decreases my appetite, so I don't attack the first piece of bread that lands within reach.

## DR. REICHMAN'S GUIDE TO ANTI-AGING EXERCISE FOR THE BUSY WOMAN

"Okay," you say, "I'm ready to change. I'll get out there and exercise every day, and cut out those evening snacks in front of the tube while I'm at it—"

Let me stop you right there. You know from past experience that a vow of total self-improvement never lasts. You'll get sore muscles, skip a day, then a week . . . and finally, you'll say, "I just can't do it!" and be back on the sofa.

Start slowly, be realistic—and remember that *some* exercise is always better than *no* exercise. If you're among the least active 20 percent of Americans, simply moving to the next-higher 20 percent confers more than half of exercise's life-saving benefits.

### Getting Started with Aerobic Exercise

#### Walking
Walking is a great way to start; it requires no special gear (just comfortable shoes), and if you don't start out at top speed, you're unlikely to get sore or injured. If you're starting from scratch, walk just a few minutes at a time, several times a day.

## Do You Have to Sweat to Get the Payoff?

We used to bombard you with "do it right" charts and target heart rate zones. Authorities dictated that you must exercise vigorously for thirty minutes, minimum, to receive any benefit. So many women joined gyms (and seldom showed up), or bought exercise machines (and used them as clothes hangers). Why? Modern schedules make it extremely difficult to reserve blocks of "sweat time" on a regular basis. And the strict admonitions of experts sometimes backfired: "If I can never get it right, why do it at all?"

The latest guidelines from the Institute of Medicine recommend getting physical for an hour a day. This extra effort can definitely pay off in greater energy and fitness. However, the greatest drop in your risk of dying—our ultimate measure of success—comes when you move from being sedentary to being a moderate exerciser.

Fortunately for the average overscheduled woman (who wants to feel and look better but has other priorities), new research supports a more flexible and realistic path to improved health. For example, a study of 1,564 college alumnae found that women who walked ten blocks or more per day cut their risk of heart disease by one-third, compared with women who walked four blocks or less. That's a huge difference for a small effort!

Also, consider this innovative study from the Cooper Institute for Aerobics Research. They randomized 313 not very active adults (aged 35 to 60) to either six months of structured exercise in a gym, or to a "lifestyle" exercise plan: accumulating at least thirty minutes of moderate-intensity physical activity on most days of the week. The lifestyle group wasn't left to manage all on their own; they met for an hour a week for the first four months (and less often thereafter) to work on overcoming obstacles and finding ways to fit exercise into their schedules—and keep it there. They also received activities calendars, quarterly newsletters, and a series of tailored manuals. (They didn't change their diets.)

How did it turn out? After six months, both groups were significantly more active and fit. While they spent about the same amount of time exercising, both groups had similar improvements in HDL/LDL cholesterol ratio, blood pressure, and body fat percentage. Cardiovascular fitness also improved (though the gym group had an edge here, since their exercise was more intense).

Did it last? At twenty-four months, the researchers found that the lifestyle fitness group had kept more of the cardiovascular fitness they'd gained. It's also worth noting that the lifestyle group didn't gain weight from months 6 to 24, and continued to reduce their body fat percentage, whereas the structured exercise group gained a few pounds. The gym group found it harder to stick with their program long term—but remember, they didn't choose that style of exercise, they were assigned to it, and it might not have been a good fit for everyone.

The conclusion? You can do well with going to classes at a gym, or exercising on your own. The trick is to choose what works best for you, figure out what obstacles (mental, logistical, practical) interfere with regular exercise, and find ways around them.

As you gain endurance, challenge yourself by gradually *increasing the amount of time* you exercise, then *raising the intensity*. Always start at a slow pace for a few minutes to warm up your muscles.

- If you are in reasonably good health, start by *walking twenty minutes a day,* most days of the week. If that's too tiring, start with ten or fifteen minutes and work up to twenty. After the first two weeks, try to cover a little more ground every day during those twenty minutes.
- Once this is relatively easy (about week 3), *walk thirty minutes* on most days. Again, try to cover a bit more ground each day. You've achieved the goal of walking briskly if you can do a mile in fifteen to twenty minutes. If you prefer to measure distance covered rather than time, walk at least *ten blocks a day*. Or count steps, an alternative unit of "walk power." Your goal should be *10,000 steps a day*. A step-counting pedometer can track this for you. Most cost less than $30 (two brands are Digi-Walker and Accusplit).
- After about a month, you may be ready for a more intense workout. After your first five minutes of walking, try *thirty to sixty seconds of jogging or stair climbing* (or stepping up and down from the curb if no stairs are available). Then resume walking for five minutes, then jogging for one minute, and so on through your thirty-minute walk (with a cool-down at the end).

The endpoint need not be the jog. It's the regularity of the walks. If you can't schedule a solid half-hour, do ten-minute portions, which is almost as effective. This may mean writing walks into your schedule, or setting up reminders. For example, if you work at a computer, set an alarm to "ping" every hour and a half, then set out for a five- or ten-minute walk. Pace long corridors. Walk to a meeting. Park your car (weather permitting) a few blocks from your destination. Take the stairs. Get your coffee at a more distant shop. And at the end of the day, add up these breaks—which should cause no aches. Did you get your thirty minutes in? No? Then make up the difference before dinner.

Another way to measure your path to fitness is to *count calories* burned.

A review of thirty-eight studies on physical activity and mortality found that working off 1,000 calories a week is plenty to stave off premature death. To lose a pound, you must burn off 3,500 more calories than you take in. Adding regular exercise can gradually subtract weight. For example, if a 200-pound woman eats as usual but starts a walking program—working up to a brisk daily mile and a half—she'll be 14 pounds lighter in a year.

Once you've gotten used to walking, you can add some variety. If you arrange to work out or play with a friend, you're more likely to keep the appointment.

## Other no-gym aerobic workouts

*Jumping rope.* This combines high impact aerobics with heart-rate-raising arm motions, and tones your legs, deltoids, and abdominal muscles. As a bonus, the footwork improves coordination. It's best to do this on a carpeted or wood floor, landing softly. You'll need a room with a high ceiling, or go outdoors on the grass. You need not jump high. Start by jumping one minute, resting for one minute. Work up to two or three minutes of jumping. You can buy inexpensive jump ropes at any sporting equipment store; fancy ones with removable hand weights cost less than $20. They're also easy to pack.

*Swimming.* A fabulous no-sweat, low-impact aerobic exercise that's easy on your joints. It's a total body workout because so many muscles

## Walking Off the Calories (Number Burned per Hour)

| At 2 mph | 240 |
| At 3 mph | 320 |
| At 4.5 mph | 440 |

are involved. (I'll discuss swimming for strength training later in the chapter.)

*Biking.* This is a low-impact, minimal weight-bearing exercise—but check with your doctor first if you have knee or back injuries. You can gradually increase the intensity of resistance and pedal speed on stationary bikes, and mimic gently sloping hills (or small mountains). Outdoor biking is now one of my favorite ways to aerobicize—I enjoy the view, commune with nature (or at least check out the neighbors' lawns), and reach a destination.

If possible, choose a bike path or quiet road. After a mile or two of gentle warm-up on a level surface, add a few sprints, pedaling faster for two minutes, then slow down for ten, go fast for two, etc. Adjust the gears on hills so that you maintain your pace and don't have to dismount and walk the bike.

Mountain biking may be beyond many of us. As those extreme athletes pedal past me while I attempt to walk a mountain path, I envy their energy output and balance. Maybe someday . . . well, maybe not.

Note: Most calorie-burning charts assume you weigh 150 pounds. The bigger you are, the more energy it takes to move; you'll expend more if you weigh more. To calculate your personal caloric burn, divide your weight by 150, then multiply the result by the number of calories for a given activity on the chart on page 98.

For example, an hour of moderately brisk walking (at 3 mph) burns roughly 320 calories for that hypothetical 150-pound woman.

- If you weigh *120,* it's 120/150 = .80, × 320 = 256 calories burned from that hourlong walk.
- If you weigh *180,* it's 180/150 = 1.2, × 320 = 384 calories burned.

Finally, you don't have to be officially "exercising" to burn calories. Every move you make counts. An hour of light housework burns 246 calories. And when at the office, try strolling over to your colleague's cubicle rather than sending her an e-mail or using the intercom. Walk up two flights instead of waiting for the elevator. It all adds up.

### Aerobic exercise at the gym
Most gyms offer a wide variety of cardiovascular and/or strength-building exercise classes. This is not an all-inclusive list; if you seek novel techniques for motion without boredom, trendy variations (such as strip-dancing) are always emerging.

## The Sporting (and Scrubbing) Life . . .

| Sports/Recreation | Calories burned per hour |
| --- | --- |
| Ballroom dancing | 210 |
| Basketball | 450 |
| Biking, 6 mph | 240 |
| Biking, 12 mph | 410 |
| Canoeing, 2.5 mph | 174 |
| Cross-country skiing | 700 |
| Golf (twosome, carrying clubs) | 324 |
| Horseback riding (sitting to trot) | 246 |
| Ice-skating (9 mph) | 384 |
| Jogging (5.5 mph) | 740 |
| Racquetball | 588 |
| Roller-skating (9 mph) | 384 |
| Running (10 mph) | 1,280 |
| Swimming (25 yards/minute) | 275 |
| Swimming (50 yards/minute) | 500 |
| Tennis—singles | 400 |
| Tennis—doubles | 312 |
| Touch football (vigorous) | 498 |
| Volleyball | 264 |
| | |
| Gym or home workout | |
| Aerobic dancing | 546 |
| Circuit weight training | 756 |
| Jumping rope | 750 |
| Running in place | 650 |
| Scrubbing floors | 440 |

(Sources: National Institutes of Health; the President's Council on Physical Fitness and Sports.)

*Spinning.* This provides a tremendous low-impact aerobic workout, with equally tremendous perspiration. "Spinning" involves pedaling on special bikes that go much faster than regular stationary bikes. Music blares, an instructor yells out commands, and you pedal like mad. I quickly learned that this wasn't a contest, and set the resistance at levels I felt I could sustain. If my classmates "passed" me, so what? We all advance our heart rates, burn our calories, and win.

*Jazzercise.* A great way to get your heartbeat up, while expressing yourself to music, à la the sixties.

*High-impact or low-impact aerobics.* These combine kicking, jumping, or dancelike moves. Some no-impact aerobics classes are held in the pool.

*Salsa, funk, and hip-hop dance classes.* Never boring, sometimes intimidating, as you watch the younger generation go. But most gyms have classes geared to all ages, and we can go, too. The low-impact aerobic movements will make you feel like you're in *Saturday Night Fever* or at Carnivale. I used to limit my Thursday-afternoon appointments so I could get to a 6:00 P.M. salsa class at the gym. That Latin beat made me feel young and walk with a suggestive bounce.

*Cardio boxing.* Muhammad Ali meets MTV: a great cardiovascular workout that should also help your agility. In a similar vein, Tae Bo classes use high-impact martial arts and boxing moves, done to music.

*Step aerobics.* This combines stair climbing, choreographed movements, arm swinging, and jumping. You're working those major muscle groups, and your mind is stimulated (you need to be alert to follow the instructor and not fall off the step!).

*Body-sculpting classes.* These strength-building classes use dumbbells, steps, bars, and tubes in movements matched to music, and cut down on the boredom inherent in doing these things solo or on gym machines.

There are many other worthy exercise programs with their own traditions, philosophies, and benefits. I lack the space and the depth of knowledge to give them more than a mention. Yoga (from India) and tai chi (from China) are calming and spiritual, provide weight resistance, balance, and may benefit the cardiovascular system. Pilates, developed in the 1920s by Joseph Pilates, uses elaborate yoga-derived moves to strengthen and stretch your muscles (with mats and special equipment). While group lessons offer hands-on instruction and social benefits, many versions of these (and all kinds of aerobics classes) are available on home video.

## Making Sure Exercise Doesn't Hurt

If you have a chronic health problem, you may have avoided exercise. As long as the illness is in a stable phase, sitting still may be the worst thing you can do. But before you start an exercise plan, get advice and approval from your doctor and/or physical therapist.

It's also a good idea to ask for a medical go-ahead if you smoke, are very overweight, or have a family history of heart disease or diabetes.

If you have problems with your back, knees, or joints, try low- or no-impact exercise, such as water aerobics or swimming, stationary bicycling, or rowing. But if possible, alternate these with moderate-impact activities like walking or dancing, so that your bones can benefit. If you are diabetic, be especially careful not to injure your feet, and keep a carbohydrate source handy in case of hypoglycemia.

Even if you don't have a diagnosed illness, monitor yourse lf as you start working out. If you suddenly become dizzy, faint, or pale, break into a cold sweat, or feel discomfort or pressure in your upper chest, it could signal a heart problem; stop exercising and call your doctor.

Physical activity may leave your muscles a bit achy at first, but *it should not cause sharp, lasting, or worsening pain*. Also, don't work yourself until you're completely out of breath. A good rule of thumb for walk-

### Get an Okay from Your M.D.

You should obtain a doctor's permission to exercise if you're over 50 and plan to start vigorous exercise (the breathe-hard-and-sweat kind) or if you have:

chest pain

irregular, rapid, or fluttery heartbeat

severe shortness of breath

significant, ongoing weight loss for no known reason

infections (such as pneumonia) with fever

any kind of fever, which can cause dehydration and rapid heartbeat

acute deep-vein thrombosis (blood clot)

a hernia that's causing symptoms

foot or ankle sores that won't heal

joint swelling

persistent pain or problems walking after a fall (this could signal a
   hidden fracture)

eye problems such as bleeding in the retina or detached retina; after
   eye surgery

(Source: National Institute on Aging.)

ing: If you're breathing so hard that you can't comfortably converse with a friend, slow your pace.

If you're not feeling well or have missed a lot of sleep, it's better to skip a day of exercise than to risk injury. If you stop exercising for more than several weeks, cut back on your level of exertion and give yourself time to build up your endurance and strength again.

## For Muscles and Bone: Weight Resistance Exercise (Strength Training)

Don't worry that you'll develop the bulging, oiled muscles displayed on the covers of bodybuilding magazines. Unless you take steroids or male hormones, strength training won't make a woman muscle-bound. What it will do is give you a trimmer body—even without weight loss—because muscle fibers take up less space than fat. You may even need to buy smaller clothes to fit your new, leaner shape.

A regular investment in strength training pays astonishing health dividends. When generally healthy postmenopausal women lift weights for thirty minutes twice a week (with warm-up and cool-down times), their bodies develop the trim appearance of someone fifteen or twenty years younger within a year. They also have greater energy, and the ability and confidence to tackle everyday physical tasks that were once beyond them. Their inactive peers continue to lose strength—and look older.

Strength training shows significant results fairly quickly, if you continue to gradually increase the amount of weight you use. Try doubling the amount you lift after two months of regular workouts. You should see a real difference in your shape within three to six months.

Lifting, pushing, and pulling those weights also complements your aerobic exercise program, and further improves your cardiorespiratory endurance. One study of volunteers over age 60 found that doing one set of twelve strengthening exercises, three times a week, created significant gains in both strength and aerobic capacity.

Here are some basic exercises you can do without advanced training that work your muscles. I've provided a lot of options so you can choose those that best suit your interests, schedule, and current fitness level. You needn't do all of them!

My suggestion for the busy woman:

Decide on nine exercises that work your major muscle groups (three upper body, three midsection, three lower body). Do them at least twice a week for a minimum of fifteen minutes. (You'll benefit more if you do them three times a week, or for thirty minutes.) If it suits your schedule better, do upper body exercises two days a week, and legs on two different days. Ideally, vary your program for greater benefit and reduced boredom.

## Strength Training: The Options

There are four basic ways to strength train. They are using:

- Free weights (dumbbells or barbells)
- Machines or other equipment (to push or pull)
- Body weight to create resistance
- Water resistance

Always *warm up* your muscles before any workout. Simply walking in place and gently swinging your arms for several minutes, or starting your walk (on the treadmill or around the block) at a gentler pace, will do. If you do an aerobic workout before your strength training, you're already warmed up.

### Using free weights: upper body, lower body, your body

How much weight should you use? If you are very out of shape, start slowly (1-pound hand weights, 3-pound ankle weights). You should be able to do at least eight repetitions (reps) of the exercise with good form; don't jerk or rush. When in doubt, or if your muscles become very sore, use a lighter weight.

To maximize benefits and avoid injury, raise weights in a slow, controlled fashion and let them down slowly. (Lowering the weight actually does the most to develop your muscles.) Count to four while lifting, hold a moment, then count to four while lowering the weight. Remember to breathe; it may help to count out loud, or to inhale while lowering the weight and exhale while raising it. Keep the rest of your body relaxed, but maintain good posture.

Once you reach twelve reps with good form, you can increase the weight by ½ pound to 3 pounds at a time, every week or two. You may find that some exercises get easier faster than others; adjust the weight accordingly. You'll probably reach your maximum liftable weight in six to nine months. Don't try to do extra work in one part of your body to "spot reduce." It will only make you sore.

## Working your upper body with free weights: arms

1. *Arm curl*. This tones your biceps (the upper-arm area that helps you lift heavy bags). While sitting or standing, hold a dumbbell in each hand, with arms straight against your sides, palms facing out. Then slowly bend your elbow and raise the weight until your palms almost touch the front of your shoulders. Pause, then slowly lower the weights.

Alternative: Curl with one hand at a time. This gives you more energy to do each repetition, and so may be easier if you're a novice.

2. *Overhead extension*. This tones your triceps (backs of your upper arms), which get flabby with age and disuse. Holding your dumbbells, with your palms facing toward you, raise both hands over your head, keeping elbows close to your head. Slowly lower the weights behind your shoulders, then back up to the starting point by extending your elbows and squeezing your triceps.

3. *Chest flies*. Lie on your back, feet on floor, knees bent, dumbbells in hands. Extend your arms toward the ceiling, with palms facing each other; keep your arms straight, and slowly lower them to your sides (backs of hands to the floor).

4. *Triceps extension*. Lie, stomach down, on a bench, with your face off the edge, knees bent, feet crossed in the air. (If you don't have a bench, you could do this one hand at a time off the edge of a firm bed.) Bend your elbows so your dumbbells are at bench level, just below your ribs. Now, slowly straighten your arms along the line of your body, so your palms face your hips. Slowly return to the starting position.

5. *Two-wrist curl-up and curl-down*. These can be done while standing or sitting.

The curl-up: Hold weights at your sides, palms facing outward; flex your wrists, pull hands up, then back to your sides.

The curl-down: With palms facing back, flex your hands upward from the wrists and release back down.

This strengthens your forearms, prevents wrist fractures, helps with your golf or tennis game—and benefits physicians who are required to pull hard on retractors during surgery.

### Working upper body, back, and shoulders

1. *Side raises.* These help your deltoids (shoulder muscles) and rotator cuff muscles. Stand with your feet hip width apart, holding the dumbbells next to the sides of your legs with palms facing in. With elbows straight, slowly lift your arms (making a T shape) to shoulder level—no higher—then lower (slow and controlled; don't just let your arms fall).

2. *Rear delt lift.* These develop the back part of the deltoid muscle. Stance is the same as above, but put one foot in front of the other and bend slightly forward from the waist, keeping your back straight. Raise your arms out to the sides with palms extended down, then lower them.

3. *Overhead press.* Hold the dumbbells at your shoulders next to your ears, palms facing forward. Now, slowly push them up over your head, then down to shoulder level again. Don't let the weights make your arms drop down suddenly.

To work your midsection, see page 107.

### Working your lower body with free weights

You can use ankle weights to increase the resistance (and difficulty) of your regular (equipment-free) exercises, e.g., with squats. Here are other examples:

1. *Outer thigh leg lift.* Lie on your side, legs stacked on top of each other, bottom knee slightly bent. Slowly lift the top leg a few inches, then lower it—either keeping it straight or bending and extending the knee when the leg is elevated. To finish, you can elevate the leg to hip level and "pulse" it front and back, or up and down. A variation: Do this standing, holding on to a chair for balance.

2. *Inner thigh leg lift.* Bend your top leg and rest that foot on the floor in front of you. Now, gently raise your bottom leg off the floor, then lower it. You'll really feel your inner thigh muscle working.

3. *Double leg extension.* Sit on a bench or firm couch. With your hands under your thighs and holding the seat, place a dumbbell between the arches of your feet. While squeezing your feet together to hold the dumbbell in place, extend both knees until you form an L shape. Hold the dumbbell there as you squeeze your quads, then slowly lower your legs to the start position without letting the dumbbell fall.

### Building strength using exercise machines

The weight room in a gym can be overwhelming. So many machines, so many women in high-cut leotards and sports bras, awesome men with popping muscles . . . and you. Most of us react by either running out in horror (and this is not an aerobic run) or attacking the equipment with false bravado, followed by very real aches and pains.

You'll need some "gym school" time: not a graduate degree, just grammar-school level mental and muscle training before you become a machine-room regular. Schedule a preliminary session with a fitness trainer. Most good gyms provide initial training free of charge when you join; it's in their interest to have you use the machines appropriately and without injury.

Remember, most women are genetically programmed to build long, lean muscles. Unless you lift for hours each day, you won't bulk up. Weight machines are actually easier than free weights; they work specific muscles, and the machines help guide your body to perform the exercises properly.

## Using Your Body—No Equipment Needed

### Upper body moves

*Push-ups.* When done right, push-ups reward your body and do not constitute a Marine-style "drop and give me 50" punishment. There are several push-up levels (having nothing to do with Victoria's Secret!).

For beginners: Kneel on an exercise mat or carpeted floor, resting your shins and feet on the mat. Position your hands at shoulder width or slightly wider apart. Slowly lower yourself to the floor, until your elbows line up with your sides. Hold briefly, then push back up, keeping your back straight and your head in line with your spine.

If you can't do a push-up at first, just hold yourself in the "up" position for a few seconds at a time. As you get a bit stronger and steadier, lower yourself partway and then back up.

Once you've mastered the "on your knees" push-up, try crossing your ankles to raise your feet and shins off the floor.

Eventually, you can try the full, or "military," push-up, supporting your weight on your hands and toes. You can make this even tougher by angling your body and doing push-ups off a curb or anchored bench, to give you a greater range of motion.

If you have weak wrists and push-ups hurt, you can buy a semicircle-shaped push-up grip, made of metal with a rubber nonslip base. Holding the grip makes push-ups easier to do.

*Triceps dip.* This is a kind of sit-down push-up. Sit on the edge of a

## Confronting the Machine

You'll need to adjust the weight, and the seat or back angle to fit your size. (Note that some machines are not built to accommodate women under five feet three.) If the gym doesn't give you a checklist, make one yourself, noting which machines you used, the starting weight, and the machine adjustments. On each gym visit, jot down dates, amounts, and number of repetitions on your checklist as you increase the weight. Eventually, you'll know your body well enough to feel what you need to do and advance the weight accordingly. Don't be discouraged if you progress faster on some machines than others. While equipment will vary from gym to gym, *here are my ten favorites for women:*

### For the upper body

*Chest press.* This works your pectoral or chest muscles. While sitting, you push the weight out to the sides of your body.

*Seated row.* Sitting with legs bent, you grasp the handles and pull them as if you're rowing a boat. This helps nearly all of your upper body muscles and back. A variation is the upright row, done while standing.

*Shoulder press.* This works your deltoids (shoulders). Sitting, you grasp the handles and push out straight. (I like exercises where you get to sit!)

*Lateral pulldown.* This strengthens your back. You grasp a bar and pull down.

*Triceps press.* Sitting, you grasp the handles at your sides. With elbows bent, straighten your arms, pressing downward and back.

*Arm curl.* Sit, pull the handles up toward your shoulders, and return.

### For the legs

*Leg curl.* This works your hamstrings (backs of thighs). Lie facedown, curl your ankles around the padded bar, press your hips down and lift your heels toward the rear—then return. It's the closest thing to stair climbing, and one of my favorite tush-shaping exercises.

*Leg press.* Sit or lie on the machine, feet against the pad, and push your legs forward and up. There's also an opposite number to this, where your legs go on top of a padded bar.

*Leg abduction and adduction machine.* This "two-fer" is my other favorite machine, for the inner and outer thighs. Seated, you start with your legs together, then push them apart—or start with your legs apart and squeeze your thighs together.

sturdy nonsliding chair or bench, with your feet on the floor in front of you (extended beyond your knees, not under them). Place your hands next to your hips, and grasp the edge. To start, gently slide forward off the bench, supporting your weight on your hands, and lower your tush toward the floor. Now, straighten your elbows and return to your starting position. This move is harder if you keep your legs straight.

**Middle body moves**

*Abdominal crunches.* As with push-ups, there are many variations of the crunch. Lie on a carpeted floor or mat, knees bent, feet on the floor. The basic goal is to contract your abdominal muscles (pushing the small of your back toward the floor) and slowly lift and lower your head, shoulders, and upper back.

To reduce tension on your neck, put your hands behind your head—but don't lead with your head or bring your weight forward using your neck muscles! If there's no neck discomfort, you can extend your arms in front of you, place them on your thighs, or cross them over your chest. For an added challenge, try bending your knees and crossing your ankles (feet in the air) while doing your crunches. If you do crunches at a gym, use a special slanted crunch platform, which helps to isolate and work your abs.

*The crossover crunch* is a variation that improves your waist-area oblique muscles (or "love handles"). As you lift, rotate your midsection from side to side, with your upper body following but your lower body staying in place. This is usually done with the elbows behind the head. But don't try to bring elbow to knee—rather, aim your shoulder toward the opposite knee.

**Lower body moves**

*Squats.* These are great for your quadriceps (fronts of thigh muscles). Stand with your feet hip width apart, then slowly lower your body downward by pushing your rear backward, as if you are going to sit inelegantly in a chair tush first. Press down on your heels, and return to the starting position.

*Single heel raises.* You can do this even while waiting in line at the bank! Put your weight on the ball of one foot. Raise the other foot behind the supporting leg, bringing your calf toward your thigh. Squeeze your calf at the top of the lift, then let your heel come down to the floor. Repeat with the other leg.

## Pilates Exercises for Abs

These will strengthen and lengthen your ab muscles. My patients with the most toned abs and unexpanded waists are either Pilates instructors (who look amazing) or those who take the classes on a regular basis. I can't begin to cover all the exercises, and some require special equipment, so work with a Pilates instructor if you want to "exercise" this option. Just to give you a taste, here are two basic exercises for beginners:

*"The hundred."* The name signifies one hundred pumps. Lie on your back on a mat, with both knees drawn into your chest. Lift your head and shoulders slightly, and put your arms forward just above the mat. Now, partially extend your legs, keeping your knees bent, so that your toes are slightly higher than your knees. Maintaining this position, rhythmically pump your arms up and down while keeping them straight. Breathe in for five pumps, and out for five pumps. Work your way up to one hundred pumps, or ten full-breath cycles.

*Rolldown.* Sit tall with your legs hip width apart, feet flat on the mat. Wrap your hands around your thighs. Curl your pelvis under you, aiming your lower back toward the floor, while you contract your buttocks. Tilt your chin down and look at your midsection, creating a C curve. Hold this position and take three deep breaths. Then curl back to your starting sitting-up position. Repeat three times.

*Inner thigh side lift.* See the weight training section—but don't use the ankle weights.

*Scissors.* Lying on your back, extend your legs to the ceiling, and move them apart. Keep your hands behind your lower back for support; point your toes. Now, pull both legs in, squeeze them together as they cross the center of your body, then slowly pull them apart.

*Pliés.* I love these; they remind me of my ballet classes. Stand with your feet wide apart, aiming toes and knees outward. Lower your body until you feel that wonderful inner thigh stretch. Then press down on your heels and squeeze those inner thigh muscles as you rise to the starting position.

*Standing side leg lifts.* These also help with balance. Stand on one leg with the other barely touching the floor. Raise this leg out to the side, then bring it down, keeping it straight and the toe pointed. Stand near a wall or chair in case you need help balancing.

*Wall sit.* This works your quadriceps, gluteal muscles (tush), and hamstrings (back of thigh). It's like sitting in an invisible chair. Stand straight, with your back against a sturdy wall. Then, bend your knees and slide your body into a sitting position, hips level with knees. Hold this as long as you can without pain, then slide back up. Repeat.

## More moves for your tush

*Lunges.* Stand with feet together, hands on hips. Step forward with one leg, and lower your body toward the floor so your front knee is over your ankle. Keep your weight on your forward heel. Now, push yourself back to the starting position with your front foot. Repeat with the other leg. (To avoid injury, don't bend your knee more than 90 degrees.)

*Tush lift.* Lie on your back, your knees bent, feet flat on floor, hands behind neck. Press your weight up from your heels, and elevate your hips off the floor, concentrating on squeezing your gluteal muscles (buns) together. Slowly lower yourself to the floor, and repeat. Be sure to tighten your abdominal muscles as you elevate your hips. Note: This can also be done using an exercise ball placed under the small of your back.

*Rear leg lift.* This works your hamstrings and glutes. Lie on your belly, resting your forearms on the floor. Raise and lower one leg behind you, keeping it straight and elevated no higher than hip level. Then, bend your knee and raise and lower the leg with foot flexed, sole facing the ceiling. You also can do this lift with ankle weights.

## Using Water Resistance (Aquatic Exercises)

Exercising in the water is a great alternative if you have joint or back problems, are out of shape after a back or knee injury, or are quite overweight or pregnant. This low- or no-impact workout uses water to create resistance and build strength, and can also give you an excellent cardiovascular workout. Water offers at least twelve times the resistance of air, and gives a naturally balanced workout (since the pressure is even all around you). It also keeps you cool, and washes away any perspiration.

Some exercises are done in shallow water, at waist or chest level, with your feet on the pool bottom. Others are done in deep water with flotation equipment that lets you stay in a vertical position. Variations include underwater jogging, aqua aerobics, aqua yoga, and water tai chi. You may

## Have a Ball with Your Exercise

These big inflated rubber orbs, also called Swiss balls or stability balls, are often used by physical therapists. They make many exercises more challenging (and effective), and are especially good for strengthening your abs and back, and improving balance. You can purchase them at many department and exercise stores, and on the Web. Choose one that lets you sit comfortably, with your knees bent at a 90-degree angle.

I was introduced to the stability ball on the one and only cruise I ever took (it was made more wonderful by the well-equipped gym). A guest kindly showed me how to work with it. A big green ball now resides in my den, and I've been using it ever since.

Here are just a few of the exercises you can do with the ball:

*For abs.* Keeping your feet firmly planted on the floor, lie on the ball and roll it carefully to the small of your back. With your hands behind your head (or crossed against your chest), contract your abs and crunch forward and backward. Depending where you place the ball, you'll feel your lower or upper abs being "crunched." If you have trouble balancing, spread your feet farther apart.

*For upper body.* Kneel behind the ball and drape your body over it. Put your hands flat on the floor. Move forward on the ball, and when you reach a comfortable balance, do push-ups. You can also do these with your toes, shins, or knees propped on the ball.

*For lower body/quadriceps.* Stand with the ball between your lower back and a wall, feet shoulder width apart and hands on hips. Now do a partial squat, so that your knees are bent 90 degrees, allowing the ball to roll up to your shoulder blades. Then, straighten your legs and let the ball roll down to its original position. You can make this harder by holding the squat position for ten seconds.

use special equipment such as aqua-jogging belts, paddlelike dumbbells that use surface area instead of weight to increase resistance, or kickboards. I suggest you take introductory water aerobics classes before attempting this on your own in a neighborhood pool.

## Stretching, Flexibility, and Balance

Flexibility training keeps you limber, improves balance, and may help prevent injuries. Always move slowly into the stretch, extending as far as you can without pain, and hold it for ten to thirty seconds. Relax, then repeat the stretch, three to five times. With each rep, see if you can extend the stretch just a bit farther. Keep your joints loose (not "locked"), and move gracefully—don't jerk or bounce.

Here are some examples of major muscle stretches:

*Hamstring stretch* (back-of-thigh muscles). *While sitting:* Sit sideways on a bench, with one leg stretched straight out along the bench, and the other off it, with the foot on the floor. With your back straight, lean forward from the hips until you feel a stretch. Repeat with the other leg.

*While standing:* Keep one leg straight, and step forward with the other, bending your knee and resting your hands on your thigh. Tilt your body gently forward over the bent knee until you feel the stretch along the back of your straight leg. Switch legs and repeat.

*Two-way calf stretch.* Stand an arm's length away from a wall. Stretch your arms out straight and place your hands on the wall. Keeping your left leg slightly bent, foot on the floor, step back with your right leg and place that foot flat on the floor. You should feel the stretch in your right calf; if not, step back a bit farther. After holding that for ten to thirty seconds, bend your right knee slightly and hold for ten to thirty seconds. Switch legs and repeat.

*Quadriceps stretch (front of thigh).* Stand on one foot, and pull the other one up against your rear (holding the toe). This is also good for your balance, though you can rest the opposite hand against a wall for support as needed.

If this isn't comfortable, you can stretch while lying on your side, with one hip stacked above the other. Pull your top leg back against your rear. (If you can't grab your heel, loop a belt or panty hose over your foot and pull gently on that.)

*Double hip rotation (outer thighs and hips).* Lie on your back, knees bent, feet flat on the floor. Keeping your knees together, gently lower them to one side, as far as you can without pain. (Keep both shoulders on the floor.) Hold for ten to thirty seconds, then bring your knees back to the center, and repeat on the other side.

*Single hip rotation (inner thigh and pelvis).* Start in the same position as the double hip rotation, but this time lower just one leg out to the side, keeping the other leg and your pelvis in place, and your shoulders on the floor. Repeat with the other leg.

*Shoulder rotation.* Now, lie flat on the floor, your legs straight. (You can place a pillow under your head.) These stretches are done with your arms (and shoulders) against the floor. First, stretch your arms out to the side, then bend your elbows at right angles, with your palms facing down (near your hips). Hold for ten to thirty seconds. Now, bend your elbows in the opposite position, with hands near your ears, palms up. Hold.

## Tips for Staying Motivated

To make exercise a healthy habit (like brushing your teeth), look for ways to reward yourself and stave off boredom. For example, do strength exercises while listening to music or an audio book, or while watching TV. Set aside movies on DVD or video for exercise viewing only; you'll want to get back to the story, and look forward to your next session. Or schedule a workout with a friend and catch up while you walk or lift. (But don't try to compete with her; we each progress at our own rate.)

Pay attention to the myriad improvements that exercise makes in your life, such as the ability to keep up with your teenager, sprint to the train or bus, or carry heavy groceries with less effort. Notice the extra energy, the reduced stress and tension—and the more flattering way your clothes fit.

### The No-Stretching Heresy

It used to be gospel that stretching was essential to prevent sports injuries and soreness. While many hold strong opinions about how, when, and why to stretch, there's minimal scientific support for these claims. Research shows that stretching does little to prevent sore muscles. However, stretching *does* promote flexibility, and it feels good—so stretch as much as you want.

If you make stretching part of your routine, do it after exercise, so your muscles are warmed up. I don't always stretch, but when I do, it's my "you're done, and deserve this" reward after an aerobic and strength training workout.

## On-the-Road Fitness

Maintaining your exercise program while traveling just takes a bit of planning. Since you carry your body with you at all times, you can do your crunches and lifts just as you would at home.

Water bottles or hotel-room phone books can serve as impromptu weights. Or bring ankle weights that can be filled with water. A lightweight rubber exercise band offers resistance for your strength and flexibility exercises (although for everyday use, bands may not sufficiently challenge your muscles). They come in differing degrees of tension, measured in pounds.

You can also take a jump rope on the road or an exercise video for your hotel room. Finally, climb the hotel stairs, take a walk (if the neighborhood is safe), or finally (my last resort) run in place in front of the TV.

### Summing Up: My Recommendations

- Aim for a total of thirty minutes (or more) of **aerobic exercise**, most days of the week. If you can do this in one thirty-minute block, great. If not, go for three ten-minute or two fifteen-minute sessions. And plan ahead—enter this into your mental or written schedule. Otherwise, you'll reach the day's end, smack your forehead, and say, "Oh, I forgot to exercise again!"
- **Strength train** at least two (ideally three) days a week, for at least fifteen minutes. Use ankle weights and dumbbells (or gym machines) to speed your progress. (Remember to allow for some muscle warm-up and cool-down time.)
- Add **stretching** and **flexibility training** as often as you like, after you've warmed up with some walking or strength exercises. While the evidence is mixed on whether this reduces injury or limits soreness, it does help to keep you moving and balanced as you get older.

If you come away from this chapter with the motivation to slow down your clock by speeding up your body motions, you may have gained more years of life—and quality of years—than from any other chapter in this book. Now, let's move on. . . .

# 4

## *Taking a Bite Out of Time (What Should I Eat?)*

ynthia married in her twenties, had two great kids, a stable marriage, a beautiful house in Beverly Hills, and wore a size 8 dress. In her forties, she started to gain weight. In years past, a few weeks of dieting got her back "on scale," so she wasn't overly concerned as she purchased size 10 pants.

By 45, she'd gained 30 pounds. Over the next five years, Cynthia went on and off the diet du jour. She'd lose weight initially. But as she started nibbling, and then guiltily consuming, the foods she bought or cooked for her family, ate in restaurants with her husband and his entertainment industry clients, and tasted "everything" as part of their vacations, Cynthia would regain what she'd lost, and more. On her fiftieth birthday, she was 70 pounds heavier than she'd been on her fortieth.

Her husband moved out, citing "irreconcilable weight." Cynthia didn't argue, feeling she'd become a professional and social liability from which he had no choice but to divest himself. Her periods also stopped, but, as she put it, hot flashes were the least of her problems.

When I asked her about nutrition and exercise, she admitted, "Even though I'm now trying to do everything right, when I wake up at four in the morning, the only thing that helps me fall back to sleep is wolfing down a couple of Pop-Tarts." Meanwhile, Cynthia's lipid levels were abnormal. Her blood pressure was 140/88; her waist measurement was 40 inches.

I suggested she switch her 4:00 A.M. snack, which she insisted on keeping, to half a cup of cooked oatmeal; this could be quickly microwaved when she awoke, with artificial sweetener or berries if needed. A nutritionist helped her create a 1,000-calorie eating plan emphasizing vegetables and whole grains, with small amounts of fruit, protein, and polyunsaturated fat. She increased her exercise to at least an hour a day, and began taking a statin to lower her cholesterol and a diuretic for her blood pressure.

Cynthia feels better, has fewer cravings for sweets, and often sleeps straight through the night sans oatmeal. She is losing one pound a week but would like to lose weight faster. Her internist has agreed to reassess her status in three months and then consider weight loss medication. She and her husband are still living apart.

Janice has been a nutritional poster girl for most of her life. She is five feet seven, weighs 108 pounds, and just turned 48. A health food store groupie, she shops daily and studies the racks of books and pamphlets to ensure she eats only what will keep her body "pure." She's vehemently antidairy; condones no red meat, poultry, or processed food; and shuns restaurants, avoiding eating as a social activity. Her resting heartbeat is 50, her blood pressure is 90/60, and her total cholesterol is 160.

She also has osteoporosis, suffers chronic insomnia, and yearns for a loving relationship. Janice has called repeatedly, requesting prescriptions for sleeping pills. I started her on Fosamax and calcium and suggested she talk to a therapist. Does Janice have an eating disorder or "extremely ordered" eating?

## LIFE, FOOD, AND EVERYTHING

The cliché "we are what we eat" sounds so prosaic, but thousands of studies have verified this statement. Our most basic instinct is the pursuit of food, and today we pursue it with a commercial vengeance at supermarkets, delicatessens, drive-through windows, and sit-down restaurants.

In this country, what, when, and how much we eat are less a matter of survival than part of our socialization. Eating is a habit, an expression of love, and a business ritual. It relieves boredom and treats the blues. It shows our wealth, taste, and cooking skill, and honors our ethnic heritage. Finally, we eat because we get hungry.

The constant availability of food has not changed the basic laws of physics or physiology. We need the same nutrients that hunters and gatherers did, and the calories we consume must be used or end up as disease-causing excess fat. For every 3,500 calories we neglect to burn off, we accumulate one pound.

But the nutritional consensus is that some calories are more health harming than others. And here's where the arguments, the "craze" diets, and the personal fortunes of those who promote them come to the fore— the fore sometimes being our abdomens, joints, and hearts.

## WHY ARE WE GETTING FAT?

We see it as we mingle in the crowds at theme parks, or get our money's worth in "all you can eat" restaurants: More than 60 percent of us are now overweight or obese. This percentage has been steadily increasing over the past quarter-century. A quarter of our children and adolescents are getting a stomach-start on this statistic. Statisticians calculate that we now eat 200 calories a day more than we did twenty-five years ago.

Our country is also producing more food, so it behooves our food makers and sellers to move it . . . into our mouths, particularly through commercial venues. Away-from-home eating has increased from 34 percent of our food budget to nearly 50 percent. Even the sizes of our plates, muffin pans, and cookware have increased.

### What We Eat: The Outsized Results of Supersizing

Our portion sizes make a mockery of the USDA portion standards. If you have a single muffin for breakfast, and one bagel and cola for lunch, why are you gaining weight? Chances are, you're downing much more than a single. A cookie from your local bakery is 700 percent bigger than a "portion"; bagels, muffins, and pasta exceed "serving" standards by 200 to 480 percent. Our original bottles of beer and bars of chocolate have grown, as have hamburgers, French fries, and sodas, which are now two to five times larger than their original.

The food industry calls it "value marketing": giving you a lot more food for a small extra fee. It's a competitive selling point to use larger plates and fill bigger containers. Upgrading to a "medium" theater popcorn from a "small" costs roughly 71 cents but adds 500 calories to your bag. When fast food is bundled as a "value meal," it's a caloric train wreck. For example, a Wendy's Classic Double with Cheese, at 760 calories, grows to 1,360 calories when you add $1.57 and opt for an Old-Fashioned Combo Meal.

### It's Not All Your Fault . . .

Yes, we're gaining weight because we have ignored the facts of physics. But a lot of other factors expand this simple "you eat too much, you gain weight" equation. These include genetic predisposition, physiologic changes due to gender and age, lifetime hormonal conditions (which include pregnancy, postpregnancy and lactation, perimenopause, and menopause), endocrinologic diseases, and neurologic conditions. Finally, some medications can cause weight gain.

Let's start with the fact that we are women. As we go through puberty and produce estrogen and progesterone, we increase fat accumulation in our hips and thighs. We typically end up with a higher body-fat percentage than men (22 to 28 percent versus 15 to 20 percent).

During pregnancy the placental hormones increase your appetite and foster fat accumulation, meant to provide calories for the developing fetus and later production of breast milk (which is 50 percent fat). Breast-feeding expends about 500 calories a day; if you don't breast-feed, that added fat is more likely to stick with you. Women who gain more than the recommended 20 to 25 pounds during pregnancy, or who don't lose extra weight within six months of delivery, often end up with an accumulation of 20 extra pounds five years later.

At menopause, women lose muscle or lean body mass—leading to a lower metabolic rate. Meanwhile, body fat redistributes around our waists and upper bodies; we go from pear shape to apple shape.

Other weight gain culprits include Cushing's syndrome (overproduction of hormones by the adrenal gland), hypothyroidism, and neurologic disorders such as stroke. Medications associated with weight gain include steroids, certain antidepressants and antipsychotics, insulin, and perhaps super-physiologic doses (above the amounts the body would normally produce) of hormones (e.g., high-dose birth control pills).

If other members of your family are obese or gained weight with age, your genes may be partially responsible for your increased girth—affecting the amount of food you need to achieve satiety, cravings for high-fat foods, or how you metabolize calories. If everyone in the family supersizes their meals and eats junk food, the cause is also environmental.

From a Darwinian perspective, your heavy, non-*Vogue*-ish forebears did the right thing by conserving their calories to survive drought, famine, and war. This energy thriftiness has become a modern liability when food is plentiful and forced exertion is rare. Evolutionary changes take thousands of years, but in the here and now you want to maintain a healthy weight and live longer—so you may have to become both "counterevolutionary" and inventive.

## What's a "Healthy Weight"?

The "you can't be too thin or too rich" dictum was questioned by the U.S. Department of Agriculture and the Department of Health and Human Services when they jointly issued guidelines in 1990 suggesting that weight gain with age was okay: A body mass index (BMI) of between 19 and 25 before age 35, rising to between 21 and 27 thereafter, was fine. A weight gain of up to twenty pounds after age 35 was acceptable. Moreover, they stated that 17 percent of middle-aged women risked poor health because they were *underweight*. However, this view of weight and its relationship to risk of death was probably skewed by the fact that women who smoke or have chronic diseases are thinner. (Also, the Department of Agriculture may not be an unbiased observer, as it represents the meat industry and food growers.)

In fact, as the Nurses' Health Study data show, once you account for smoking, middle-aged women with the lowest death rates have BMIs of 19 or lower. Risk slowly rises with added weight, with significantly higher mortality from heart disease and cancer at BMIs of 27 and higher. In fact, death from all causes increases with weight.

In contrast to our government's reassurances, we now know that the incidence of diabetes, hypertension, and heart disease begins to increase before we get to a BMI of just 21. Even a relatively small weight gain of 10 pounds, or an increase in waist size of two inches without weight gain, can affect your health and longevity. Gaining 22 pounds or more after age 18 is linked to significantly higher middle-age death rates. Unfortunately, we are so used to obesity and poor health as an American way of life that only half of the heavy ever hear a doctor suggest that they do something about it!

If you are an average American size (152 pounds and not quite five feet four, i.e., your BMI is over 26), you're probably really depressed now. If you are already overweight, you may not be able to get down to the re-defined "healthy size." This doesn't mean you should give up and attack a pint of Häagen-Dazs. A weight loss of just 5 to 10 percent, whatever your size, can improve your blood pressure, lipid levels, and glucose tolerance, significantly decreasing your risk of diabetes, hypertension, heart disease, and osteoarthritis.

## Apples and Pears

Health depends not just on how much fat you have, but where you store it. As we age, many of us find that our shapes evolve from comfy "pears" into more dangerous "apples." If your waist measurement divided by your hip measurement (waist-to-hip ratio) is above 0.8, you are at an in-creased risk for heart disease. (For example, if your waist is 34 and your hips are 40, your ratio is 0.85.)

Or just look at your belt size. A 2002 review using NHANES III data (a sample of over 33,000 Americans) found that a larger waist circumfer-ence—above 35 inches for women—is an independent marker of in-creased health risks, no matter what your size or BMI. Other studies show that even a girth of 32 inches puts you at added risk for heart disease.

## Fat Is a Longevity Issue: What Rubens Did Not Portray

Weight-related medical conditions are our second leading cause of death. A two-decade study of 900,000 people sponsored by the American Can-cer Society found that excess weight was responsible for one in five cancer deaths among women—and that weight loss would prevent most of these deaths. If you expand into "android" obesity (translation: a male-like pot belly), you are at increased risk for developing insulin resistance, type 2 diabetes, abnormal lipids, hypertension, and coronary artery disease.

Obesity promotes or worsens just about every chronic condition and disease. Here's the expanded list, in alphabetical order:

Cancer
    breast
    cervical, uterine
    colorectal
    esophageal

> gallbladder
> Hodgkin's lymphoma
> kidney
> leukemia
> liver
> multiple myeloma
> ovarian
> pancreatic

Cardiovascular disease

Carpal tunnel syndrome

Congestive heart failure

Deep-vein thrombosis

Dyslipidemia (high triglycerides; high LDL and low HDL cholesterol)

Gallbladder disease (stones)

GIRD (gastroesophageal reflux disease—which can lead to esophageal and stomach cancer)

Gout

Hernias

Hypertension

Immobility

Impaired breathing (respiratory function)

Impaired immune response

Impaired wound healing

Infertility

Insulin resistance

Liver disease

Low back pain

Obstetrical complications (including higher rate of Cesarean section)

Osteoarthritis

Pulmonary embolism (clot)

Rheumatoid arthritis

Sleep apnea

Stroke

Surgical complications

Type 2 diabetes

Urinary stress incontinence

Varicose veins

# What's My BMI?

The days are past when weight and height tables developed by life insurance companies showed us what we ought to weigh. We now use the body mass index (BMI) to "measure up."

**BMI classifications** *(from the International Obesity Task Force)*

| | |
|---|---|
| Healthy | 18.5 to 24.9 |
| Overweight | 25.0 to 29.9 |
| Class 1 obesity | 30 to 34.9 |
| Class 2 obesity | 35 to 39.9 |
| Class 3 obesity | 40 or higher |

*To determine your BMI, multiply your body weight in pounds by 704, and divide that by your height in inches squared. For example, if you're 5'5" and weigh 136 pounds:*

136 × 704 = 95,744
65 inches squared = 4,225
95,744 ÷ 4,225 = a BMI of 22.7

For the math-phobic, here's a handy weight chart:

| Height | Normal weight (at or lower) | Overweight (at or above) | Obese | Extreme obesity |
|---|---|---|---|---|
| 4'10" | 115 | 119 | 143 | 191 |
| 4'11" | 119 | 124 | 148 | 198 |
| 5'0" | 123 | 128 | 153 | 204 |
| 5'1" | 127 | 132 | 158 | 211 |
| 5'2" | 131 | 136 | 164 | 218 |
| 5'3" | 135 | 141 | 169 | 225 |
| 5'4" | 140 | 145 | 174 | 232 |
| 5'5" | 144 | 150 | 180 | 240 |
| 5'6" | 148 | 155 | 186 | 247 |
| 5'7" | 153 | 159 | 191 | 255 |
| 5'8" | 158 | 164 | 197 | 262 |
| 5'9" | 162 | 169 | 203 | 270 |
| 5'10" | 167 | 174 | 209 | 278 |
| 5'11" | 172 | 179 | 215 | 286 |
| 6'0" | 177 | 184 | 221 | 294 |

(Note: Ideal BMIs may differ slightly postmenopause, when we tend to carry less muscle and more fat.)

Are you motivated yet? Don't despair . . . even a small weight change can pay off big. Keep on reading. . . .

## DIET PLANS THAT PROMISE INSTANT SVELTENESS AND ETERNAL HAPPINESS

On every magazine cover, we're faced with "perfect" images of five-foot-ten models who weigh 110 pounds. Most of us are unlikely to grow that tall (given our average height is five feet four inches) and will never weigh so little.

Research shows that when starting a "diet," obese women often have overambitious weight loss goals. They expect to lose about 32 percent of their body weight, and are disappointed when they lose 17 percent—even though they look better, feel more energetic, and move more comfortably. Unless you've had surgery (see page 135), a realistic goal is to lose no more than 10 to 15 percent of your body weight over a period of six to twelve months.

Losing just 5 to 10 percent of your initial body weight lowers blood pressure; improves lipid profiles and inflammatory markers (such as CRP and IL-6) linked to heart disease; and helps with blood sugar control. Diet specialists feel that once this level has been reached, more ambitious weight loss goals can be considered. Your energy expenditure decreases at lower weights, and the rate of weight loss plateaus with time.

The most important thing is to *keep the lost weight off*. Even though I'll refer to the following eating programs as "diets," realize that long-term weight loss will not be achieved by periodically "going on" said diet. Weight yo-yoing causes ever higher ups and downs, and actually increases disease and death rates. Ultimately, what you need to do is make a lifestyle change in your food quantities and choices. Later in this chapter, I include those I feel are most healthful, and that are my personal choices.

### Comparing Apples and Oranges, Steak and Wheatgrass

What packs on pounds: too many carbs or too much fat?

The anticarb gospel was first preached to the U.S. masses in the early 1970s by Dr. Robert Atkins. Forget potatoes, bread, and pasta: Go for steak, bacon, eggs, and cheese. To many people, this is a yummy-sounding alternative to the usual diet plan. ("High protein" is defined as 20 percent or more calories from protein; a very-high-protein/very-low-carbohydrate diet contains 30 percent protein, 55 percent fat, and 15 percent carbohydrates.)

These popular diets show a fast payoff on the bathroom scale: The drop in carb intake and the spike in protein and fat trigger loss of water weight as well as loss of some muscle mass. As your body tries to get rid of the extra waste products (ketones) from the overload of protein and fat, you end up in a state called "metabolic ketosis." This can affect your appetite, as can eventual protein boredom.

A review of low-carb research published in the *Journal of the American Medical Association* confirmed the truth behind high-protein diets: You lose weight because you end up eating fewer calories. And when you go off this rigid eating plan (as most people do sooner or later), the weight comes back. Consider a new one-year comparison of the Atkins diet and a low-fat diet (with fewer than 25 percent of calories from fat). After initial instruction, subjects were mostly left to fend for themselves, like real-world dieters. The results? At three months and six months, the low-carb group had lost more weight—but at the end of a year (after some weight regain), both groups had lost the same amount. And they all had trouble sticking to their diets; nearly 40 percent dropped out of the study.

There are also health concerns about high-protein/low-carb diets. While they probably won't hurt you in the short term, a spike in fat and protein consumption can leave you tired, dizzy, nauseated, and dehydrated—not to mention exuding bad breath from ketosis. An unbalanced diet can lead to deficiencies in vitamins, minerals, and fiber, which create other problems, including constipation. You should avoid these diets if you are pregnant, or have kidney or liver problems or diabetes. When it comes to heart health, an overload of fat is a medical oxymoron. Decades of data show the damage caused by high saturated-fat diets.

If you are extremely overweight, the benefits of low-carb *may* be worth the risk. When 132 severely obese people (most already suffering from diabetes or metabolic syndrome) were assigned to a low-carb diet (30 grams or fewer per day) or a low-fat diet, after six months the low-carbers had lost more weight. They also showed more improvement in their triglyceride levels and insulin sensitivity than would be expected for their actual weight loss. The researchers were not sure they had proved the low-carb point; as usual, they cautioned that more and longer studies are needed.

Overall, there's no question that losing weight on either a high- or low-fat diet can improve your blood pressure and insulin sensitivity. But, given the many long-term studies demonstrating the safety and health benefits of a balanced diet with no more than 30 percent of calories from fat (the right fat), I think the choice is a "better-hearter" and a no-brainer.

**The Zone variation**
The Zone diet, developed by biochemist Dr. Barry Sears, is supposed to help people who tend to overproduce insulin in response to carbohydrates; he believes 75 percent of the population falls into this category. While it is often referred to as a high-protein diet, it is not supposed to induce ketosis. It does, however, strictly limit starches such as bread and pasta. Sears recommends that each meal consist of one-third low-fat protein (a serving no larger than the palm of your hand) and two-thirds fruit and vegetables, with a small amount of monounsaturated fat. The diet is supposed to promote consistent blood sugar levels and thereby help limit hunger. Certainly, if you cut sweets and carbohydrates in favor of ten to fifteen servings of fruit and vegetables a day, you ought to lose weight!

While we don't yet have long-term data on the health effects of the Zone diet, it may be helpful for women with insulin resistance (see chapter 6), especially if the protein is low-fat (such as fish) and complex carbohydrates are included in moderate amounts. Strictly following an ideal Zone diet with so few carbs requires unusual discipline and planning in our American eating environment.

**The "But it's low fat!" trap**
In the wake of changes in the USDA's Dietary Guidelines for Americans, suggesting that we take in no more than 30 percent of our calories from fat, the food industry rolled out "fat free" or "low fat" goods, including ice cream, cookies, and crackers. The average proportion of fat in our diets declined from 40 percent to about 33 percent. Correspondingly, cholesterol levels and heart disease deaths declined.

Unfortunately, Americans' average weight did not go down—quite the contrary; since 1976, obesity has grown by one-third. One reason is we replaced high-fat foods with carbohydrates. Those low-fat goodies were packed with sugar: Intake of sugar and other sweeteners increased from 120 pounds per person in 1970 to 150 pounds in 1995. We were so busy counting fat grams that we forgot: Total calories are what count.

Can a low-fat diet that avoids this sugar trap help you lose weight? The best-known low-fat standard-bearer is Dr. Dean Ornish. Primarily for heart disease prevention, but also for weight loss, he prescribes a very-low-fat diet (less than 10 percent of calories), emphasizing complex (unrefined) carbohydrates and cutting out meat. (This requires supplementation with vitamin $B_{12}$.) Ornish views a traditional Asian diet as close to ideal, and notes that a plant-based diet has no cholesterol, is low in saturated fat and oxidants, and high in antioxidants and fiber. When patients with coronary artery disease followed this diet—and stopped smoking, exercised, and practiced a stress management routine—narrowing of coronary arteries was partially reversed.

This diet has almost certainly saved lives, but it's a bit like entering a monastery of eating. Many find a very-low-fat diet extremely rigid and difficult to live with. Also, a diet low in total fat can reduce LDL ("bad") cholesterol, but it also tends to reduce HDL ("good") cholesterol; a low HDL level is strongly linked to coronary heart disease. (We now understand that "what's your cholesterol level?" is not the right question; rather, it's "what's the ratio of LDL to HDL?")

If you have heart disease, your doctor may suggest that you try a modified Ornish plan. If your risk factors are not better in six months, she or he will probably recommend medications.

### Is there a middle way?

While the argument continues, evidence seems to be mounting in favor of a Mediterranean-style diet combined with sensible portion control, for overall health and for doable lifetime weight management. See my comparison of food pyramids on page 137, and my "ideal diet" (starting on page 152).

## WHAT REALLY WORKS FOR
## WEIGHT LOSS?

The only way to lose weight permanently is to change your energy equation: Burn off more calories (move around more), or take in fewer calories (eat smaller portions and/or lower-calorie foods), or both. Since it takes time to gain weight, it makes sense to lose it at a gradual, steady rate—unless you want to gain it right back.

### *How Many Calories Do I Need to Maintain My Current Weight?*

Here's a formula to figure out a maintenance calorie goal. For the purposes of this example, you are a 150-pound woman who walks briskly for a half hour several times a week.

First, figure out your *body weight in kilograms*.
(divide pounds by 2.2., e.g., 150 pounds divided by 2.2 is about 68 kilograms)
Next, *multiply that by 7* (68 × 7 = 476), and *add 800* (1,276).
Finally, *factor in your activity (exercise) level:*
Not very active (1.2), moderately active (1.4), or very physically active (1.6).

This gives you 1,276 × 1.4 = 1,786, or roughly 1,800 calories a day to maintain your weight.

## How Many Calories Should I Subtract to Lose Weight?

This is simpler: *To lose a pound a week, subtract 500 calories a day* (7 days × 500 calories = 3,500 calories, or 1 pound of fat). If you have a lot of weight to lose, you can subtract 1,000 calories to lose 2 pounds per week.

Obviously, *adding exercise* makes you lose faster and is critical for maintaining the weight loss (see chapter 3).

## Getting Ready to Change

It might be an upcoming high school or college reunion, a looming milestone birthday, a new job, the end of a relationship, or the premature death of a friend or relative. It could be a little thing: an unflattering photo, a nagging pain in your knee, a hurtful comment, or catching a glimpse of yourself in a store window. Whatever it is, it sparks your determination to treat yourself better and change the way you eat. (Research shows that if you try to lose weight only to please other people, it won't last long.)

Here are some proven strategies:

- *Set small, achievable goals.* Nothing's more motivating than success, but don't measure it solely by the number on the scale. Think of other things that will make you feel good: fitting more comfortably into a chair, climbing two flights of stairs without panting, playing tennis again, zipping up a slightly-too-small pair of jeans.
- *Have realistic expectations.* Most experts recommend a goal of losing 5 to 10 percent of your current weight. Beyond pounds or dress sizes, note the many improvements in health and reductions in risk factors that you're likely to achieve. Also, many women are surprised at how much more energetic and self-confident they feel after even a moderate weight loss.

## Will It Shrink Your Waistline . . . or Just Your Wallet?

How can you tell if a weight loss program or product is a good health investment—or a health risk?

### What to look for in a weight loss program

*Specific and comprehensive services.* Ask about what you'll do, where, with whom (group or individual sessions), and for what reasons. What kinds of materials will you take home? Is there a plan to help maintain weight loss (the toughest part)? You may prefer or reject the use of premade meals or prescription medications, but all programs should include nutritional counseling. Group meetings are useful for motivation and idea sharing: A two-year study of adults randomly assigned to a self-help weight loss program or Weight Watchers found that the structured program worked better, especially with faithful attendance.

*Staff qualifications.* Ask about education, certification or licensure, and experience helping people with needs similar to yours.

*Program goals.* A realistic goal is losing one or two pounds (or 1.5 percent of body weight) per week. A promise to lose more weight faster is high-fat baloney and may put your health at risk—one reason that very-low-calorie diets are medically supervised (see page 134). A good program will also explain the substantial health benefits of even a 5 to 10 percent loss in body weight.

*Potential risks.* You should hear about the risks of the recommended medications or supplements, as well as planned exercises. If you have particular health problems, find out how the program can be safely adapted to accommodate them. You should also be told about symptoms (e.g., dizziness) that merit a physician visit. (Note: You should check with your doctor before starting any weight loss program if you regularly take prescription meds, have a chronic health problem, or want to lose more than 15 or 20 pounds.)

*Costs.* A good program will tell you what costs are up front, including entry or renewal fees, ongoing services, special foods, and any optional services (such as medical tests).

*Show me the data.* The best programs collect and share information on how much weight clients lose and how many keep it off. They should also tell you that exercise will help maintain weight loss.

*(continued)*

*A brand name or affiliation with a reputable medical center.* Programs such as Weight Watchers help you plan a balanced diet using everyday foods. Jenny Craig uses its own line of prepared food but also guides you to future wise diet choices. Hospital-based programs may start with more drastic calorie containment such as liquid diets, then let you advance to "regular food."

### What to avoid

According to a 2002 report by the Federal Trade Commission, 55 percent of weight loss ads featured at least one false or unsubstantiated claim. Skip products or programs that use these kinds of come-ons:

*"Lose weight without diet or exercise!" "The more you eat, the more you'll lose!"* The über-scam. If there really were a way to lose weight while sitting on the sofa and wolfing down pizza, someone would have won a Nobel prize!

*"Lose 15 pounds in a week!"* This is not only highly unlikely, but losing a lot of weight quickly can cause gallbladder disease and other health risks. And starvation-style weight loss is usually followed by weight rebound (the infamous "yo-yo" dieting cycle).

*"Success guaranteed … or you don't pay a cent!"* The FTC has sued many companies over dishonest money-back guarantees.

*"Proven 100 percent safe!" "Not a prescription drug—no dangerous pills to take!"* Since most ads don't tell you what's in their product, you have no way of assessing this claim. If this "natural" product is an herbal supplement, no testing of safety and effectiveness is required before it can be marketed (see chapter 5).

*"Speeds up your metabolism!" "Helps your body burn fat!"* The only way to "burn" fat is by moving muscles. Supplements that make these claims often contain caffeine or other stimulants to give you a temporary high.

*"Clinically proven!" "Doctor-recommended!"* Almost 40 percent of ads in the FTC survey claimed some kind of scientific or clinical proof—often coming from a "leading" or "respected" (but strangely anonymous) medical center. Another 25 percent claimed that a product was discovered or endorsed by a doctor (usually fictional, unlicensed, or with a financial interest in the company).

*"The secret to permanent weight loss!"* There is no good evidence that over-the-counter diet supplements help keep weight off; exercise and lifestyle changes are a far better bet.

*"I lost 57 pounds and saved my marriage!"* Ms. Before slumps behind unkempt bangs and baggy sweats; smiling Ms. After has a great haircut and sleek dark-colored suit. While we all like a good story, testimonials are not proof.

In fact, the FTC recently sued a company called Body Solutions that was promoted by hundreds of local radio personalities. Their "it worked for me!" results were due to creative ad copywriting, not use of the product.

*"Prescription weight loss—order from the comfort of your home!"* This one is really scary, especially if you remember the "fen-phen" diet drug deaths. If you want prescription medication, get it from your doctor as part of a supervised weight loss program (see page 131). A shady Internet site may send you sugar pills, or something doctored with who-knows-what chemicals and contaminants.

If you have doubts about a claim, or want to file a complaint, check the Federal Trade Commission's Web site, *www.ftc.gov,* or call 1-877-FTC-HELP. The FTC has also issued voluntary guidelines for providers of weight loss products and services.

- *Review your track record.* If you had some weight loss success in the past, what worked? What undermined your efforts? Think about particular places, foods, people, or emotions.
- *Find your trouble spots.* Keep a "food diary" for a week. Most people eat a lot more than they think they do. One clever study at the University of Arizona compared what people said they ate with the contents of their trash bins. Candy intake was underestimated by 80 percent, overall sugar intake by 94 percent. Conversely, healthy foods like fruit were overreported; cottage cheese was inflated by 311 percent! A diary can reveal foods or times of day where you can cut out calories. (A few high-calorie snacks can quickly add up.) Write down not only what and how much you eat, but where, with whom, and how you are feeling at the time—useful for spotting unhealthy-eating triggers.
- *Make gradual changes.* If you want to make permanent alterations in your lifestyle, it's easier to do this gradually than all at once. For example, each week choose one of your usual recipes and find a way to make it healthier (chicken instead of beef, olive oil instead of butter, replacing potato with other vegetables). If you don't want to give up meat, use less of it; cut a small portion into chunks and add it to a vegetable stir-fry.
- *Find ways to build confidence and stay motivated.* An ongoing support group (formal or informal) can be helpful. Talk about little changes that worked, and get kudos and strategies from your diet cohorts. Get together regularly for healthy activities.

- *Consider help from health professionals.* A dietitian can help you modify recipes and cooking techniques, spot hazards in food labels, brainstorm ways to handle relapses, and track and celebrate your progress.
- *Treat yourself with care.* Give up fantasies of "everything will be wonderful when I'm thin." Do all of the thin people around you look happy all of the time? You will actually have greater success at weight loss if you stop beating yourself up and find things to like about your body as it is. Would you ever treat, or insult, someone else's body the way you do your own?

## Trigger Foods

These are high-calorie foods eaten not because you're hungry but because you're bored, depressed, or seeking nurturing and comfort. The "munch parade" includes:

- cakes, pastries, cookies, candies
- chips and processed snack foods
- cheese, cheese pizza
- ice cream or frozen yogurt with yummy add-ins (fudge swirls, chocolate chips)
- fries or onion rings

With some thought and planning, you can often find substitute foods to calm your particular cravings.

- For sweet cravings: Try piece-at-a-time fruits such as berries or grapes, tangerine or orange sections, a cut-up apple—or a spoonful of chocolate chips eaten one at a time.
- For crunch cravings: Cut up carrots or other crunchy vegetables, and perhaps mix in a few almonds or peanuts.
- For smooth-and-cold cravings: Nonfat yogurt, regular or frozen; add a few berries, a spoonful of fruit spread, or a small amount of sweetener or melted chocolate.
- For cheese: Try part-skim mozzarella string cheese; peel the "strings" and slowly enjoy.
- For salt (if you're not salt-sensitive): Air-popped popcorn; mix in a touch of vegetable oil so the salt will stick. Take or make a reasonable serving, and put the rest away.
- For fries or onion rings: Steamed or fresh vegetables with mustard or

salt; a small amount of nuts (in the shell is best—cracking them open slows you down).

## When Your Health Calls for a Drastic Solution: Medical or Surgical

More drastic measures are sometimes needed in our fight to control the mounting weight epidemic. For each aggregate pound we abolish, we save thousands of dollars and lives. Here's what's available:

### Weight loss medications

In the 1990s, many of my patients joined the millions who used the "off label" combination of fenfluramine (Pondimin) or dexfenfluramine (Redux) with phentermine. "Fen-phen" caused serotonin levels to rise, creating a sense of satiety and well-being. Unfortunately, high doses used long-term promoted leaky heart valves and the possible risk of severe heart and/or lung disease. The "fen" drugs were withdrawn from the market in 1997. (Phentermine is still available as a solo act.)

Doctors are now medically and legally leery of prescribing antiobesity drugs, but there is a time and place for the right medication. If your BMI is greater than 27 and you have what we call co-morbid conditions (such as hypertension, diabetes, or heart disease), or if your BMI is greater than 30 even without diagnosed disease, diet drugs can be used to augment diet, exercise, and lifestyle modifications. If you fail to achieve a 10 percent weight loss, or cease to lose weight after three months, it's considered reasonable to prescribe these meds, especially if you are postmenopausal. (At this point, your BMI may underestimate your percentage of body fat, because you've lost muscle mass.)

Two drugs are approved by the FDA specifically for weight reduction and weight maintenance, for use up to two years:

*Sibutramine (Meridia)*. This prolongs the activity of two neurotransmitters in the brain, serotonin and norepinephrine, so you feel full sooner and are more able to control your portions. The dose is 5 to 15 mg daily. It has been found to lead to a permanent weight loss of 5 to 8 percent (when used with appropriate diet and exercise). If you have a history of coronary heart disease, congestive heart failure, arrhythmias, or stroke, use sibutramine only with close medical monitoring. Side effects include a very slight increase in heart rate, usually just four to five beats per minute—and on rare occasions, a significant elevation in blood pressure (if this is going to happen, it usually shows up within the first four weeks of treatment). Dry mouth, headache, insomnia, and constipation are also common. If you don't lose 4 pounds within the first four weeks, this medication probably won't work well for you, and you'll need to try another drug or method.

*Orlistat (Xenical).* This drug binds to lipases in your gut, causing a 30 percent reduction in the amount of fat in your food that is absorbed through your intestine—so you "get" fewer calories than you consume. The unabsorbed fat is excreted in the stool. In studies, those who took orlistat for a year lost an average of 9 percent of their body weight. It also limits weight regain. Type 2 diabetics, who generally have a harder time losing weight, may improve their success by adding this medication.

The dose is 120 mg taken with, or within an hour of, breakfast, lunch, and dinner. Orlistat blocks absorption of the fat-soluble vitamins in your food, especially vitamin D, so make sure you take a multivitamin supplement at least two hours before or after taking it. Side effects—frequent oily stools, flatulence, and the embarrassment of fecal incontinence—depend on how much fat you eat and therefore excrete. One potential plus of this drug is that it may help "train" you to eat a lower-fat diet.

*Other drugs.* Several other prescription meds that can be used for short-term (generally twelve weeks) treatment of obesity suppress the appetite by activating certain receptors in the brain's hypothalamus. They are chemically related to amphetamines, but changes in their molecular structure make them less likely to stimulate the central nervous system and reduce the risk of addiction.

Unfortunately, there are few studies demonstrating their safety or efficacy for six months of use or beyond, and their appetite-blocking effect tends to wear off after a few weeks. To avoid a long list of generic names, I'll just give their trade names: Tenuate, Tenuate Dospan (slower-acting form), Adipex-P, Fastin, Ionamin (phentermine, the safer half of the "fen-phen" program), Bontril, Plegine, Prelu-2, and finally Sanorex and Mazanor.

These drugs may help "kick start" a weight loss program, and keep you motivated as you adapt to new eating and exercise habits. All can cause side effects, including dry mouth, constipation, nervousness, headache, sweating, irritability, sleeplessness, nausea, palpitations, and increased blood pressure. They should only be prescribed by physicians experienced in what's now called "bariatric" (weight loss) practice. In general, these drugs are contraindicated if you have advanced arteriosclerosis, significant coronary vascular disease, glaucoma, hypertension, or overactive thyroid. Tell your doctor what other medications you are taking, because many are not compatible with appetite suppressants; in particular, these should never be used within fourteen days of taking an MAO inhibitor (a type of antidepressant).

### "Off label" prescription drugs

Other medications have been tried to aid and abet weight loss, even though they're not FDA-approved indications (reasons for use).

*Fluoxetine (Prozac).* Although fluoxetine has been shown to promote weight loss in nondepressed obese patients, the pounds tend to creep back—sometimes more than before—within six to twelve months.

*Bupropion (Wellbutrin).* This antidepressant helps control appetite for cigarettes (see page 259), so why not for food? In studies of bupropion prescribed for treatment of depression, some patients reported losing weight. A sustained-release form is now being tested to see if this weight loss is true and ongoing. I have prescribed it, with limited success, in my patients who seem to eat because they're depressed (but not depressed because they eat). Avoid this drug if you have a seizure disorder.

*Topiramate (Topamax).* Doctors found that patients who used this drug to control epileptic seizures also reduced their food intake and lost weight. It's being tested in obese patients who do not have seizures, and may be particularly helpful for those with binge-eating disorders. Side effects include kidney stones, tingling sensations, dizziness, fatigue, and sleepiness.

*Metformin (Glucophage).* This was approved to treat type 2 diabetes by decreasing glucose production in the liver and improving insulin sensitivity (see page 251). In so doing, it can cause minor weight loss, or at least prevent weight gain. Since insulin resistance is often the end result of obesity, and obesity increases insulin resistance, this medication may help prevent more serious disease as well. About 5 percent of adults who try to take metformin can't, however, because of the side effects: nausea, flatulence, bloat, and diarrhea.

### No-prescription-needed "diet pills"

We've all heard and seen ads for Acutrim, Dexatrim, Control, Mini Slims, Permathene, Pro-Trim, Thinz Back-to-Nature, Thinz-Span, and more. These svelte-sounding pills contained phenylpropanolamine, the only over-the-counter (OTC) product approved for treatment of obesity. In 2000, these pills were withdrawn due to concerns about potential side effects such as hemorrhagic (bleeding) strokes. That leaves us with just the "natural" products found in the alternative section of the drugstore or supermarket or on the Internet. I'll cover most of these in chapter 5. Here's a quick overview:

*Chromium picolinate.* Purported to enhance weight loss and improve glycemic control, it probably doesn't do much at standard doses—and high doses can damage your kidneys.

*Ephedra (ma huang).* This dangerous herb (causing abnormal heart rhythms, heart attacks, and seizures, to name a few) was popular before the FDA ban. Any weight lost came right back once ephedra use was discontinued.

*5-Hydroxy-tryptophan (5-HTP).* Though this is promoted for disorders ranging from headaches and depression to obesity, there's little evidence of its effectiveness. In 1998, samples of this metabolite of l-tryptophan were found to have low levels of a potentially harmful contaminant called "peak-x," which can cause chronic muscle pain, blood cell irregularities, and even death.

## Meal Replacement (Liquid "Shakes" and Food Bars)

Meal replacement has become a fairly tasty way of filling up, and knowing what you get, without getting very much. It enables consumption of a very-low-calorie diet (VLCD), defined as 800 calories or fewer per day—a difficult task with conventional foods. Patients who use VLCD in conjunction with behavior therapies for thirteen to sixteen weeks can lose 30 to 50 pounds.

Meal replacement got a bad rep because in the 1970s, liquid diets were 75 percent protein with no vitamins. Today, these liquid diets, whether available without a prescription and/or through a doctor's office, have a healthier combination of carbs, protein and fat, vitamins and minerals, and usually almost half the daily requirement of calcium. Now they are truly food replacements. Nutritionally, they surpass what you get at fast-food restaurants.

The OTC products (such as Ultra Slim Fast) contain approximately 36 grams of carbohydrates; prescription products generally contain only 7 grams. An OTC liquid can replace one or two meals a day; this can be very effective in combination with a low-fat lunch or dinner. Even the prescription replacements are generally not used for all meals. You are a candidate for a prescribed liquid diet if you have diabetes, need to lose weight rapidly before a surgical procedure, or if your BMI exceeds 30. (If it's lower, you're much more prone to lose lean body mass than fat when on a very-low-calorie diet.)

The general consensus is that you can use a liquid diet for up to three months. After the initial weight loss, slowly start adding solid food. You are more likely to maintain the loss if you use a drink for one meal a day and work on behavioral strategies to change your eating habits. A Wisconsin study showed long-term weight loss of 10 pounds when an OTC shake (Ultra Slim Fast) replaced one meal daily for five years; by contrast, a control population gained 16 pounds over five years.

## Bariatric Surgery: When All Else Fails

Although even a little excess poundage, especially around the middle, can be dangerous to your health, "morbid" obesity means that your risk of dying within the next ten years is drastically higher.

You are a candidate for weight-reduction surgery if you:

- Have a body mass index (BMI) of 40 or higher—or a BMI of 35 or higher with significant health problems, *and*
- Have tried to lose weight through other methods and failed
- Have no endocrine abnormalities that caused the weight gain
- Do not abuse alcohol or drugs
- Understand how the surgery works
- Understand that there may be complications, and there are no guarantees
- Understand and accept the need for a new post-op eating pattern
- Are psychologically healthy.

Under optimal conditions, appropriate surgery will allow for quick, effective weight loss in many patients and provide some amazing improvements in their multiple medical conditions. The goal is not to become svelte but to achieve a healthier—albeit probably higher than ideal—weight.

### Staple, cut, remove . . . and how?

To reduce weight by restricting the size of the stomach, gastric bypass using the *Roux-en-Y* technique is the preferred method. It bypasses 95 percent of the stomach, and part of the upper intestine—restricting the amount of food that *can* be eaten, and preventing some of what *is* eaten from being absorbed. This gives the best weight loss results, averaging a

35 percent loss of initial weight (65 to 75 percent of the excess). There may be some weight regain after three to five years.

With experience, doctors have learned how to limit surgical complications (now seen in about 7 percent of cases) and perioperative deaths (less than 1 percent). Complications from this procedure included clots in deep veins (probably due to the combination of obesity and bed rest), leaks where the stomach connects to the small bowel, and wound infections. Since this surgery reduces the absorption of nutrients, iron and vitamin $B_{12}$ deficiencies can occur over time.

A common, uncomfortable side effect called "dumping syndrome" causes nausea, bloating, abdominal cramps, and diarrhea as food passes quickly from the reduced stomach into the small intestine. "Late dumping symptoms" (lightheadedness, palpitations, and sweating) may occur within two hours of eating large or carbohydrate-heavy meals. Knowing this can happen, patients tell me they have learned to reduce their food intake to small portions and to limit sugars and carbs—a self-imposed caloric restriction to accommodate their stomach restriction. A certain amount of "dumping" seems to be associated with better weight loss success.

A second approach to surgical weight loss, *biliopancreatic bypass (BPB)*, leaves a larger stomach pouch but bypasses much more of the small intestine—creating weight loss by preventing absorption of nutrients. This procedure causes a large weight loss (75 to 80 percent of excess weight) that seems to be maintained over time. However, a third to half of patients may develop metabolic problems within the first year, such as anemia or fat-soluble vitamin deficiencies; 3 to 5 percent are hospitalized for treatment of protein-calorie malnutrition. (That's why most doctors reserve this operation for the extremely obese, who are hundreds of pounds overweight.) BPB's intestinal alterations can also cause ongoing diarrhea and foul-smelling stools.

Most of these procedures can be performed through a laparascope (small incision, less hospital time), but they are not simple "Band-Aid" surgeries; despite the small incisions, they entail major rearranging of the G.I. tract and digestive process. So this clearly remains the technique of last resort. But for the right patient, there can be impressive improvements in obesity-associated insulin resistance, hypertension, lipid levels, cardiovascular problems, and sleep apnea. When type 2 diabetes is a complication of morbid obesity, bariatric surgery has actually led to normal plasma glucose levels in over 80 percent of patients—even within days of the surgery. For women, weight loss from bariatric surgery has also been shown to have a positive effect on hormone balance, menstrual irregularities, fertility, and urinary stress incontinence.

Now that some well-known personalities have had obvious success with bariatric surgery (including my *Today* show colleague Al Roker and singer Carnie Wilson), popular demand has increased—and so has the number of surgeons and centers offering the procedures. But these procedures have a steep learning curve, and you don't want the surgeon to learn on you. Do your homework and go to a facility that specializes in bariatric procedures and offers long-term nutritional follow-up.

## FINDING A BETTER WAY TO EAT

### Comparing the Pyramids: A Monument to the Past— or a Pointer to a Longer, Healthier Life?

In the 1950s, we had the four food groups: milk, meat, fruits and vegetables, and breads and cereals. Then, in 1992, the "food pyramid" was unveiled by the U.S. Department of Agriculture (not the National Institutes of Health or another medically oriented agency). At the time, the overriding concern was to reduce saturated fat and cholesterol and their damaging effects on the heart—and to keep advice as simple as possible so the public would "get it." So, the pyramid pointed upward to the lowest suggested component, fats, and replaced them with carbs, including bread, potatoes, rice, and pasta (and, to a lesser extent, with fruits and vegetables).

While the intentions were laudable, unfortunately some critical nutritional realities were entombed. A pyramid of research evidence now shows that:

- Refined carbs, such as white rice, potatoes, and white bread, are metabolized too quickly into glucose, causing unhealthy spikes in blood sugar and consequently in insulin levels (see the section on glycemic index, page 149). These overprocessed carbs should be replaced by grains processed the old-fashioned way: stone-ground breads, steel-cut oatmeal, and whole grain pasta.
- Some fats and oils—monounsaturated and polyunsaturated—actually *reduce* deaths from heart disease and cancers. Moreover, trans fats (the hydrogenated ones—see page 149) are even more dangerous than the saturated fats in butter. (It also turns out that the "no more than 30

percent of calories from fat" dictate was not based on science but just agreed upon by committee.)

- While potatoes are technically vegetables, their starch acts like a processed carb and rapidly raises blood sugar levels. Using them to meet your daily vegetable serving goal crowds out the truly healthful vegetables.
- All protein sources are lumped together. Research is clear that fish, low-fat meats, and nonanimal sources, such as nuts, legumes, and tofu, are the preferred protein providers. This is also true for dairy, where nonfat or low-fat sources should get emphasis.

Since the food pyramid is a political product, efforts to update it based on research findings have drawn protests from special-interest groups, including the meat and dairy industries. (In fact, their lobbying delayed—and kept animal products prominent in—the original pyramid.) Nongovernment groups have developed a series of apolitical, competing

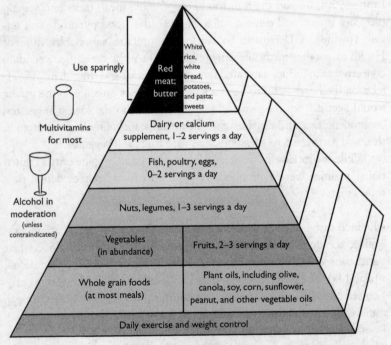

**Healthy Eating Pyramid**

(© Adapted from *Eat, Drink and Be Healthy* by Dr. Walter C. Willett, Simon & Schuster, 2001.)

pyramids—Asian, Latin American, vegetarian, Californian, South Beach. Perhaps the most easily followed alternative is the Healthy Eating Pyramid, promoted by Dr. Walter Willett and colleagues at the Harvard School of Public Health and Harvard Medical School.

The Healthy Eating Pyramid is based on the traditional eating pattern of Mediterranean countries, where the locals have low rates of heart disease and cancer, live long lives, and look great!

This pyramid is significantly different, from base to tip:

- Whole grains and healthy plant oils form the foundation.
- Vegetables are encouraged without limit.
- Nuts and legumes are separated from fish, poultry, and eggs—which are in turn separated from red meat and butter.
- The "use sparingly" apex is now shared by red meat and butter, and refined carbohydrates.
- Moderate alcohol consumption is noted as an option (unless health problems prohibit it), and a daily multivitamin is suggested.

## COFFEE, CHOCOLATE, AND WINE: DO I HAVE TO GIVE THEM UP?

Lest the chefs, food critics, the Food Network, and my patients who enjoy cooking and eating label me "anticulinary," let me hasten to add some good news. We don't have to take a vow of self-deprivation in order to maintain good nutrition and health.

### Coffee and Caffeine

Caffeine is an amazing psychoactive drug. I know it helped get me through the rigors of medical school and residency, and allowed me to stay awake during the many nights when I delivered babies. At coffeehouses in the sixties, we read poetry; today we hold business meetings, study, and log on to the Web. It was at a café that a caffeine-sparked journalist emoted on the evils of monarchy and set off the French Revolution.

The coffee plant has been lovingly grown for hundreds of years. Even if you don't drink coffee, you may be "on" caffeine; it's present to some degree in over sixty human-cultivated plants and trees. Caffeine is closely related to other stimulants, such as theophylline (in tea) and theobromine

# Caffeine Is Everywhere

| Coffee | Serving size | Caffeine content |
| --- | --- | --- |
| Coffee (drip) | 8 oz | 135 mg |
| Coffee (instant) | 8 oz | 95 mg |
| Espresso (depends on brand) | 1 oz | 50 mg |
| Coffee (decaf drip or instant) | 8 oz | 3 mg |
| **Sweet drinks** | | |
| Classic and Diet Coke | 12 oz | 46 mg |
| Pepsi and Diet Pepsi | 12 oz | 36 mg |
| Sunkist Orange | 12 oz | 40 mg |
| Mountain Dew | 12 oz | 54 mg |
| Java water | 8 oz | 62 mg |
| Chocolate milk | 8 oz | 8 mg |
| **Tea** | | |
| Black tea (3-minute brew) | 6 oz | 35 mg |
| Instant tea | 6 oz | 25 mg |
| Green tea | 6 oz | 25 mg |
| **Sweets** | | |
| Ben and Jerry's nonfat coffee fudge frozen yogurt | 1 cup | 85 mg |
| Starbucks low-fat mocha ice cream | 1 cup | 60 mg |
| Häagen-Dazs coffee ice cream | 1 cup | 58 mg |
| Hershey's Special Dark chocolate | 1.5 oz | 31 mg |
| Baking chocolate | 1 oz | 25 mg |
| Chocolate-flavored syrup | 1 oz | 4 mg |
| **Coffee-flavored food** | | |
| Dannon coffee yogurt | 8 oz | 45 mg |
| Dannon light cappuccino yogurt (where did the coffee go?) | 8 oz | 0 mg |

| *Over-the-counter medications* | | |
| --- | --- | --- |
| No Doz, maximum strength | 1 tablet | 200 mg |
| Excedrin | 2 tablets | 130 mg |
| Anacin | 2 tablets | 64 mg |
| Midol, maximum strength | 1 caplet | 60 mg |
| *Prescription medications* | | |
| Cafergot (migraines) | 1 tablet | 100 mg |
| Fiorinal (tension headaches) | 1 tablet | 40 mg |
| Darvon Compound 65 (pain reliever) | 1 capsule | 32.4 mg |

(in chocolate). Our average daily consumption of caffeine is about 280 mg, equivalent to 2½ six-ounce cups of brewed coffee a day.

Let me insert a disclaimer in this coffee encomium: I own no stock in Starbucks or other coffee chains (no thanks to the advice of my stockbroker). As I enjoy my own coffee (of undisclosed brand), let me consider caffeine's benefits from a medical and dietary perspective.

Caffeine prevents sleepiness and sharpens thinking by blocking the action of the neurotransmitter adenosine, lifts mood by affecting dopamine, and "revs you up" by promoting release of adrenaline—starting at doses lower than 50 mg, about the amount in a serving of black tea or cola. It has been shown to improve muscle coordination and strength if consumed just prior to exercise or an athletic event; it also increases energy expenditure and, to a very small extent, helps us burn calories.

Because it helps relax the airways of the lungs, caffeine is associated with fewer asthma attacks in asthmatics. And here's an effect that we've all noticed: It increases peristalsis, and may act as a laxative; in fact, many women rely on that morning coffee to keep them "on schedule" from both a gastrointestinal and daily activity perspective. Two or 3 cups a day may lower the incidence of Parkinson's disease (according to the Nurses' Health Study data) and seems to decrease gallstone formation (at least in men, who are generally less likely to get gallstones than women).

However, I also have to warn you about the negative effects of caffeine—because when all is said and "drunk," we shouldn't all be ingesting it.

*Caffeine and pregnancy.* There may be as much as a 30 percent increase in early miscarriage of normal pregnancies for women who drink just 1 to 2 cups of coffee a day; this goes up to 40 percent with 4 cups. Pregnant women metabolize caffeine much more slowly; it readily passes through the placenta, and the fetus can't metabolize it, so caffeine intake during pregnancy should be radically diminished or stopped. There is also concern about caffeine consumption while trying to conceive. Some studies have shown infertility rates double for women who drink more than 2½ cups of coffee a day.

*Caffeine and cancer.* While some early studies suggested a caffeine-cancer connection, this turned out to be true only if you inhaled tobacco while imbibing your coffee (the researchers forgot that most smokers are coffee drinkers).

Traditionally we've told women who have lumpy, painful breasts to cut caffeine consumption. In my experience, some find this helpful. But a review of randomized, controlled studies found that caffeine restriction failed to provide a benefit for fibrocystic breast conditions.

*Caffeine and osteoporosis.* Caffeine can block absorption of vitamins and minerals, especially calcium and iron. It's also a diuretic, causing us to urinate more and secrete calcium in our urine. Thus, it would be reasonable to assume that overconsumption could increase our risk of osteoporosis. But a recent study from Penn State University found that habitual caffeine intake did not lower bone density, and the National Osteoporosis Society has stated that there is no conclusive link between caffeine consumption and thin bones.

Concerns should probably be focused on adolescents, who consume caffeinated beverages, especially colas, in lieu of milk, and forgo their major source of calcium. As we get older, we can probably compensate for any caffeine-related calcium loss by either drinking milk, taking calcium, or in the best of all worlds, having a caffè latte (with low-fat or nonfat milk).

*Caffeine and hypertension.* Caffeine can raise your blood pressure for a few minutes and, in some cases, hours. However, coffee consumption does not seem to cause an ongoing hypertensive disorder. If you already have hypertension, a cup of coffee can raise your blood pressure, especially in high-stress settings, which could ultimately increase your risk of stroke.

*Caffeine and heart disease.* Caffeine can cause palpitations, irregular or fast heartbeat, and if you have an existing abnormal heart rate or heart disease, this could be a problem. One study found an increased risk of cardiac arrest in nonsmokers who consumed 6 or more cups of coffee a day. But in general, we don't blame heart disease or heart attacks on "reasonable" caffeine consumption.

*Caffeine and headaches.* While caffeine can increase the effectiveness of headache medications, these combined products can actually cause re-bound headaches. To avoid creating this "take a pill, feel better—then worse" cycle, do not use over-the-counter medications with caffeine for more than two days at a time.

*Caffeine and PMS.* Caffeine acts as a diuretic and should theoretically decrease the discomfort of bloat. It can also cause a fall in blood sugar, which may potentiate the symptoms of PMS. Some studies have shown a threefold increase in PMS when we drink 3 to 4 cups of coffee a day.

*Caffeine and bladder conditions.* Caffeine speeds the kidneys' pro-cessing of fluid, so we have to go more frequently. It can also irritate the bladder, causing urge incontinence (your bladder contracts, causing a sometimes unsuccessful race to the toilet). Women with urge inconti-nence are urged to give up caffeine (together with spicy foods, sugar, and too much citrus). The dehydrating effects of caffeine are especially unwel-come on an airplane, which combines dry air and only two bathrooms for two hundred people.

*Caffeine and sleep.* A caffeinated brain is not one that easily falls into sleep cycles. Caffeine also affects levels of melatonin, which promotes sleep. It takes four to seven hours to metabolize caffeine; the older we are, the longer it takes. If you're on birth control pills or take estrogen, the half-life of caffeine may be doubled—so an afternoon cup of coffee can cause late-night insomnia.

*Caffeine and anxiety or panic attacks.* High doses of caffeine increase the levels of brain chemicals associated with anxiety and exacerbate panic attacks.

*Caffeine and heartburn.* Even decaffeinated coffee can increase stom-ach acid production and affect the closing of the valve between the stom-ach and esophagus, leading to reflux and heartburn. If you're currently on Nexium, Prilosec, or another proton pump inhibitor medication for re-flux, you not only need to decaffeinate, you need to de-decaffeinate.

## Caffeine: Are We Addicted?

Caffeine, like nicotine, amphetamine, ephedrine, or even cocaine, can af-fect neurotransmitters that activate reward systems in your brain. At high doses (defined as anywhere between 200 and 800 mg), there can be nega-tive effects, such as nervousness, anxiety, and rapid heartbeat. As little as 1 cup, or 100 mg, can be addictive, causing withdrawal symptoms if you try to stop suddenly after just a few days of "habituating" use. Withdrawal symptoms include headache, fatigue, irritability, depressed mood, inability to concentrate, and even flulike symptoms. All this can last for one or even two weeks, especially if you stop cold turkey.

So, yes, we're addicted. And one of the problems for pre- and postoperative patients is the presence of these symptoms when they stop their caffeine consumption. Doctors now allow most patients (who are not in the cardiac ICU) to have black coffee before surgery or resume it as soon as possible after the procedure.

**Should you put down your cup of joe? Say it isn't so!**
Two to 3 cups a day should be your limit. But if you're planning a pregnancy, are currently pregnant, or suffer from rapid heartbeats, anxiety, panic attacks, chronic high blood pressure, heartburn, or bladder conditions, wean yourself off coffee—and warn family and friends that you may feel out of sorts for a couple of weeks.

## Alcohol and the Medical Whine

What other fluid made from natural products can distill romance, mellow our minds and moods, and heal our hearts? Alcohol has medical origins; in fermenting grains, vegetables, fruits, and honey, our foremothers brewed protection from infections in the generally nonpotable waters of the Olde World.

Before I become too heady in my praise of Bacchus (and join his frolicking maenads), I should issue the strong medical warning that alcohol is, as we all know, the cause of inebriation, auto accidents, and traumatic death. It may also increase our risk of breast cancer. Alcohol-related illnesses constitute the third leading cause of death for women between the ages of 35 and 55.

**Temperance vs. moderation**
Women are far more susceptible to the wrath of fermented fruits and grains than men. Because we are generally smaller than men and have a greater percentage of body fat, we have less body water to dilute the alcohol—giving us a higher blood alcohol concentration from the same amount of alcohol. We also produce fewer of the stomach enzymes that break down alcohol's most potent form, ethanol. Finally, women's cerebral perfusion (flow of blood and nutrients to the brain) is more rapid than that of men: food for thought, but also a cause of speedy inebriation.

## Judging the Alcohol (and Calorie Count) in a Drink

| Type of drink | Grams of ethanol | Calorie count |
|---|---|---|
| 12 oz beer | 12 | 150 |
| 12 oz light beer | 10 | 110 |
| 5 oz glass of wine | 12.5 | 90 |
| 1.5 oz distilled spirits (e.g., vodka, rum) | 14 | 90 |
| 1.5 oz liqueur (e.g., Kahlúa) | 14 | 160 |

Simply put, one drink for a woman has an effect roughly equal to two drinks for a man. Women taking birth control pills or hormone replacement absorb alcohol even faster and it stays in their bodies longer. And, of course, there is the issue of calorie and sugar content; each gram of alcohol contains 7 calories.

How much and how fast we drink has more to do with inebriation than what we drink. If a woman who weighs 150 pounds has two drinks in two hours, her blood alcohol level will be at least 0.05. In some states, this approaches "legally drunk." The less she weighs, the more easily she'll reach that limit.

The terms "alcoholic" and "serious alcohol abuser" are medically appropriate for women who regularly have four or more drinks a day—or five-plus drinks on five or more days per month. According to the NIH, women represent one-third of the roughly fourteen million Americans who abuse or are addicted to alcohol. Other than smoking, heavy drinking is the most effective way to speed forward your clock, age rapidly, and die.

## Alcohol-Related Diseases

Women who are heavy drinkers significantly increase their risk of:

- Cirrhosis and liver disease
- Hypertension
- Brain damage
- Stroke
- Heart disease (cardiomyopathy)
- Gastrointestinal hemorrhage
- Anemia and malnutrition

- Colorectal cancer
- Pancreatic cancer
- Breast cancer
- Suicide
- Victimization (rape and assault)
- Accidents

The National Highway Traffic Safety Administration predicts that three in ten of us will be involved in an alcohol-related car accident at some point in our lives. Other conditions exacerbated by heavy alcohol consumption include menstrual irregularities, infertility, sexual dysfunction, and fetal malformation (affecting a baby's brain, face, and body). Too much alcohol also decreases women's ability to absorb calcium, leading to osteoporosis. And while men may drink for twenty-two years before health damage is evident, women suffer the same effects after just thirteen years of alcohol abuse. The ultimate result: The life expectancy for women who drink heavily is cut short by an average of fifteen years.

**Why some of us face a higher risk for alcohol abuse**
Like obesity, alcoholism has complicated genetic, biologic, and environmental contributors. If a first-degree relative (parent or sibling) is an alcoholic, you are four times more likely to be at risk. Certain genes affect how you metabolize alcohol, as well as how much alcohol it takes to stimulate the pleasure centers in your brain. And women who suffered childhood sexual abuse, started drinking before age 15, were heavy college drinkers, or had clinical depression are more likely to become alcoholics.

## Moderation: Is It Good for Our Hearts at the Expense of Our Breasts?

The oft-cited Nurses' Health Study showed that women aged 35 to 59 who consumed one to three drinks a week had a 17 percent lower mortality from heart disease than did women who were teetotalers. However, note this caveat: The only women who benefited from light to moderate drinking were those who had at least one risk factor for coronary heart disease. In other words, they had high cholesterol, diabetes, or high blood pressure, smoked, or had a parent who had a heart attack before the age of 60. For women without risk factors, moderate drinking didn't seem to help or hurt.

The study did show a worrisome correlation between alcohol and other diseases. Nurses who consumed more than 3 drinks a week had a *higher* mortality rate, primarily due to an increase in breast cancer and cirrhosis, and those downing 1.5 drinks per day at least five days per week faced a 44 percent greater risk of hypertension.

Touting the positive research findings, the wine and beer industries began a PR war over which beverage is more heart-healthy. Actually, the risk of death did not differ significantly among beer, wine, or hard-liquor drinkers. There was a small trend toward greater protection with wine, but this may be because wine is more often drunk with meals. (Some data suggest that antioxidant polyphenols from the skin and seeds of grapes make red wine a cancer fighter.) On the other hand, small amounts of beer seem to be associated with less hypertension. The bottom line: Depending on your health and genes, a little alcohol may be good—but a lot can be disastrous.

### Breast cancer

To better instill the less-is-better idea, a pooled analysis of approximately 322,000 women (including the Harvard-study nurses) showed that two to five drinks a day increased breast cancer by 41 percent compared with non-drinkers; each extra drink increased the risk by 9 percent. One factor here may be that alcohol can increase estrogen levels by either raising production or decreasing breakdown. (And because the plants they are made from contain phytoestrogens, alcoholic beverages can have estrogenlike effects.)

My final recommendation: An occasional glass of wine or beer for celebratory and special events is okay, but rationalizing drinking as beneficial to your health and well-being just doesn't wash. If you feel your culinary life or stress management is incomplete without a drink to go with dinner, don't go beyond that one, and sip it slowly.

### *Cheers for Chocolate*

When the Europeans discovered America, they also found chocolate, and predictably went nuts for it—attributing curative powers for dozens of ailments, from fever to kidney stones, to the cacao bean. They also believed chocolate could spark appetite for food and sex—anticipating current research, which shows that chocolate increases the activity of neurotransmitters involved in mood regulation.

Chocolate also contains cancer-fighting antioxidants called "flavonoids"—such as those found in healthy fruits and vegetables (see the box on page 150). Much of chocolate's fat content comes from stearic acid, which works in the body like a healthy monounsaturated fat. And to the consternation of dentists, there's some evidence that this fat may help protect against cavities.

Nonetheless, chocolate foods come with hefty doses of calories. Milk chocolate and ice cream contain a lot of animal fat and sugar, with most flavonoids processed out. To get the most from chocolate, buy the good stuff: high-quality dark chocolate (perhaps with some added healthy nuts). White chocolate is but a pale excuse, usually containing cocoa butter, milk, sugar, and flavorings.

## AN EATING PLAN YOU CAN LIVE WITH—FOR A LONG TIME

These food choices can keep you deliciously feeling younger, looking better, and living longer: whole grains for carbs, legumes and nuts for protein, and lots of fruits and vegetables, "entréed" with fishy omega-3 fatty acids. Whether you aim for 20 or 30 percent of total calories from fat, emphasize the "good" fats (nonhydrogenated, unsaturated).

### Do the "Right" Fat

Limit saturated fats: the kinds found in red meat, cheeses, butter, and poultry that are hard at room temperature—and, of course, the trans fats. Trans fats are more insidious in the rise they cause in our triglycerides and lipoprotein a, and in the promotion of insulin resistance.

The Nurses' Health Study showed that higher intake of the right fats (nonhydrogenated, polyunsaturated, and monounsaturated) decreased the risk of coronary heart disease (CHD) and cancer—and was more important than *total* fat intake. Two other studies have shown that when women eat two or more servings of fish a week, they lower their risk of coronary heart disease by 30 percent. On the vegetable side, alpha linoleic acid (ALA) and omega fatty acids found in flaxseed, canola, and soybean oils are converted in our bodies to the two active components found in fish oil: EPA (eicosapentaenoic acid) and DHA (docosahexaenoic acid).

It's been found that those women who frequently consume oil and vinegar salad dressing (a major source of ALA) have a decreased risk of

## What's a "Trans Fat"?

For years, we heard the lectures about heart-harmful animal fats, and virtuously ate our margarine. Now we hear that margarine contains "just as bad" trans fatty acids. What's the story here?

While a few trans fats occur naturally in meat or dairy products, most are human created, when vegetable oil is hardened by adding hydrogen (hydrogenated) to create margarine or shortening. These fats are even worse for your arteries than butter; they raise LDL cholesterol *and* lower protective HDL cholesterol. The harder the margarine, the more trans fats it contains. (Another reason to avoid fried foods in restaurants: They often use hydrogenated oil.)

But don't substitute butter; soft tub margarines without trans fats are now available. Check labels: The first ingredient should be liquid vegetable oil. Seek unsaturated oils such as canola, corn, safflower, olive, sesame, sunflower, soybean, or peanut.

Trans fats are also popular with snack makers, because they stay "fresh" longer. That box of crackers with the proud banner NO CHOLESTEROL! probably has trans fats lurking inside. The FDA recently issued a rule requiring that trans fats be listed on all food labels by 2006. As a result, some companies are seeing the light and switching from hydrogenated oils to "pure" liquid vegetable oil.

The best advice: Read labels carefully, or make your own snacks.

developing or dying from CHD. And studies have shown that women with heart disease who ate fish twice weekly or took fish oil had a 29 percent lower mortality after two years. When we try to cut calories by skipping nuts or oil-based salad dressings, we miss out on healthful fats.

### Carbohydrates . . . The Glycemic Index Story

Sugar, even without the spice, may make things taste nice, but it also gives an immediate directive to your pancreas to produce and secrete insulin— and increased insulin levels ultimately result in increased triglycerides, fat accumulation, damage to small arteries, atherosclerosis, and coronary heart disease (see page 248). Ultimately, the pancreas may become exhausted, refuse to respond to sugar overload—and diabetes develops. The glycemic index (GI) ranks foods based on the rise they cause in blood glucose.

Carbohydrates vary considerably in their GI grade. Foods with compact granules, such as spaghetti and oatmeal, or soluble fiber, such as barley, oats, and rye, are digested quite slowly and hence don't cause a sudden rise in blood glucose (i.e., they have a lower GI). Unfortunately, potatoes, white rice, and especially white bread are in the high-GI category. In over 75,000 women followed for ten years, it was eating large quantities of high-GI foods that increased their risk of CHD. In other words, one piece of white bread or roll before a healthy dinner is not going to automatically create an insulin overload, but if the dinner consists of rolls, pizza, and Coke, you're in insulin hell. What's more, the rapid rise and drop of blood sugar from refined carbs can make you feel hungry and lead to overeating.

The GI value of your food is not printed on its "table of contents," but you can get a sense of its starch effect by looking for the terms "whole" or "refined" grains. The latter is one of the biggest misnomers: "Denuded" is more like it! Processing any cereal grain strips it of its fiber,

## Add Healthy Color—with Fruits and Vegetables

Perhaps the simplest (and most delicious) anti-aging remedy is to eat more fruits and vegetables. These aren't just crunchy or juicy vitamin pills; their complex combinations of phytochemicals (plant nutrients) fight cancer, heart disease, hypertension, diabetes, and macular degeneration (a major cause of blindness). Supplements cannot copy nature's marvelous mix of phytochemicals, vitamins, and minerals, making vegetables and fruits the most potent antioxidants ever produced.

The Nurses' Health Study found each additional daily serving of fruit or vegetables was linked to a 4 percent lower risk of coronary heart disease and a 6 percent lower risk of stroke. Green leafy vegetables, cruciferous vegetables (broccoli, cabbage, bok choy, cauliflower), and citrus fruits gave the greatest cardiovascular benefit. Studies have also shown that high consumption of fruits and vegetables reduces the risk of cancer.

Five servings a day is your minimum goal; nine are even better. A serving is $1/2$ cup of cut-up fruit, or raw or cooked vegetables; 1 cup of raw leafy greens; a glass of juice; or a medium piece of fruit. To get the full array of benefits, it's best to eat a variety of produce. Fortunately, the color of your food can give clues to the health goodies within (e.g., beta-carotene—which your body converts to vitamin A—tints vegetables and fruits orange). Aim for a bright palette: red, orange-yellow, green, and blue-purple. For greatest benefit, buy fresh fruit, wash it well, and eat it with the skin on.

essential fatty acids, and phytochemicals, making it the highest form of starch with a soaring glycemic index.

## When It Comes to Protein . . .

Both the type and amount of protein we eat matter. Too much can lower your absorption of calcium, leading to osteoporosis, and can stress your kidneys. The consensus is that the right proteins, forming 15 to 20 percent of your diet, will help prevent coronary heart disease, especially if you also consume less saturated fat. Protein from vegetables, nuts, and legumes is fabulous, in part because of all the other nutrients in these plants.

Nutritionists have now become nuts over nuts, and the monounsaturated and polyunsaturated fat, fiber, and magnesium they contain. Magnesium may decrease insulin resistance, and despite their fairly high caloric content, nuts have a low glycemic index. At least six studies of nut eaters have shown a decrease in risk of CHD by as much as 50 percent. If you're worried about the calories, use nuts to replace red or processed meat, or refined starches. One compensation: Nuts are more filling.

Other studies have clearly shown that replacing red meat with skinless chicken or fish reduces CHD. And in 1990, the Nurses' Health Study found a two and a half times higher risk of colon cancer in women who consumed red meat as a main dish daily compared with those who ate it less than once a month. I personally gave up red meat fourteen years ago, but I realize that may be too austere for many individuals (including my husband, who craves an occasional steak or hamburger). Just make sure the meat portion is small, lean, and appropriately cooked.

## When It Comes to Weight . . .

I want to weigh in with a contradiction to a belief we've accepted for decades: that decreasing total dietary fat is *the* major path to eternal slimness. It's probably far more effective to change the *type* of fat you eat, along with the type of carbs and total calories. Portion control, together with healthy choice control, is our best way to weight control. These changes, plus regular exercise and not smoking, will do more to slow our clock down than any quick-fix supplement or over-the-counter or prescription medication.

# THE SLOW YOUR CLOCK DOWN "LIFELONG" DIET

This is my personal ideal diet. I've found it fairly easy to stick to as long as once a day I add a treat—something eaten not for pure nutritional value but because it tastes good, comforts me, or satisfies a craving. If you're forced to veer "off plan" because you're eating out, traveling, or cooking for family members who protest, try some of my secrets for social eating (see pages 156–61).

## Get Going: Breakfast

Whatever you do, don't skip breakfast! Studies show that long-term, low-blood-sugar levels caused by the fourteen-plus hours of fasting between dinner and tomorrow's lunch can shorten your lifespan. This forced hypoglycemia plays havoc with subsequent insulin production (it "overshoots") and will lead to increased hunger, weight gain, and perhaps atherosclerosis. Here are my daily breakfast choices:

1. *An egg-white omelet* (use two to three eggs, but if you need that yellow from the yolks, either add a bit for color or treat yourself to a whole egg three times a week). Cook with olive oil spray, and add diced vegetables (mushrooms, tomatoes, avocado, broccoli, or spinach) plus small amounts of grated low-fat or nonfat cheese for flavor (part-skim mozzarella, reduced-fat cheddar or Swiss, or feta).

   On the side, add two pieces of whole-grain *toast;* top with soft spread containing no trans fats (such as Smart Choice or Fleischmann's light margarine; check the labels), and/or fruit spread.

2. 1 cup cooked (not instant) *steel-cut oatmeal* with nonfat milk or high-calcium soymilk. Add berries, sliced apple, crushed walnuts, or cinnamon for flavor.

3. 1 cup *whole-grain cold cereal.* Look carefully at the package label; it should read very little or no added sugar, and contain at least four grams of fiber. Add 1 cup nonfat milk or high-calcium soymilk, and perhaps berries or other fruit.

4. 1 cup *nonfat yogurt* with ¼ cup blueberries (or other berries in season), or chunks of melon. Add one to two slices of whole-grain *toast* (as in choice number 1).

Beverages, for all of the above:

- 1 glass of orange juice or tomato juice.
- If desired, 1 cup of coffee with nonfat milk, or 1 cup of tea (black or herb). If it has to be both hot and sweet, use artificial sweetener or just a pinch of brown sugar.

If you don't take your vitamins or other medication with breakfast, you can drink grapefruit juice (or eat half a grapefruit) in lieu of orange juice. Grapefruit can interfere with the metabolism of some medications and vitamins. If you purchase ready-made orange juice, get the calcium-fortified kind.

## Timeout: A.M. Snack

Of course you get a snack! Noshing through the day keeps hunger for the wrong foods away. . . .

Choices:

1. ½ to 1 cup nonfat *yogurt,* with berries or chopped walnuts (if you didn't choose this for breakfast)

2. ½ cup nonfat cottage cheese (this has less calcium than yogurt, so you may need to increase your supplement)

3. A piece of fruit (a sliced apple with a tablespoon of peanut butter is delicious and satisfying)

4. 1 Wasa cracker (they're big) with peanut butter or soy nut butter

## The Halfway Meal: Lunch

Choices:

1. *A salad* featuring dark greens (not iceberg lettuce).

    Add any raw vegetables you wish, including up to one-quarter of an avocado.

    You may also add 3 ounces of water-packed or fresh tuna or salmon, skinless white-meat chicken, or turkey.

    Other salad ingredients can include nuts, 1 ounce of goat cheese, cooked soybeans, or tofu.

    Dress lightly (2 tablespoons should do it) with healthy oils (olive, canola, corn, and vinegar). If the dressing is premade, Italian or vinaigrette is usually okay.

2. *A sandwich* on whole-grain (dark) bread, containing: peanut butter and fruit spread; or water-packed tuna, sliced white-meat chicken, or turkey (best if baked or grilled).

    Pile on veggies, greens, tomato, avocado in moderation, or sprouts. For condiments, use mustard, nonfat fruit-based relish, or small amounts of canola-oil mayonnaise or light margarine (with no trans fats).

3. *A "luncheon"*
    - 3 ounces of fish (preferably salmon or other cold-water fish), or
    - 3 ounces of skinless white-meat chicken or turkey (baked or grilled)

    If you crave a hamburger, try a low-fat chicken or turkey burger, or an extremely lean beef burger. A 3-ounce portion of meat should resemble a deck of playing cards; it should not be spilling over a white bun. Use a whole-grain bun or, better yet, substitute whole-grain bread. (You can also just take half the bun off and eat the rest.)

    Add ½ cup each of two different steamed or grilled vegetables (see dinner menu) and/or a green salad.

    *Beverage choices:*

    Water, or one glass of nonfat milk, or a glass of iced or hot tea (add artificial sweetener if needed).

*Dessert choices:*

If you must have it (try to skip or keep it for a later snack), choose a piece of fruit, a cup of fruit salad, or ½ cup nonfat frozen yogurt or sorbet.

Note: A cup of cut-vegetable soup or vegetable-puree (cream free) soup, preferably homemade, can replace a vegetable, a dinner appetizer, or a lunch, depending on the serving size.

## A Late Break: P.M. Snack

Choose from the morning snack list.
If you hit a four o'clock low and must have something sweet, allow yourself:
- a small piece of chocolate, preferably dark (e.g., a "fun size" or "snack-size" chocolate bar—about 50 to 100 calories), or
- ½ cup nonfat chocolate frozen yogurt, or
- if you've had no more than a cup or two of coffee so far, a cappuccino made with nonfat milk and a sprinkle of chocolate, or
- ½ whole wheat pita with hummus spread lightly in the middle (this can also be a morning snack).

## The Last Repast: Dinner

Start with:

- a green salad featuring raw veggies, with healthy oil-based dressing (see lunch salad); may add tofu, goat cheese, olives, or nuts; or
- a cup of soup (see Note above).

*Main-course choices:*

The same foods listed in a "luncheon": 3 to 6 ounces of grilled, steamed, baked, or sautéed-in-olive-oil *fish* (preferably salmon or other cold-water fish), *poultry* (remove the skin), or *lean meat*. (I don't eat meat, but if you do, you may choose it two or three times a week.)

*Side-dish choices:*

- two portions (½ cup each) of lightly cooked *vegetables*. Go for a colorful mix: dark green, orange, yellow, or purple, and

- a *carbohydrate* that makes you feel your meal is complete. Instead of mashed potatoes or French fries, substitute sweet potatoes or yams, pasta in amounts equal to your vegetable, or ½ cup whole-grain rice.

If now and then you really crave potato, allow yourself a portion equal to ¼ to ½ of a medium spud (best if baked or boiled with skin). Top if desired with mustard, lemon juice, nonfat yogurt, salsa, or nontrans-fat spread—or sprinkle with Parmesan cheese.

### Dessert choices:

Skip dessert if you're full; the healthier food in this daily diet may be more than your stomach is used to. Or select berries, fruit salad, or sorbet. If other desserts are served, just taste them; 2 to 3 spoonfuls should make your taste buds happy. (The first few bites are always the best anyway.)

### Beverage choices:

Same as at lunch, or up to 1 glass of red or white wine—depending on your risk factors (see page 146) and, naturally, your main course.

## A Bedtime Snack?

If you brush your teeth before you see the evening news, you may not need this. But if you feel deprived, consider postponing your fruit dessert until now, or fix a half-bowl of whole-grain cereal or oatmeal to make you carb-sleepy.

### Personal asides

Spicing and dressing up these foods with a wide selection of oils, tasty herbs, and condiments can give you many delicious variations on the basic theme. Using these menus as a template, you can achieve caloric control and portion control. When you do your own cooking, or (like me) influence those in your household who do it, it's fairly easy to direct this sort of mix among the Mediterranean, Ornish, and, yes, Reichman diets.

## My Secrets for Away-from-Home Eating

Here, too, I've honed some eating skills that I feel provide good nutrition without taste deprivation or excess, useless calories.

## On-the-job eating skills

*Bring your own!* Take fresh fruit, yogurt, cottage cheese, and/or home-made sandwiches to work. Either store them in a small office refrigerator, or in an insulated lunch bag or food container. Stock nuts, peanut butter, and whole-grain crackers (sans trans fat) in a drawer for snacking—but limit this to a one- or two-week supply, and don't restock before the allot-ted time.

*Bring leftovers.* You've cooked a healthy dinner—so cook a little extra and take a lunch portion to work where you can reheat it or eat it cold. If you had a restaurant dinner the night before, eat a reasonable portion (usually less than half of what's served) and take the rest "to go" for your next day's lunch. Now you've had two good meals for the price of one.

## Restaurant skills

My personal secret: Eat some nuts or a piece of fruit before you head to the restaurant, so you don't arrive famished and attack the first thing they put in front of you, which is usually white bread. When bread is served, remember there's a lot of food to come; just break off a little piece. If you need something on it, ask for olive oil. If that's not available, use a small amount of butter, or ask for mustard—it's a great way to spice up bread.

If you order wine, save most of it to sip with your main course. Be sure to also order a nonalcoholic, nonsugary thirst quencher: water, iced tea, or diet soda.

Salads should be ordered with dressing on the side, so you can deter-mine amounts.

See if someone at your table will share an entrée, or consider ordering two appetizers. Otherwise, plan to eat no more than 6 ounces of fish, meat, vegetables, and salad, and take the rest home. I'm not anti-pasta in Italian restaurants, but start with the antipasti, in which case you'll prob-ably only want one-third to one-half of the pasta portion served—and again, take it home. Stay away from foods cooked with butter (margarine is no better) or cream, or fried in nonvegetable oil.

Whenever possible, order fish (fresh wild salmon is best) or grilled chicken breast (cut the skin off). If you order duck, make sure it's an inner piece without the fatty skin. Should you splurge on a steak, cut away the fat and eat only a deck-of-cards portion, taking the rest home for tasty leftovers (or for the dog).

When ordering vegetables, ask if you can have them steamed, or cooked with olive oil rather than butter. Avoid mashed potatoes and French fries, but if they land on your plate, taste rather than consume them.

For dessert, ask for fresh fruit. If you feel that will cause supreme unhappiness, consult the others at your table and get a dessert to share; your share should not exceed several teaspoonfuls. If you want to finish this off with something warm, herb tea is lovely. If you believe the waiter's decaf promise, consider coffee: A cappuccino with nonfat milk makes you feel like you've had a yummy dessert.

My prandial motto: You've failed your restaurant experience if you don't walk out with a bag of your leftover food.

### Ethnic restaurants

*Chinese food.* An exposé of take-out Chinese food by the Center for Science in the Public Interest (CSPI) reported that many dishes contain a huge amount of calories or fat: For example, a large Chinese chicken salad had 1,014 calories with 61 grams of fat.

Some Chinese restaurants do serve brown rice. If you order the white rice, use it as an accent rather than the staple of your meal. Anything that's fried or batter-coated will be calorie-laden (that covers fried wontons, egg rolls, and most sweet-and-sour chicken). Steamed dishes are best, or ask that the chef wok your vegetables plus chicken or shrimp (or beef) with as little oil as possible. If you add soy, use the low-sodium kind.

If you want a taste of your companion's kung pao chicken (1,275 calories and 75 grams of fat), fine, but satiate your hunger with more healthy choices. Some menus now feature little hearts next to lower-fat dishes.

*Japanese food.* Try the delicious tofu dishes. Go light on the white rice. If you're having sushi with uncooked fish, make sure it's fresh and served in a restaurant that does a bustling business, with fast turnover. Start out with edamame, a wonderful soybean appetizer, and/or miso soup with tofu and seaweed. Grilled dishes are preferable to fried (tempura). Use low-sodium soy sauce, and limit amounts. Rather than ordering green tea ice cream for dessert, have the sushi chef make a beautifully carved orange—an excellent end to a protein-rich Japanese meal.

*Mexican food.* You don't have to add sour cream or thick cheese sauces to enjoy Mexican cuisine. Find out ahead of time if the restaurant uses lard or oil; the latter is obviously preferable. Don't fill up on chips and salsa (I just take a couple of chips and taste the salsa or guacamole). Most restaurants will grill their chicken, fish, or beef. Food is often served with refried beans (usually not low-fat), but some restaurants will give you whole beans that may bear less cooking fat.

Use as much salsa as you like, and order corn rather than flour tortillas. If you must have a margarita, don't salt the rim, and get a plain rather than a fruit-flavored sugary calorie bomb. Olé! (Note: A light beer will have far fewer calories.)

*French and Continental food.* This is a tough one. It's hard to ask a French chef to forgo foie gras or butter. So if you must, taste the former and order the food that you think may have the least of the latter. The French no longer frown upon your asking for the sauce on the side. They do grill some of their fish and meat, and they generally have wonderful salads. If you're faced with one of those six-course tasting menus, do exactly that: Taste a little bit of each dish (believe me, you'll be filled—"*C'était délicieux!*"). Enjoy it, but don't do it too frequently!

When the cheese course comes, ask for *chèvre* (goat) rather than *vache* (cow). It's lower in fat, and just as delicious.

*Italian food.* For a wonderful appetizer, choose *tricolore* salad or half a portion of tomato and mozzarella. If you order pizza, limit yourself to two pieces (share the rest) and go for one with veggies instead of sausage or pepperoni. If you order pasta, choose one made with wine, tomatoes, or olive oil—nix the Alfredo and cream sauces. Half portions of pasta are often available, or order the appetizer size.

Most Italian restaurants will grill fish, shrimp, and chicken breast. Ask them to substitute olive oil for butter. The Italians love marinated vegetables and veggies cooked in olive oil. These, along with fish and fresh fruit, may be the tasty secret to the healthy rewards of the Mediterranean diet.

*Fast-food dining.* Even though McDonald's has changed their French-frying formula, they and all the other major burger restaurants give you an awful lot for your money, and we now know it's way too much. In the mid-1950s, McDonald's served one size of fries—equivalent to today's "small," and one-third the weight of the now largest size. A king-sized pack of Burger King fries has 590 calories and 30 grams of fat.

But to their credit, some chains now serve salads (watch the dressing), grilled chicken, and "light" tacos; a serving of Burger King chunky chicken salad has only 142 calories. If you are a frequent fast-food eater, check the Web for ways to minimize the damage. The Wendy's Hamburgers chain, for example, features a "build a meal" nutrition calculator on its site that gives ingredients, calories, total and saturated fats, sodium, carbs, and protein for any meal combination you enter.

Don't forget about the alternatives: an array of fast-service salad and sandwich shops (some that originated in Europe, and others that spread from the coasts), as well as Mexican restaurants that serve fresh, no-lard dishes. Unfortunately, you can't make caloric assumptions here, either; the *Wall Street Journal* reported that Fresh City's chicken teriyaki wrap contained 968 calories, and Baja Fresh's chicken salad had 857 calories. Again, check the Web or ask the manager to be sure you've made a healthy selection.

Often, the issue is the side orders: the mashed potatoes, creamed spinach, and macaroni-and-cheese. Try to find yams, steamed vegetables, baked beans, or salad. If you crave pizza, have a few thin-crust slices.

And forget the 64-ounce, 800-calorie Coke; quenching your thirst can end up expanding your abdomen and thighs. A venti-sized Starbucks white chocolate mocha has 600 calories, the same as a Big Mac. Go for the double-tall, nonfat cappuccino, a diet drink (my last choice), or cool fresh water.

### Eating skills for travel

Room service is so convenient; just make sure you request the same healthy foods you fix at home. A Continental breakfast usually includes about 800 calories in pastries. Substitute whole wheat toast, fruit, and yogurt, or a whole-grain cereal with nonfat milk. When I order eggs, I specifically request egg whites only, prepared with a minimum of oil. Finding an alternative to butter is nearly impossible, so either use it sparingly or reach for the marmalade. Ask to substitute sliced tomato for the ubiquitous hash browns.

If you must lunch on the run, find out at your hotel where the closest salad or sandwich shop is, and choose a non-French-fry, non-cheese-laden, nonoversized lunch. At a business meal in an upscale restaurant, choose as you would at your local restaurant or at home.

### When you're a guest

This is a challenge, because you don't want to insult or inconvenience your hosts. If you don't eat red meat (like me), call ahead and relate this, perhaps with an upbeat "but I love vegetables, so I don't mind just eating those you prepare to go with the meat." If the food looks extraordinarily rich, say you're a light eater and ask for small portions, while showing an eagerness to try and extol everything. If you know you're going to have a

## Airborne Eating

I spend a lot of time on planes commuting between New York and L.A. to do the *Today* show, to give talks in cities throughout the United States, and even occasionally go on vacation. On long flights in any class, you are presented with high-calorie foods designed to keep you quiet, diminish boredom, and hopefully even cause a postprandial nap. The best thing you can do is take along your own food; that's what I do.

For lunch, pack a sandwich and some fruit. Note: If you don't have time to make them at home, or you're leaving from a hotel, you can often get good sandwiches made on whole wheat bread or rolls, as well as yogurt, at the airport before boarding the plane.

At dinnertime you can either make do with that sandwich or, if you're familiar with the city, get a take-out salad, antipasti, or even an entrée-sized meal that won't go bad if you put it in an overhead bin for a few hours.

Most airlines will also let you call ahead and order a special meal. You can choose between seafood, vegetarian, low-fat, and kosher.

When all these options have failed because you didn't have time or didn't plan, eat the nuts served on the plane. Order whatever looks least processed: the dry cereal with nonfat milk in the morning, the salad with chicken or the sandwich at lunchtime (eat just half the bread, and scrape off the spread), and anything not in cream sauce or under cheese for dinner. Try to kill boredom by consuming a good book instead of more than one alcoholic beverage, or ice cream and packaged cookies. Remember, at the end of your journey, normal food awaits.

Flying is extremely dehydrating due to the low air moisture and diminished oxygen. So drink much more than you would on the ground. My rule of "drink": 6 ounces of water for every 60 minutes of flying.

really "naughty" dinner, go light on your breakfast and lunch consumption, either that day or the next.

If you have medical dietary concerns, call ahead and say, "You know, my doctor has me on a low-salt, low-fat diet, so there may be certain dishes you serve the other guests that I might have to pass on." If you know your hosts well, they will know your preferences, and likely will serve alternatives to the lamb chop entrée if you're a vegetarian (and will skip pork or shellfish if you keep kosher).

## Eight Glasses a Day: Does It Really Hold Water?

There is a prevailing opinion that there's no such thing as too much water. The more we drink—especially that which comes in designer bottles—the less we'll eat, the more we will "flush" toxins from our bodies, and the moister and dewier our skin will be. Countless magazine articles have recommended eight glasses a day (two quarts) as the gold standard for health.

None of this bears medical scrutiny. A diligent review, published in the *American Journal of Physiology*, could locate neither the origins of this edict nor any evidence to support it. The moisture in your skin will suffer only if you meet the medical standard for dehydration.

There's no need to monitor the color of your urine or count your empty water bottles. We have a marvelous built-in hydration control—it's called thirst—which works through multiple hormones and sensors in our vascular system. (Note: Your thirst "control" may become less reliable as you age.) Also, much of what we consume contains liquid, even though it's not water. And despite what you've heard, coffee, caffeinated soft drinks, and other fluids do count (and—to a point—even dilute alcoholic beverages such as beer).

Finally, there are good reasons not to overdo fluids. Many women complain of incontinence problems simply because their overfilled bladder contracts before they reach the toilet. As with most vitamins, a deficiency of water is bad, but excess is unhelpful or even dangerous: If you take in fluid faster than your kidneys can process it, you could end up with "water intoxication," causing confusion, coma, and even death.

# 5

## *Supplements: Herbs, Schmerbs, and Verve*

From an early age, I was conditioned—by my father the theoretical physicist, my college math and science professors, and finally, my traditional medical training—to be skeptical of any belief, practice, or therapy not supported by scientific evidence. Yet I have to admit that, like many of my patients, I am drawn to the myriad claims made about the remarkable effects of supplements, herbs, and nontraditional potions. I want them to be true. I want to find that magical blend of herbs, minerals, and vitamins that will help me thrive, look great, and live forever!

Alysha, 42, came to me with complaints of fatigue and PMS. When I asked her if she was taking any medications, she replied, "Oh, no—I don't believe in drugs."

"What about herbs and vitamins?" (Forty percent of patients who take herbal medications don't tell their doctor.) She proudly produced a Saks shopping bag filled with bottles, and proceeded to line them up on my desk for my perusal (and approval). Alysha was taking *forty* herbs and vitamins daily: evening primrose and St. John's wort for PMS, ginseng for general well-being, dong quai and black cohosh for hot flashes, soy tablets for breast health, coenzyme $Q_{10}$ for heart health, ginkgo for brain health, three multivitamin pills (plus extra B complex, vitamins E and C, calcium, and magnesium), echinacea and goldenseal to prevent colds, and valerian so she could sleep.

Blood tests showed that Alysha's liver enzymes were abnormally elevated—but she didn't have chronic hepatitis nor did she abuse alcohol. We negotiated a "cease supplement" agreement (except for one multivitamin and 1,000 mg of calcium) for the following twelve weeks. At that point, I rechecked her liver enzymes; they had returned to normal. Her fatigue had also diminished, and she was sleeping through the night.

"But these were high-quality, expensive natural products," she protested. "They must have been doing *some* good. . . ."

## TRUTHS AND MYTHS
## ABOUT SUPPLEMENTS

For those who manufacture and sell vitamins, minerals, and herbs, 1994 was a very good year. Congress passed the Dietary Supplement Health and Education Act, decreeing that supplements should be considered in the same category as food—not drugs. There was thus no need to demon-

---

### The U.S. Government's Definition of a Dietary Supplement

"A product (other than tobacco) intended to supplement the diet that bears or contains one or more of the following dietary ingredients:

a vitamin,

a mineral,

an herb or other botanical,

an amino acid, or

a dietary substance for use by man [or woman] to supplement the diet by increasing the total dietary intake, or a concentrate, metabolite, constituent, extract, or combination of the above ingredients."

Try saying that in one breath!

strate a supplement's safety, purity, or effectiveness or to obtain FDA approval to market it.

This means that anyone can concoct a product and tout its potential benefit, as long as they refrain from making statements that the product acts as a drug and prevents or treats disease. But they are free to proclaim that it promotes, enhances, and supplements our physiologic processes and well-being: "Our product has been shown in studies to . . ." In small print, you'll find the qualifier "This statement has not been evaluated by the Food and Drug Administration." This free-for-all and all-for-supplements call to sales has enriched the vitamin, mineral, and herb industry as we spend an astounding *$18 billion a year* in the hope that what is said or implied on the bottle is true.

Lest I be considered the supplement Scrooge, I also want to acknowledge those who have persisted in their quest for natural compounds shown to help women in cultures throughout the world. Traditional alternative therapies have been used for hundreds, even thousands of years— and although unrecorded in modern scientific parlance, they may have worked. If they helped women in other times and places, they have the potential to benefit us. Because most of these compounds cannot be patented, the cost of developing them and obtaining the same FDA approval now needed for prescription drugs would be prohibitive. Should centuries of wisdom be ignored because there is no foreseeable big payoff?

It's time for collaboration and a conditional acceptance that adding vitamin and herbal supplements to our "what to take" list can help us in our quest to maintain well-being and forestall symptoms and progression of disease. The National Institutes of Health created the Center for Complementary and Alternative Medicine, which does research and provides information and recommendations on many of these therapies. Medical schools and hospitals have developed programs integrating complementary medicine with traditional approaches.

And we do have some official guidelines, as well as due process. The Federal Trade Commission can prevent companies from making misleading or deceptive claims. The U.S. Pharmacopoeia is now putting its USP mark on supplements to verify that the product contains what the label says, was manufactured in a clean, professional facility, is free of common contaminants, and is in a form that can be absorbed and used by your body. Companies must pay the USP for the testing, so this mark will probably be found only on the products of large manufacturers that can afford it. Another organization, ConsumerLab.com, examines certain categories of popular supplements without charging their makers. Companies not so "chosen" can also pay between $2,500 and $4,000 to have their product tested—and if it passes, receive the ConsumerLab seal of approval. Finally, the Good Housekeeping Institute reviews manufacturing processes and conducts limited testing. A caveat: Only companies that agree to buy ad space in the magazine can get the Good Housekeeping seal. But Good Housekeeping does require that manufacturers submit evidence from scientific journals to back up their health claims.

In this chapter, I'll profile the most commonly used vitamins and supplements. I've tried to balance the facts presented in controlled medical studies with those proffered by less traditional but respected experts.

## VITAMINS

Vitamins attach to and facilitate enzymes that "run" our metabolic processes so they, and we, don't succumb to wear and tear. These co-workers—or to be more precise, coenzymes—are necessary for the vital chemical reactions in our bodies. So, can we "vitamin" our way out of aging? A thirteen-year study of over ten thousand Americans reported in 1993 by the Centers for Disease Control and Prevention (CDC) found no evidence that longevity was increased among the vitamin and mineral supplement users, not even those with nutritional deficiencies resulting from alcoholism, smoking, and chronic diseases. A more recent five-year British study published in *The Lancet* followed over twenty thousand adults with heart disease or diabetes—some of whom were randomly assigned to take antioxidant vitamins—and came to a similar conclusion: Vitamins did not reduce the incidence of any type of vascular disease, cancer, or other major disorder.

On the other hand, review-of-research articles published in two of the most prestigious medical journals—the *New England Journal of Medicine* and the *Journal of the American Medical Association*—concluded that every adult should take a daily multivitamin. Before I address the "multi," let's look at the functions of, and claims made for, each vitamin separately.

## THE ANTIOXIDANTS

Most of the chemical reactions in our body require oxygen. During this oxidative process, free radicals are formed. These are not political entities, but they *are* unstable: These molecules have given up an electron during oxidation, which they now want to retrieve. They bombard the intact cells in our bodies, attempting to bond with the missing electron. This constant assault eventually damages DNA, causing abnormal function, improper division, and mutations, which can lead to cancer and other major diseases.

Here are some examples:

- Oxidized LDL cholesterol forms plaque and atherosclerosis, which can lead to heart disease and stroke.
- When our brain cells (neurons) are oxidized, amyloid plaque may be deposited, leading to Alzheimer's disease.
- Oxidized skin cells and connective tissue lose collagen and become pigmented, thin, and wrinkled.
- Oxidative damage in joints leads to arthritis.
- Oxidation in our eyes can cause cataracts.

Into the fray march the antioxidant vitamins to neutralize the roaming radicals. When these antioxidants are present in our food, there is good evidence that they do this. The seven-billion-dollar question (that's about what we spend on vitamins and minerals every year!) is whether we need or benefit from the extra helping proffered in capsules, pills, sports drinks, and vitamin waters.

### Vitamin A and Carotenoids

Vitamin A is a fat-soluble vitamin (stored in body fat and excreted in stool, not urine). It's essential for reactions that control your vision (especially night vision), bone growth, cell division and differentiation (what a cell will become "when it grows up"), and reproduction. It helps keep the lining of your lungs, intestines, and bladder intact, and protects the surface of your skin and mucous membranes, preventing infection. It also helps your immune system fight infection.

## Food sources of A

Completely preformed vitamin A, ready for your body's use, is called *retinol*. It's found in animal foods, especially beef or chicken liver, eggs, and the fat portion of milk products. (Most fat-free and dried nonfat milk solids are fortified with vitamin A.)

We needn't rely on meat and dairy to get our A. The pigments in fruits and vegetables, called *carotenoids*, are *provitamins*: In our bodies they are transformed into retinol. There are over six hundred carotenoids in food; the most convertible and famous of these is beta-carotene. Many are also marketed in a bottle. Some, such as lycopene, lutein, and zeaxanthin, are not converted by your body to A but have other health properties, possibly helping prevent cancer mutations and promoting vision.

The most colorful foods have the most carotenoid pigments: carrots, leafy green vegetables, yellow vegetables, sweet potatoes, peaches, and cantaloupes. Nearly one-third of the carotenoids you consume are converted to vitamin A, some of which is stored in the liver for future use.

## How much vitamin A do you need?

The recommended dietary allowance (RDA) is 4,000 IU (international units) in nonpregnant women over the age of 19. Eating 3 to 6 milligrams (mg) of beta-carotene daily (five or more ½ cup servings of colorful fruits and vegetables) will give you this amount. It doesn't seem that hard. But less than 20 percent of us get our A the food way.

*Vitamin A deficiency.* In developing countries, 500,000 children become blind every year due to lack of this vitamin in their diet. It also hampers immune response, making infectious diseases devastating.

Do we Americans need to be concerned about our A-levels? Only in cases of chronic malabsorption problems due to diarrhea, sprue (gluten intolerance), or pancreatic disorders—or after stomach-reducing surgery for weight loss. Vegetarians who don't eat eggs or dairy products need to make sure they consume enough dark green leafy vegetables and orange and yellow fruit to A-up.

## Disease and anti-aging protection with vitamin A?

*Naturally, in food.* Diets rich in beta-carotene and vitamin A are associated with a lower risk of cancer, including breast and lung cancer. Why? A fruit- and vegetable-heavy diet provides multiple carotenoids and vitamins, and leaves less room for meat and fat—a pattern that promotes health and longevity.

*As supplements.* The bad news is that vitamin A supplements render negligible benefit, and can even do harm. A twelve-year study found that beta-carotene supplements didn't decrease cancer or heart disease in half of 22,000 physicians who took them. Nor did pills help some 29,000 Finnish smokers beat lung cancer; indeed, after five to eight years, those who took this supplement had *higher* rates of lung cancer. (I would certainly advise any woman who is still smoking not to attempt to counteract its oxidative damages by supplementing with this antioxidant.) Supplements also don't seem to help fight breast cancer or colon cancer.

## Megadoses of A

Retinoids are potent and potentially dangerous substances. A synthetic form, isotretinoin (Accutane), used to treat severe acne, is known to increase fetal malformations twenty-fivefold. When natural retinoid, in the form of vitamin A supplements (over 10,000 IU per day), is taken in early pregnancy, it can lead to birth defects in one of every fifty-seven exposed pregnancies. (The damage can be done even before a woman knows she's pregnant.) Fortunately, this only occurs with preformed vitamin A, and not with beta-carotene. Other overdose side effects include liver abnormalities (the liver is where the vitamin is stored), loss of bone density, osteoporosis, hair loss, skin disorders, and even psychiatric symptoms. So make sure that the vitamins you take—especially when you attempt to combine several, or if you eat a diet rich in organ meats and dairy products—do not put you over that 10,000 IU of A per day.

*My recommendation:* Eat fruits and vegetables, and don't take additional vitamin A beyond that contained in a "standard" multivitamin.

## Vitamin C

This water-soluble vitamin is eliminated from your body in urine within three to four hours of ingestion, so you need to get some on a daily basis. However, the more you take, the less you absorb. You also absorb less if you smoke, have a high fever, or take aspirin, antibiotics, or steroids.

We've been told since childhood that we need our C, especially if we're catching a cold. Perhaps our mothers instinctively knew that once we were sick, less C was getting into our bodies; hence, we needed to drink that orange juice.

Since this vitamin is a cofactor in reactions that synthesize collagen, many "make your skin younger" products use vitamin C in an effort to pump up collagen production. (See chapter 7 for more on this.) Collagen is also an essential component of our bones, teeth and gums, and connective tissue, so C helps hold us together. We also need vitamin C to absorb iron, and to form our red blood cells, heal our wounds, and help our immune systems fight off bacterial infections.

## Food sources of vitamin C

The best food sources for C are citrus fruits (orange juice again—and if it's calcium fortified, a glass will also give you one-fourth of your daily calcium requirement), strawberries, melons, tomatoes, broccoli, and peppers.

Cooking, storage, and long-term exposure to air can decrease these foods' vitamin C content. Hence, you should try to get fresh products.

## How much do you need?

The RDA for women has been increased from 60 to 75 mg, and many feel it should be 90 mg. This goal is easily reached with five portions of the appropriate fruits and vegetables. After 200 mg, our tissues are saturated, and more C will simply give us vitamin-rich urine.

*Vitamin C deficiency.* This causes scurvy, a disease common among sailors before they stowed lemons and limes on board. Their symptoms included easy bruising, bleeding, loose or lost teeth, and reduced ability to fight off infection. Life at sea lacked C.

## Disease and anti-aging protection

A healthy person will do better getting her vitamin C from fruits and vegetables. Absorption of C from supplements varies widely depending on how the pills were manufactured, when you take them, and how much you take.

*Colds.* Taking extra C in supplements to ward off colds will not work, despite what our mothers said, unless the individual normally gets very little C in her diet.

*C and heart disease.* A scientific review of vitamin use, published in the *Journal of the American Medical Association* in 2002, found that the evidence that vitamin C supplementation prevented coronary heart disease was "unconvincing"—although C and E together *might* yield benefit for preventing CHD. Randomized trials are ongoing to check this hypothesis.

*C and cancer.* Studies show that the higher the intake of C, through consumption of fruit and vegetables, the lower the rates of oral, esophageal, and stomach cancers. This was also found to be valid for premenopausal breast cancer, especially among women with a positive family history for this disease. No studies, however, have given evidence that C *supplementation* actually decreases cancer risk.

## Megadoses of C

At doses of 500 mg or higher, extra C is excreted via urine. At doses of 1,000 mg, oxalate and uric acid levels increase in the urine, which may promote kidney stones if you are susceptible. Large supplemental doses also blunt the beneficial effects of chemotherapy for breast cancer, and may actually act on DNA to encourage cancer cell growth. And vitamin C megasupplements have been found to free up ferric iron stored in the body and convert it to ferrous iron, which can damage the heart and other organs.

*My recommendation:* I don't encourage my patients to, nor do I, supplement C beyond what's provided in a multivitamin. I do suggest that we

### The Power of the True Natural Vitamins: Fruits and Vegetables

A 2002 article in *The Lancet* quietly demonstrated this power. In a study of a group of 690 healthy individuals between the ages of 25 and 64, half increased their fruit and vegetable intake by an average of 1.5 portions per day. Over six months, this group's average systolic blood pressure fell more than 4.0 mm Hg, and the diastolic, more than 1.5 mm Hg, compared with the less-fruit-and-vegetabled control group. Ultimately, this very small dietary change (just three-quarters of a cup!) would be expected to reduce their future incidence of stroke and hypertension by 15 percent, and heart attack by 6 percent.

Another reason to favor fruits and vegetables over supplement pills: Foods contain thousands of compounds that may affect our biological functions, including hundreds of antioxidants, flavonoids, and carotenoids. We can't begin to put all of these into pills, let alone combine them for optimal health benefits.

make an effort to drink orange juice and eat C-rich fruits and vegetables so that our bodies "C" the benefits without the risks.

## Vitamin E

Vitamin E is fat soluble. There are eight different E compounds, called tocopherols, identified with letters of the Greek alphabet, from alpha to zeta. Each serves slightly different functions in the body, but alpha seems to be the most active form.

Vitamin E is a grand antioxidant protector, helping prevent destruction of other vitamins, namely, A, B-complex, and C. It also plays a role in blocking the oxidation of LDL cholesterol; decreasing the stickiness of platelets so clots are less likely to form; and keeping muscle cells from proliferating and thickening and closing off blood vessels—all contributors to atherosclerosis and heart disease.

Vitamin E protects cell membranes from oxidation and damage, and stimulates immune reactions. It blocks the formation of cancer-causing substances called *nitrosamines,* which are produced in the stomach from nitrates we consume (as in hot dogs and processed lunch meats). Vitamin E has also been shown to reduce the chromosomal damage from radiation and chemicals.

### Food sources of E
One primary source is vegetable oils, especially wheat germ oil, but also safflower, corn, soybean, olive, and canola oils. Nuts, legumes, and green leafy vegetables provide E; the highest concentration is found in almonds. Mangos and kiwi are lesser sources.

### How much E do you need?
The RDA for women is 22 international units (IU) or 15 mg of alpha-tocopherol. Note that E supplements can either be synthetic, labeled as dl-alpha-tocopherol, or natural, labeled d-alpha-tocopherol. The natural form appears to be more potent than the synthetic, although synthetic E was used in many of the studies cited below.

*Vitamin E deficiency.* This is rare but may occur with certain conditions such as cystic fibrosis, fat malabsorption, or chronic liver disease. The issue is not disease from E deficiency per se, but whether inadequate E puts you at higher risk for chronic diseases.

## Disease and anti-aging protection

*Heart disease.* The ongoing Harvard study of ninety thousand women nurses found that those with the highest intake of E, through nutrition and supplements, had a 40 percent lower risk of heart disease than those with the lowest intake. Just 100 IU or more of vitamin E supplements over two years provided this protection. The amount in a standard multivitamin (usually less than 30 IU) also helped. But a 4½-year prospective trial of ten thousand patients at high risk of heart attack or stroke found that 400 units of daily vitamin E did *not* reduce the incidence of heart attack, heart failure, or stroke. (Prospective studies follow people forward in time, instead of relying on their memories of what they ate.) Likewise a study of twenty thousand British adults with coronary artery disease or diabetes who were given antioxidant supplements (400 units of E, 250 mg of C, and 20 mg of beta-carotene versus a placebo) found there was no difference in the occurrence of heart attacks or risk of death from any cause.

These results present an E conflict: Either more time is required in order to see any positive effects, or it's possible that we need to start E supplements before we develop heart disease—as prevention, rather than treatment.

*Cancer.* Once more, study results are mixed. Higher intake of vitamin E, in the Harvard study of 90,000 women, and another in New York State with 18,000 women, did not show a reduced risk for breast cancer. But an Iowa study of over 35,000 women showed that use of E supplements did decrease colon cancer risk.

*Alzheimer's disease.* Consumption of vitamin E in food has recently been found to lower the risk of Alzheimer's in a prospective study of over 3,100 women who were 55 or older and were followed for six years. Also, a study that followed 6,000 people aged 65 and older for over three years found that intake of vitamin E, from food or supplements, was linked to reduced cognitive decline (memory and speed of perception).

Many neurologists and psychiatrists who research memory loss suggest that E supplements at doses between 400 and 1,000 units may be helpful, especially for those at risk for Alzheimer's (see chapter 8).

*Cataracts.* Vitamin E supplements may decrease cataract formation, but studies did not find this benefit in those who smoke.

*Skin.* There does not seem to be good evidence that vitamin E, when applied as a cream, lotion, or beauty product, either is absorbed or protects the skin from sun damage and aging.

*Hot flashes.* Documented studies are few and far between, but anecdotally many women attest that they obtained hot-flash relief through use of 800 daily units of vitamin E, plus 1 gram of calcium.

*Breast pain.* While there is no solid research to back this up, I and other physicians often recommend taking vitamin E (together with caffeine reduction) for breast pain due to fibrocystic changes (lumpiness that worsens during hormonal cycles).

## Megadoses of E

So far, we know of no adverse side effects from taking vitamin E in doses up to 800 units. The Institute of Medicine has set 1,000 mg to 1,500 units as an "upper tolerable intake limit" for alpha-tocopherol (the E found in most supplements). At higher levels, vitamin E can prevent normal blood clotting and increase the risk of bleeding. Note: For this reason, you should stop taking vitamin E supplements two weeks before surgery. Combining high doses of E with aspirin, other blood thinners, and herbs such as ginkgo can increase bleeding tendencies. In addition, high doses can cause headache, fatigue, nausea, diarrhea, stomach cramps, weakness, blurred vision, and even abnormal ovulation.

*My recommendation:* Whereas many antioxidants can be obtained through consumption of fruits and vegetables, it's hard to do so when it comes to vitamin E. The best sources (oils and nuts) are calorie-dense. Here's my "it won't hurt, and may very likely help" proviso: Because a multivitamin usually has 30 units of E or less, add a supplement of 400 to 800 units of vitamin E per day.

## The B Vitamins

These water-soluble vitamins work together to help convert the carbohydrates you eat into glucose, aid in metabolism of fat and protein, and are essential for the functioning of your nervous system and the muscles that propel food through your gastrointestinal tract. Although they are often present in the same foods, the Bs are separate entities.

## Folate (folic acid)

Folate is necessary to make DNA and RNA. It is crucial for the formation and growth of new cells during pregnancy and infancy. It is concentrated in spinal fluid and brain cells, and "proper" amounts are required for brain development and function. Folate helps prevent damage to DNA that can lead to cancer. It helps form *heme,* the iron-containing protein found in red blood cells. With vitamins $B_6$ and $B_{12}$, folate helps enzymes metabolize and break down homocysteine, an amino acid harmful to the vascular system and considered a marker for increased risk of heart attack and stroke.

### Food sources of folate

Folate is present in leafy green vegetables, especially spinach and turnip greens, dried beans, and peas, as well as papaya, avocados, and tomato juice. As of 1998, folic acid has been added to breads, breakfast cereals, pasta, rice, and other grain products. (Note: The synthetic folic acid in these fortified foods and in supplements has a simpler chemical structure than natural folate, and is actually absorbed more easily. Once in your body, it's identical to the folate you get from unfortified foods.)

### How much folate do you need?

The RDA for nonpregnant women over 19 is 400 mcg (micrograms); it's 600 to 800 mcg during pregnancy.

*Folate deficiency.* Now that folate's been added to commonly eaten foods, deficiency is much less of an issue. However, in some situations you may need more, lose more, or absorb less. These include:

- Pregnancy and breast-feeding
- Excessive alcohol intake (indeed, the Nurses' Health Study showed that the increased risk of breast cancer associated with alcohol was attenuated in women who took multivitamins containing folic acid)
- Chronic diarrhea and malabsorption
- Liver disease
- Some types of anemia
- Taking certain medications (anticonvulsants, metformin, sulfasalazine, triamterene, methotrexate)

If you are on a high-protein/low-carb diet, you may not get enough folate from vegetables or fortified grains. Moreover, animal protein has large amounts of methionine, which without folate is likely to be converted to homocysteine (see below). Signs of folate deficiency can include diarrhea, loss of appetite and weight loss, weakness, sore tongue, headaches, heart palpitations, and irritability. Folate deficiency in pregnancy increases your child's risk of neural tube defects (such as spina bifida).

## Disease and anti-aging protection

*Heart disease, stroke, Alzheimer's: the homocysteine connection.* Homocysteine is a vessel-unfriendly amino acid. It injures the cells lining the arteries and stimulates overgrowth of muscle cells in their walls, interrupting blood flow and increasing clot formation—all of which fosters coronary vascular disease (CVD), heart attack, stroke, and perhaps dementia from Alzheimer's. High homocysteine levels are a risk factor for CVD.

Will lowering homocysteine with additional folate prevent heart disease? A series of studies has shown that 800 mcg of folate, together with vitamin $B_{12}$ and probably vitamin $B_6$, lowers homocysteine levels by as much as 25 percent. However, a 2002 article in the *Journal of the American Medical Association* noted that high homocysteine levels are not as good a marker for heart disease risk in women as they are in men. As of this writing, we're not absolutely certain that homocysteine itself is the culprit in CVD, or whether it's a marker for something else that does the heart damage. We also don't know if lowering levels with extra folate will ultimately prevent heart disease. Several large studies are under way to answer these questions.

*Folate and cancer.* The Nurses' Health Study found that women who took a multivitamin containing folate (usually 400 mcg) for fifteen or more years had a 75 percent reduction in their risk of colorectal cancer. Higher folate levels may also reduce the chance of developing breast cancer, particularly in women who regularly consume alcohol. This, however, is not considered sufficient evidence to recommend folate supplements for cancer protection.

## Megadoses of folate

There doesn't seem to be such a thing as folate toxicity. However, when given alone, high levels (more than 1,000 mcg per day) may mask the anemia that can occur with $B_{12}$ deficiency. Untreated $B_{12}$ deficiency can cause permanent neurologic damage (see page 178).

*My recommendation:* Take a multivitamin that contains 400 mcg of folate (most do). If you are at high risk of coronary heart disease (including a family history of early CHD), take up to 800 mcg a day. However, if you are age 50 or older, have your doctor check your $B_{12}$ status before you take that higher level of folate.

## *Vitamin B₆*

Vitamin B₆ exists in three chemical forms: pyridoxine, pyridoxal, and pyridoxamine. This vitamin is needed for the more than one hundred enzymes involved in protein metabolism. B₆ helps make hemoglobin and enhances its oxygen-carrying capacity. It also aids in the creation of white blood cells and antibodies. In the brain, it assists in the production of neurotransmitters such as dopamine and serotonin. What's more, B₆ is involved in converting stored carbohydrates into glucose to maintain normal blood sugar levels. And it aids the function of a fatty acid called *linoleic acid,* which some researchers suggest helps combat PMS symptoms.

### Food sources of B₆
The good news: B₆ is found in almost everything we consume, from proteins to produce. It's also added to fortified breakfast cereals.

### How much B₆ do you need?
The RDA for women between ages 19 and 50 is 1.3 mg, and 1.5 mg for women over 50.

*B₆ deficiency.* True deficiency is rare. However, older women may have low blood levels of B₆ and, over an extended period of time, this can cause skin inflammation, a red, sore tongue, depression, confusion, and even convulsions. It's a not uncommon cause of older-age anemia, with subsequent fatigue.

### Disease and anti-aging protection
*Nervous system disorders.* Low levels of serotonin are correlated with depression and migraine headaches, and B₆ helps synthesize serotonin. However, adding B₆ supplements has not been shown to relieve these conditions.

*Carpal tunnel syndrome.* Doses of 100 to 200 mg of vitamin B₆ have somehow become popularized, without the appropriate randomized studies, for the treatment of carpal tunnel syndrome. This falls in the realm of megadosing, and may cause side effects.

*PMS.* Here again, the popularity of B₆ supplements for this problem has not been supported by supplemental scientific evidence. Doses up to 600 mg have been touted—causing increasing numbers of women to develop neuropathy (abnormal nerve sensations).

*$B_6$, homocysteine, and heart disease.* As mentioned, a deficiency of $B_6$, folate, or $B_{12}$, together or separately, may increase levels of homocysteine. We're still not sure whether lowering homocysteine levels will reduce the risk of heart disease.

## Megadoses of $B_6$

Here, "mega" begins at more than 100 mg a day. Too much $B_6$ has been shown to cause nerve damage to the arms and legs. Thankfully, it's reversible when supplementation is stopped.

*My recommendation:* Your multivitamin should give you more than enough $B_6$. If you take a B-complex supplement in order to get more folate, make sure you do not exceed 100 mg of $B_6$ per day. Unless you have a clear medical need, there's no reason to consider separate $B_6$ supplementation.

## Vitamin $B_{12}$

Another water-soluble vitamin, $B_{12}$ is found only in animal products (milk, eggs, poultry, fish, meat). It is necessary for fat and carbohydrate metabolism, production of red blood cells, and protein synthesis.

## How much $B_{12}$ do you need?

The current recommended daily allowance for $B_{12}$ is 6 mcg per day.

*$B_{12}$ deficiency.* Vegetarians, especially vegans who avoid all animal-derived foods, could end up $B_{12}$ deficient. Risk is also increased in any disorder that creates poor intestinal absorption of $B_{12}$. Elderly persons often have poor $B_{12}$ absorption, and can develop a specific type of anemia as well as neurologic abnormalities such as changes in sense of body positioning and balance.

## Disease and anti-aging protection

*Deficiency correction.* Correcting low $B_{12}$ levels will prevent or reverse the anemia and neurologic changes noted above. When folate is given alone, deficiencies or their side effects may be masked, so it's now recommended that $B_{12}$ levels be checked, or extra $B_{12}$ be included with folate supplements.

*Homocysteine/heart disease.* Adding $B_{12}$ to folate increases its ability to lower homocysteine levels by about 7 percent.

## Megadoses of $B_{12}$

The popularity of $B_{12}$ shots has extended from actors who feel tired to executives who need an extra "push." One two-week study of $B_{12}$ injections found some benefit for back pain; otherwise, there is no scientific evidence that this intramuscular shot works to increase energy, vitality, or health. High doses, however, don't seem to cause adverse effects.

*My recommendation:* You should get all the $B_{12}$ you need in your multivitamin. But as you get older, or if you develop anemia, your $B_{12}$ level should be checked. In general, if you are over 65, or if you follow a vegan diet, it's a good idea to at least double the recommended daily dose (i.e., add another 10 mcg).

### The Rest of the Bs

The other B vitamins are listed below. Even though it's possible to have deficiencies in these (and this would likely happen in conjunction with deficiencies of all the Bs), there is little evidence that taking supplements will prevent chronic disease or prolong life. (The possible exception, niacin, should not be taken without medical supervision.)

- **Niacin ($B_3$)** can raise HDL, lower LDL, and reduce triglycerides, and is often "prescribed" in addition to statin drugs. The RDA is 14 mg. However, if your doctor recommends higher doses, you can take 1 to 4 grams as long as your liver function is monitored and stays normal. At doses over 1,000 mg (1 gram), there are often annoying side effects such as flushing (like hot flashes), stomach problems, itching, or headache. Slow-release niacin may be better tolerated.
- **Thiamin ($B_1$)** is a coenzyme involved in carbohydrate metabolism and nervous system functioning. The RDA is 1.1 mg; it's found in brewer's yeast, legumes, and grains. We usually see deficiencies only in people who take certain diuretics (e.g., for congestive heart failure), who have Crohn's disease, or severe eating disorders (anorexia), or are alcoholics. For these patients, extra $B_1$ may make sense.
- **Riboflavin ($B_2$)** is a cofactor for $B_6$ and folate, and often found in the company of other B vitamins (in organ meats, vegetables, legumes, and brewer's yeast). The RDA is 1.1 mg. Marginal deficiencies are occasionally seen in older people, but the $B_2$ in a multivitamin should be enough to correct them.

• **Pantothenic acid (B$_5$)** (from the Greek for "from everywhere") is found in "everywhere" foods, so very few people become deficient. Vitamin makers have bottled one of its derivatives, pantethine, purported to lower LDL and raise HDL, but the studies behind this claim are very small.

## Vitamin D

Vitamin D (calciferol) is a fat-soluble vitamin, which we can actually make ourselves if we get enough sun. D is needed for proper absorption and use of calcium and other nutrients important for bone health, and for maintaining healthy levels of other minerals such as phosphorus.

### Sources of D: sun and food

Ultraviolet (UV) rays from sunlight trigger vitamin D synthesis in your skin. Fifteen minutes a day of summer sun (not blocked by sunscreen, clouds, or smog) provides sufficient vitamin D. If you routinely use sunscreen with factor 8 or greater, the UV that produces D is blocked, so you'll need to get your D through food or supplements.

There are a few food sources of vitamin D$_3$—a prohormone version, which your liver and kidneys turn into usable D: cod-liver oil (1 tablespoon contains over 1,300 IU of D) and saltwater fish, as well as D-fortified milk. (Note that other dairy products, such as yogurt, cheese, and ice cream, are not D fortified.)

### How much D do you need?

The current RDA is 400 IU. If you are over 65 or out of the sun most of the time, most experts advise 800 IU per day, through food and/or supplements.

*Vitamin D deficiency.* In children, lack of D causes rickets (malformed bones). In adults, it can cause osteomalacia (soft bones and muscle weakness); an ongoing D deficiency can contribute to osteoporosis and the risk of fractures. Inadequate D can also cause secondary hyperparathyroidism, with the same bone results. Over 25 percent of postmenopausal women are deficient in vitamin D; that number rises to 50 percent in women with known osteoporosis.

## Disease and anti-aging protection

*Osteoporosis and osteopenia.* Vitamin D supplementation (with calcium) has been shown to decrease bone loss and fractures. Among elderly women with osteoporosis, supplementation decreased the rate of new hip fractures by 43 percent. At least 800 IU of D should be added to calcium for women at risk for, or under treatment for, osteoporosis.

*D and cancer.* Studies have shown that increase of dairy foods, or diets high in calcium and vitamin D, lower the incidence of colon cancer. It's not yet clear whether supplementing with D can reduce your colon cancer risk.

## Megadoses of D

D toxicity causes nausea, vomiting, poor appetite, weight loss, and weakness. Too much D can cause blood levels of calcium to rise, resulting in heart rhythm abnormalities, kidney stones, and mental confusion. It's hard to overdo vitamin D through diet alone, unless you consume large amounts of cod-liver oil. Stay below 2,000 IU per day.

*My recommendation:* If you are healthy, active, not at high risk for osteoporosis, and under the age of 65, take 400 IU of vitamin D a day via your multivitamin. If you are older, at risk of osteoporosis, or have already developed it, add additional vitamin D so that your daily dose is 800 to 1,000 units.

## Vitamin K

A fat-soluble vitamin, K is best known for its role in helping blood clot normally. It's also important for healthy bones.

## Food sources of vitamin K

Dark green vegetables, especially spinach, are good sources of K. But your body can actually make its own K, with the help of normal intestinal bacteria.

## How much K do you need?

The recommended daily dose for women is 90 mcg.

*K deficiency.* Long-term use of antibiotics, which destroy the bacteria that produce K, can cause deficiency; so can kidney or liver disease, or any form of malabsorption. As a result, bleeding can occur with the slightest trauma, or in the G.I. tract. If you are taking anticoagulant drugs such as Coumadin (warfarin), which works by inhibiting a vitamin K clotting process, you may need special instructions about what you can and cannot eat, and vitamin K supplementation.

### Disease and anti-aging protection

*Osteoporosis.* There is preliminary evidence that vitamin K might help prevent bone fractures, but there is currently no recommendation that you should take K to prevent or treat osteoporosis.

### Megadoses of K

There's no known toxic level of vitamin K intake, but there's also no reason to take megadoses.

*My recommendation:* Eat your spinach, and take your multivitamin—unless you are on an anticoagulant.

## MINERALS

Minerals are nonorganic compounds found in food. That may not sound appetizing, but minerals are vital to health. The amount of minerals in

Unless you have one of the medical conditions or risk factors mentioned above, your vitamin needs should be amply met by a daily multivitamin. The contents of a typical multivitamin:

| Vitamin | Amount per pill |
| --- | --- |
| Vitamin A (20 percent from beta-carotene) | 5,000 IU |
| Vitamin C | 60 mg |
| Vitamin D | 400 IU |
| Vitamin E | 30 IU |
| Thiamin (B$_1$) | 1.5 mg |
| Riboflavin (B$_2$) | 1.7 mg |
| Niacin (B$_3$) | 20 mg |
| Vitamin B$_6$ | 2 mg |
| Folic acid (folate) | 400 mcg |
| Vitamin B$_{12}$ | 6 mcg |
| Pantothenic acid (B$_5$) | 10 mg |

your food depends in part on the mineral content of the soil where that food is grown. Soil can be depleted by years of farming, and mineral content may differ from place to place. (This is one reason that some experts encourage the use of a multivitamin with added minerals.)

I'll begin with the four minerals that women are most likely to be low on: iron, calcium, magnesium, and zinc.

## Iron

This essential mineral is necessary for the formation and function of hemoglobin in red blood cells (which transports oxygen to all of your tissues), as well as myoglobin, which supplies oxygen to muscles. Women lose iron with their monthly periods; after menopause, we lose very little iron unless we have health problems that involve chronic bleeding.

You maintain your iron status by absorbing it through food. Fifteen percent of your body's iron is stored for future needs, and mobilized when intake is inadequate. (Note that vitamin A deficiency limits this ability to store iron.) When your "rainy day" supply is gone, anemia can result.

**Food sources of iron**
The iron we consume comes in two forms: animal (heme), found in fish, meat, and poultry; and vegetable (nonheme), found in lentils and beans, with lesser amounts in spinach and tofu. The nonheme type of iron is less easily absorbed, meaning that vegetarians generally need to get twice as much iron as omnivores. Flour, cereal, and grain products are now fortified with nonheme iron, as are infant formulas.

Nonheme iron absorption can be improved if you take it at the same time as vitamin C and/or meat protein. On the other hand, calcium, the tannins found in tea, and phytates present in plant foods such as legumes, rice, and grains can decrease absorption of iron. (Avoid taking iron supplements, even the ones in multivitamins, together with your calcium.) The protein in soybeans has also been found to interfere with iron absorption (another concern for vegetarians).

**How much iron do you need?**
Women still having periods need 18 mg of iron daily. After age 50, if there's no cyclical bleeding, your requirement goes down to 8 mg a day. (Note: With cyclical HRT, bleeding can continue, in which case you

should also continue premenopausal doses of iron.) If you're pregnant, you need more: 27 mg. If you exercise intensively (e.g., long-distance running), your iron requirement may be 30 percent higher. A reduction in stomach acidity due to age, medication, or disease can reduce iron absorption and thus increase your need.

There are two forms of iron supplements: ferrous and ferric. The ferrous form is better absorbed. It's very common to experience side effects with supplemental iron, including nausea, constipation, dark-colored stools, bloating, or diarrhea. I suggest that, if you need it, you take iron in divided doses with food, and start with a low dose to see how you react and help your body adjust. Slow-release iron such as Slow-fe and Chromagen may be easier to tolerate.

*Iron deficiency.* Surveys have shown that during their childbearing years, most women don't get enough iron from food alone. The World Health Organization considers iron deficiency humanity's number one nutritional disorder.

The first step toward deficiency is iron depletion: Your body uses up its stored iron but has not yet reached a point where red blood cell count or hemoglobin levels are low. Depletion is diagnosed by checking levels of ferritin (a form of iron in the blood) and iron saturation. If iron is not added, you become anemic: Hemoglobin levels fall, causing fatigue, weakness, problems maintaining body temperature, poor concentration, hair loss, and—most worrisome—decreased immune function and lack of resistance to infection. In pregnancy, iron deficiency can increase the risk of premature delivery and low-weight babies, and can pose health risks to the mother as well.

Iron-deficiency anemia can also be a *warning sign* of "silent" bleeding anywhere in the body, but especially in the gastrointestinal tract—from ulcers, polyps, or hemorrhoids. Don't just pop iron supplements without a medical workup; you could be ignoring, and delaying treatment of, a life-threatening illness.

**Disease and anti-aging protection**
This presents a dilemma. Once you become menopausal and stop bleeding, you're losing less iron, and taking extra iron may cause harm (see below). On the other hand, as you get older, you are likely to absorb less iron. So the compromise is to have your blood count and iron levels checked every two years after age 55. Ask your doctor if you should take a multivitamin that includes iron, or even add extra amounts of it.

## Megadoses of iron

Iron supplements are the most common cause of poisoning deaths among children, and overload is dangerous at any age. If you are not anemic, doses over 45 mg can cause constipation, vomiting, nausea, or diarrhea. Note: If you are anemic, you may need to take as much as 100 to 300 mg a day until your iron stores are restored.

One reason for a conservative approach to iron supplementation is that you may have a genetic disorder called *hemochromatosis*. (Hemochromatosis affects one in 250 people of northern European descent, but is also found in persons of other ethnic backgrounds.) In this case, your iron absorption is so efficient that there is a buildup of excess iron in your body's organs, which can cause serious liver, heart, thyroid, and joint problems, as well as liver cancer. Since most women menstruate for thirty or forty years, this problem may not show up until after menopause.

Iron may also aid the formation of free radicals, those unstable age- and disease-promoting molecules. In fact, one theory of why younger women have less heart disease than men is that prior to menopause, women's mild iron deficiency acts as a cardiac shield against free radical damage. (This has not been proven.)

*My recommendation:* While you're menstruating, a multivitamin that contains small amounts of iron should more than suffice, unless your periods are heavy and/or your doctor has diagnosed iron-deficiency anemia.

Be careful to take your iron separately from nutrients such as calcium, zinc, or copper, since it may decrease their absorption, especially if you take them on an empty stomach. If you're postmenopausal and not iron deficient (have this checked every year or two), don't take iron supplements—and choose a multivitamin that is iron-free.

## Calcium

Calcium is the cement of our bones, and we need a constant supply. We lose 250 mg of calcium every day through urine, stool, and perspiration—and absorb only 25 to 30 percent of the calcium we consume. Depending on age and health, a woman needs 1,000 to 1,500 mg a day just to keep up.

Most of us are calcium deficient from childhood. This inadequacy is the major cause of osteoporosis. See the osteoporosis section of chapter 6 for details on types of calcium supplements and calcium's effect on your health.

## Foods containing calcium

Our traditional calcium source is dairy products. To give you a rough idea of how much calcium you're getting: A cup of low-fat or nonfat yogurt has 400 mg of calcium (once fruit is added, you lose about 100 mg), and a glass of nonfat milk has 300 mg. An ounce of sliced cheese averages 200 mg—but surprisingly, ½ cup of nonfat cottage cheese only has 80 mg. (A lot of my patients think that cottage cheese is a great low-calorie, high-calcium food. They're only right about the calories.)

Those who don't like, or prefer not to eat, milk products can get their calcium in other ways, but it's tough. A cup of broccoli only gives you 170 mg of calcium. Collards and dried beans do better, at 270 mg per cup. But 3 ounces of canned sardines with bones (it's "in dem bones") has 370 mg, and the same portion of canned salmon has 200 mg.

*My recommendations:* Depending on your calcium-rich food intake, add supplements so that you reach a total of 1,000 mg a day if you are aged 25 to 50, or 1,200 mg if you are over 50. You need 1,500 mg if you are not taking hormone replacement therapy, are older than 65, or have low bone density. But don't take more than 2,500 mg a day, as this can cause kidney stones and damage. Never take more than 500 or 600 mg at once; it won't be absorbed. Try not to take your calcium together with iron, concentrated dietary fiber, or foods that contain oxalates (spinach, rhubarb, tea)—all of which interfere with its absorption.

## Magnesium

This is a mineral required by every cell of your body. It's necessary for muscle and nerve function, for steady heart rhythm, and to help calcium in the support of your bones.

### Food sources of magnesium

Since the center of the chlorophyll molecule contains magnesium, you'll get it in every vegetable that's green. It's also found in nuts, seeds, and whole grains.

### How much magnesium do you need?

The recommended daily amount of magnesium for women is about 320 mg. If you are healthy and eat a varied diet, you don't need a magnesium supplement.

*Magnesium deficiency.* This is rare but can occur during treatment with diuretics, some antibiotics, and chemotherapy, or result from chronic vomiting or diarrhea, uncontrolled diabetes, or alcoholism. Signs of severe magnesium deficiency include disorientation, loss of appetite, depression, muscle cramps, tingling, numbness, abnormal heart rhythms, heart damage, or seizures.

## Disease and anti-aging protection

*Osteoporosis.* There are some data that calcium is better absorbed with magnesium, and this mineral is often combined with calcium in supplements.

*Blood pressure.* Magnesium has a role in regulating blood pressure. Diets that contain fruits and vegetables, which are good sources of potassium and magnesium, are associated with lower blood pressure. But note that this is diet, rather than pill, management.

*Heart disease.* Higher magnesium intake (from food sources) has been shown to lower risk of coronary heart disease and stroke.

## Megadoses of magnesium

High doses of magnesium (often added to laxatives and antacids) can cause diarrhea. Excess magnesium may damage your kidneys; this is more likely to occur as you get older and kidney function declines. The signs of magnesium toxicity are similar to those of magnesium deficiency. If you're already getting extra magnesium (check the labels of any laxatives, antacids, or calcium supplements you take), make sure it's no more than 350 mg or at most 500 mg daily.

*My recommendation:* Try to get your magnesium through foods. Monitor the amount of magnesium in supplements, so you don't overdose. If you are taking calcium and estrogen and develop leg cramps, it may be helpful to add 250 mg a day of magnesium.

## Zinc

This essential mineral stimulates over one hundred different enzymes, and is key to protein function and normal growth and development. It also supports your immune system, helps wound healing, and maintains your sense of taste and smell.

## Food sources of zinc

Oysters are very rich in zinc, but most of us achieve our zinc goals with red meat or fortified breakfast cereals. It's also present in chicken, beans, nuts, and milk products. A diet high in animal protein aids in zinc absorption (so vegetarians need to plan their zinc intake).

## How much zinc do you need?

The daily zinc recommendation for women is 8 mg. Vegetarians may need twice as much because of their lower rate of absorption.

*Zinc deficiency.* Signs include hair loss, diarrhea, eye and skin lesions, loss of appetite, weight loss, delayed wound healing, lethargy, and changes in taste (in food, not fashion). Deficiency can occur with very-low-calorie diets, alcoholism, and some digestive diseases.

## Disease and anti-aging protection

*The common cold.* Can zinc lozenges shorten or reduce the severity of a cold? Some studies suggest that the zinc ions released in the mouth and throat after sucking on a lozenge help decrease the length of your suffering from cold symptoms. Zinc gluconate glycine lozenges were more likely to be effective than zinc acetate lozenges. So you might give zinc a chance, but check the label. In 1999, the Federal Trade Commission announced that manufacturers of zinc lozenges had agreed to stop making claims that the product could prevent colds or relieve allergy symptoms.

*Other infections and wound healing.* Your immune system will get a boost from supplemental zinc only if you are zinc deficient.

## Megadoses of zinc

Although zinc is needed for immune function, too much can have the opposite effect. Also, high doses may lower HDL ("good" cholesterol) and promote atherosclerosis, and they may interfere with absorption of other minerals, especially iron. The suggested upper limit for zinc is 40 mg a day. Zinc toxicity occurs at 150 to 450 mg.

*My recommendation:* Most of us don't need added zinc. Small amounts are present in most multivitamins; this should suffice.

## Other Minerals

Our bodies need many minerals—some only in trace amounts, with no ideal dose specified as yet. For space reasons, I can't go into all of them. Here is information on a few that my patients often ask about, or that have known disease protection properties.

### Iodine

This mineral is stored in the thyroid gland, and is used by your body to make thyroid hormones. The RDA for iodine is 150 mcg; the upper limit is much higher, at 1.1 mg (1,100 mcg). Most food sources have little iodine; iodized salt is our chief and cheap dietary source. Some authorities have encouraged people who live near nuclear power plants to keep iodine tablets on hand. If a radiation accident occurred, megadosing could protect the thyroid from damage and cancer. But consistent intake of four hundred times the recommended daily dose can cause a goiter or hyperthyroidism.

*My recommendation:* Don't take added iodine beyond what you get through table salt and/or your multivitamin tablet.

### Selenium

Selenium, an essential trace mineral, helps antioxidant enzymes protect cells against the effects of free radicals. It is found in grains and vegetables, but the amount depends on how much selenium was in the soil in which that food was grown. Selenium is also present in some animal-derived foods; amounts depend on the soil where their fodder grew. The selenium RDA is 55 mcg. Selenium deficiency seems to be much more common in China than in the United States.

An oft-quoted study completed in the early 1990s, in which 1,300 patients were given selenium supplements for ten years in the hope of reducing the occurrence of skin cancer, showed that their skin cancer rates were unaffected; however, these patients had a significant reduction in cancer mortality as well as in lung, colon, rectal, and prostate cancers.

However, in the Nurses' Health Study, toenail clippings were sent in for selenium analysis; after 3.5 years, when the nurses with high and low selenium levels were compared, no cancer prevention benefit was found.

Selenium has also been considered an antioxidant, with the potential to limit oxidation of LDL cholesterol and thus prevent coronary heart disease. But the evidence is not considered sufficient to recommend selenium supplements for prevention of CHD. There have also been suggestions that selenium's antioxidant activity may help control arthritic symptoms.

Can you have too much selenium? Selenium toxicity is rare in the United States. If high blood levels do occur, a condition called *selenosis* may develop; symptoms include G.I. upset, hair loss, white blotchy nails, and nerve damage. The recommended upper daily dose for selenium is 400 mcg.

*My recommendation:* Most of us haven't a clue about the composition of the soil whence our food cometh. So, it might be worthwhile to tap selenium's antioxidant powers with supplements up to—but not exceeding—200 mcg a day. Check the dose in your multivitamin/multimineral pill before you take extra selenium.

## Chromium

This essential trace mineral has attracted media attention with claims that it could promote weight loss and improve body composition. It does stimulate insulin action in the body, but we don't know what the daily chromium requirement is, or whether supplementation has a positive effect on glucose levels. One trial of 180 people with type 2 diabetes suggested that 1,000 mcg a day of chromium might help with glucose control. On the other hand, the American Diabetes Association does not endorse the use of chromium supplementation.

In the late 1990s, the Federal Trade Commission sued several manufacturers of chromium picolinate supplements, saying that their claims of weight loss were unsubstantiated and deceptive. Depending on whose studies are cited, it seems that there may be some decrease in body fat and added muscle mass, but much of the medical/scientific community feels the only mass increased by chromium is the bank accounts of chromium supplement makers.

Chromium is present in much of the food we eat, and 25 mcg a day is considered an adequate intake. Little is known about the possible adverse effects of chromium from supplements, so an upper limit has not been set.

## Copper

Found in organ meats, seafood, nuts, and seeds, this mineral is necessary for development and function of connective tissue, nerves, and skin pigment. The recommended daily allowance is 900 mcg. Liver damage can occur with supplement intake of more than 10 mg a day. With normal nutrition, there is no need to take additional copper.

## Manganese

Bone and protein formation depend on manganese, as do fat and carbohydrate metabolism. You should get enough manganese if you consume nuts, legumes, and whole grains, and/or drink tea. The RDA is 1.8 mg; there don't seem to be adverse health effects up to 11 mg. There is no need to take separate supplements of manganese.

### Boron, nickel, silicon, and vanadium

These nutrients seem to play a role in promoting good health, but we don't yet know exactly what they do, or how. Thus, there are still no recommended intake levels. In animal studies, harmful effects have been seen in intakes of 20 mg a day for boron, 1.8 for vanadium, and 1 mg for nickel. (My only suggestion at this point—I'm sorry—is, don't suck on change or computer chips.)

## Other Supplements

These supplements are neither vitamins nor minerals, but are either building blocks of proteins or function as enzymes for protein synthesis and action. The question is: Is it vital, helpful, or potentially harmful to try to enhance these reactions? (And remember, supplements are not regulated as drugs—so whatever the claimed or "scientifically proven" benefits, the product at your drugstore may not be the same as the one used in the study.)

### Coenzyme $Q_{10}$

Coenzyme $Q_{10}$ ($CoQ_{10}$) is present in the mitochondria (the energy-forming units of all of our cells) and aids the cell's energy production. It also has antioxidant properties. This ubiquitous substance, also known as ubiquinone, is abundant in beef, soy oil, sardines, and peanuts.

$CoQ_{10}$ supplements are touted as a natural way to increase overall energy and endurance; improve blood pressure, heart health, and immune function; treat cancer, stroke, and gum disease; even block wrinkles and slow aging. It's clear that all this is too good to be true. Here's what we do know:

## "Cliffs Notes" on Vitamins and Minerals
## What *Should* I Take?

In most cases, you don't need to take individual supplement pills for different nutrients. *Take one daily multivitamin supplement.* If you are postmenopausal and don't have periods, buy multivitamins that are iron free.

Add

one vitamin E capsule (400 IU)

calcium (multiple doses, adding up to 1,000 to 1,500 mg)

400 mcg of folate (*if* you plan to become pregnant)

10 mcg of vitamin $B_{12}$ (*if* you are over 65, or if you are a vegan)

400 IU of vitamin D (*if* you are over 65 or you have osteoporosis)

When you go supplement shopping, keep in mind:

There is no evidence that "natural" vitamins are more bioavailable or otherwise superior.

"House brand" supplements are fine, as long as the house brand is from a well-established company or chain—so it's more likely that you'll get what it says on the label. Be wary of small producers without a track record.

More expensive does not mean better.

Have realistic expectations. Unless you have a real deficiency, vitamins will not give you more energy. Nor will they guarantee youth or longevity.

*CoQ₁₀ and heart disease.* Concern has been voiced (especially by the $CoQ_{10}$ makers) that certain prescription drugs cause depletion of this substance—and that without supplementation, you risk developing or worsening heart disease. The most publicized drugs of concern have been the cholesterol-lowering statins. Some studies have shown that $CoQ_{10}$ levels decline by 30 to 50 percent with statin use, and that taking 100 to 200 mg a day brought levels back to normal.

There is weaker evidence for $CoQ_{10}$ depletion with beta blockers, oral glucose-lowering drugs (sulfonylureas), tricyclic antidepressants, diuretics, and antihypertensives. Low levels of $CoQ_{10}$ have been seen in patients with congestive heart failure, the theory being that $CoQ_{10}$ is "used up" during the excessive heart muscle exertion associated with this disease. $CoQ_{10}$ might lower blood pressure in people with hypertension, and perhaps promote recovery of the heart muscle after cardiac surgery. Should people who take these drugs, or have these medical conditions, use $CoQ_{10}$ supplements? The final answer is still hidden in our mitochondria.

*CoQ₁₀ and Parkinson's disease.* Low levels of $CoQ_{10}$ have been noted in blood cells and brain mitochondria of people who suffer from Parkinson's disease. A 2002 NIH study involving eighty patients with early-stage Parkinson's disease found that the group given high doses of coenzyme $Q_{10}$ (1,200 mg a day) had significantly less decline in mental and physical function, and in their ability to carry out daily activities, than the group given lower $CoQ_{10}$ doses or none at all. Please note: It's premature to suggest that we all go on $CoQ_{10}$ to protect our brains, or that the half-million-plus Americans affected by Parkinson's use it; larger studies are needed. There is also interest in studying $CoQ_{10}$ supplements for patients with Huntington's disease.

Commonly used and sold doses of $CoQ_{10}$ range from 30 to 120 mg a day.

Possible side effects include heartburn, nausea, stomachache, diarrhea, fatigue, and skin reactions.

## Omega-3: Will a Spoonful of Fish Oil Protect Your Heart?

I always believed that the cod-liver oil my mother gave me when she thought I was getting sick worked—as a threat and a placebo. If I had to take it, I was damned if I'd get sick! The polyunsaturated fats from the liver of the cod, as well as those from other oily dark-meat fish (such as mackerel, salmon, sardines, bluefish, swordfish, and canned tuna), may be true health boosters.

It wasn't just our mothers who noticed that people who eat a lot of fish—such as Alaska natives, Greenland Inuits (Eskimos), and Japanese living in fishing villages—had a much lower incidence of heart disease than the rest of us. Scientists found that the fish they consumed contain fatty acids (*eicosapentaenoic acid,* or EPA, and *docosahexaenoic acid,* or DHA) that reduce triglyceride levels and the stickiness of platelets, and "smooth out" cardiac rhythms, helping prevent irregular heartbeats. These healthful fats also help prevent abnormalities in the cells that line blood vessels, and may reduce vessel spasms, essentially lowering blood pressure.

Do all these lab data translate to non-Eskimos, who either have heart disease or are at risk, and are told to increase their fish consumption? And, for those who don't like or eat fish, would it help to take omega-3 capsules or even the foul-tasting (lately improved with artificial flavors) cod-liver oil?

A 1999 trial, including over eleven thousand individuals who'd had heart attacks, did find that those who took fish oil capsules had a lower risk of death, subsequent heart attacks, and stroke. (Note: High doses can give your breath a fishy smell, and you may notice loose stools.) A dose of 1 gram daily gave clinically important benefits.

However, another, more recent double-blind study of three hundred people who'd had a heart attack showed no positive results, even after taking 4 grams of concentrated omega-3 fatty acids daily for twelve to fourteen months—although their HDL went up and triglycerides went down. (Perhaps if the study had continued longer, they would have seen benefits.) Also, a twenty-four-week double-blind placebo-controlled trial of three hundred people who'd had heart attacks found no reduction in adverse heart events in the fish oil group, compared with a group taking corn oil.

Fish oil has also been suggested as a way to reduce the symptoms of rheumatoid arthritis. The theory is that the omega-3 fatty acids reduce production of prostaglandins, which cause inflammation and pain. Thirteen different double-blind studies of over five hundred individuals showed this to be the case. After several months of supplement taking, patients often felt they could decrease the doses of drugs they used to quell joint stiffness and swelling. Unfortunately, there are no data to show that fish oil slows joint destruction.

Standard daily doses of fish oil capsules contain 3 to 9 grams, providing 1.8 grams of EPA and 0.9 gram of DHA (be sure you read the label to know what's in your fish oil capsule). Taking cod-liver oil is not the best way to go for these fatty acids, since it has a high content of vitamin A.

Is it better to get your oil by dining on salmon, mackerel, halibut, or other cold-water fish? I believe that consuming nutrients naturally rather than through a pill is almost always preferable, and eating fish does appear to be effective in decreasing coronary heart disease in women: The Nurses' Health Study showed that those who had the highest fish and shellfish consumption had a 33 percent decrease in their rate of CHD compared with the fish-averse.

Unfortunately, we power our world with coal, and contaminate our atmosphere and water systems with mercury. This is processed through the ecosystems of plants and ingested by little fish, which are eaten by bigger fish, where the mercury gets concentrated in the very fatty areas of the fish that we hope will bestow good health on humans. High levels of mercury, at least in men, have recently been shown to increase heart disease.

Once mercury enters the human body, it stays put. During pregnancy, it's passed to the fetus, where it can harm the developing brain and heart; by some estimates, high mercury levels have lowered the IQs of 10 percent of our newborns. PCB contamination of fish is also a concern. Women who are not pregnant but intend to be should limit their intake to 12 ounces of cooked fish a week, about two or three portions; when they are pregnant, their intake should be only one portion a week. Small plant-eating fish are likely to be the safest; we know that the most mercury-laden fish are the large, top-of-the-food-chain ones such as shark, swordfish, king mackerel, and tilefish. Eating a variety of fish may reduce your odds of overexposure to particular contaminants.

Finally, because fish oil capsules affect platelet stickiness, they may increase the effect of blood-thinning medications, even aspirin. (Regular aspirin users did not see a benefit from extra fish intake in the Nurses' Health Study, perhaps because the aspirin was sufficient as a heart helper.)

## Glucosamine and Chondroitin

These two supplements are often sold together, and on the bottle you'll see the claim that they promote "the health and resilience of joints." (On the back, there's a note that these statements have not been confirmed by the Food and Drug Administration.)

Glucosamine, found in our joints, is important for the production and function of cartilage. Supplements are made either from chitin extracted from ground-up crab or lobster shells, or from synthetically produced glucosamine. Chondroitin is also found in cartilage, keeping it moistened and more elastic. It blocks certain enzymatic reactions that damage cartilage. Supplements can either be synthetically produced or extracted from cow or shark cartilage. The combination of these two supplements has become popular as a remedy to alleviate joint pain and stiffness due to osteoarthritis. What's the evidence for these claims?

### Osteoarthritis

In a National Institutes of Health review of fifteen-plus studies, there was evidence that these supplements can "modestly" improve symptoms such as pain. Chondroitin seemed to help slow cartilage damage, and the combination created virtually no side effects. However, it takes several months of use to see results.

**Commonly used and sold doses**
A typical dose of glucosamine is 1,000 to 1,500 mg a day in divided doses. For chondroitin, it's up to 1,200 mg in divided doses.

The bottom line: If you have arthritic pain, it's reasonable to try this supplement. First, see your doctor for appropriate diagnosis. If your joint health is fine, there's no reason to use this supplement "just in case."

Remember, these are unregulated supplements, not drugs: In recent tests, one-third to one-half of the bottles did not contain what their manufacturers claimed they did. You can check to see if your chosen brand has a seal of approval from the U.S. Pharmacopoeia (USP mark), ConsumerLab. com, the Good Housekeeping Institute, or *Consumer Reports*.

### Amino Acid Supplements (Creatinine, L-lysine, Tryptophan, SAMe)

Of the twenty-two amino acids our bodies need to make protein, we self-produce all but eight. These eight "essential" amino acids have to come from an outside source—namely, our food. Most meat and dairy products contain them; it's also possible to combine vegetable protein sources, such as nuts and legumes, to get the right amino acid combinations.

Between what your body makes and what you eat, you should have enough to maintain the protein component of your tissue. Spurning this self-reliance, the supplement industry has industriously produced add-on or "make better" products in the form of tablets, capsules, liquid, mixes, and the ubiquitous energy bars.

To get sufficient amino acids for our everyday body needs, we should consume 0.24 gram of protein per pound of body weight—about 55 grams for a 130-pound woman. Note: Six ounces of meat, fish, or poultry gives you 40 grams; a cup of nonfat yogurt, 13 grams; and a cup of almonds, 25 grams.

Consider increasing your protein intake (and calories) if you're involved in rigorous or endurance sports; roughly double your intake per pound. Consuming high-protein food should do it. But this is not the advice you'll get at your gym, in fitness magazines, or at the health food store—which all proclaim your American-consumer right to enlarge your muscles, lose weight, and promote energy through amino acid supplements and protein formulas. Is there any evidence to back up these claims? In the case of the amino acid called creatinine, perhaps.

## Creatinine

While studies vary in size and the consistency of results, creatinine seems to build strength and increase muscle size, but only if you consistently work out. Most studies have been conducted on men, but one small study of women showed increased muscle strength with exercise after ten weeks of use. Creatinine may also help athletes who need energy for intense but brief exertions—sprinters, short-distance swimmers, and weight lifters. But this has not been shown to be the case with longer, low-intensity activities such as long-distance running, cycling, or walking.

*A typical dose:* 1 or 2 mg a day. Sometimes athletes will take a "loading dose" of 20 to 30 mg for seven days.

*Side effects and risks:* Most studies were short-term and involved young, healthy, athletic individuals (and few women). Side effects such as muscle cramping, G.I. distress, and unwanted weight gain have occurred. And because creatinine is excreted by the kidneys, there may be a risk for renal damage when taking high doses over long periods.

## L-lysine

Another well-known amino acid, l-lysine, has been touted not for muscle building, but for relief of type 2 (genital) herpes outbreaks—the thought being that it stops the virus from replicating. That's been shown to happen in a test tube, and may work in actual women, but the results are not stellar. If you have a chronic herpes infection (and 20 percent of us do), high doses (1,250 to 3,000 mg daily) may make recurrent outbreaks fewer and less severe. But l-lysine has not been shown to help with a first outbreak or with sporadic use when symptoms appear.

*Side effects* of long-term l-lysine high doses are unfortunately unknown. Note: There are prescription antiviral medications, such as Valtrex and Famvir, which can be taken for just three to five days to facilitate rapid recovery from an acute herpes infection. Moreover, daily use will protect against recurrence and viral shedding, and will reduce infections of partners by at least 80 percent. These medications are FDA approved and are what I prescribe for my patients with recurrent herpes type 2 infections.

## Tryptophan

Supplements of l-tryptophan were popular in the 1980s as treatments to promote sleep and diminish anxiety and depression. The FDA mandated that they be taken off the market in 1990, after 36 users died and over 1,500 became seriously ill with blood cell and muscle disorders. This amino acid disaster was traced to multiple contaminants in the product, which was produced by a Japanese chemical company. Subsequent to this ban came a chemically similar, and supposedly noncontaminated, supplement: 5-hydroxy-l-tryptophan (5-HTP). This product has been touted as a "drug free" way to combat depression, due to its conversion into serotonin in the brain. So far, study results are equivocal.

*A typical dose:* 100 to 300 mg three times a day. (In some clinical trials, lower maintenance doses were used after a starting high-dose period.)

*Side effects and risks:* In 1998, a few samples of 5-HTP were found to contain the chemical contaminant that caused the problems with l-tryptophan. While the FDA has not, to date, called for the removal of 5-HTP, I would be leery of its use.

## S-adenosylmethionine (SAMe)

This substance is formed by combining the amino acid methionine with adenosine triphosphate (ATP), an energy source in our cells. You don't get SAMe through food: Your body relies on its homemade supply, and this seems to suffice. SAMe is part of many biochemical reactions, and helps protect, manufacture, and repair cartilage.

SAMe has become a popular dietary supplement reputed to treat joint pain, muscle pain, and depression. Unfortunately, much of the success quoted in studies came through use of injectible SAMe; the amount you get through pills, after breakdown in the intestine, may not be enough for a therapeutic effect. The product that is sold in the United States calls for doses three to four times lower than the dose used in studies. An oral dose high enough to potentially achieve a therapeutic effect (1,200 to 1,600 mg a day) would cost as much as $200 a month.

The best evidence so far for the effectiveness of oral SAMe supplements comes from a one-month study of 732 people with osteoarthritis. They noted reduced pain, but the effect was equal to 750 mg a day of naproxen (Aleve, an inexpensive over-the-counter NSAID). Studies of SAMe's potential antidepressant effects have been small. There are anecdotal reports of success, but the evidence does not suffice to currently recommend its use in the treatment of depression.

*Side effects:* While oral doses up to 1,200 mg did not trigger side effects in short-term studies, the effects of long-term use at these doses are not known.

## SO-CALLED YOUTH SUPPLEMENTS: SLOWING TIME BY PRESCRIPTION?

### Human Growth Hormone

In 1990, a research report appeared in the *New England Journal of Medicine,* and became the Holy Grail for the anti-aging commercialization complex. The study included twenty-one healthy men (aged 61 to 81); twelve received injections of biosynthetic *human growth hormone* (hGH) for just six months, while nine served as controls. The results of this tiny study were proclaimed as legitimizing a therapy that would increase lean body mass, decrease fat mass, increase bone mass, and even increase skin thickness. What followed was an extraordinary "growth spurt" in the use of this expensive hormone, which heretofore had been reserved for children and adults with congenital or disease-caused growth hormone deficiencies.

Will injections keep us thin and buff, and out of gyms? Can we have our cake and eat it, too?

Multiple hormones are involved in growth regulation. *Growth hormone-releasing hormone* (GHRH) is produced in the hypothalamus area of the brain, and stimulates production and release of hGH by the pituitary gland. Subsequently, hGH induces the liver to produce *insulin-like growth factor 1* (IGF-1); it's this hormone that triggers the growth of bones and other body tissues. High levels of IGF-1 result in negative feedback (like a shutoff valve), which reduces pituitary production of hGH and prevents overload. These hormones are influenced by stress, sleep, exercise, food intake, and blood sugar levels.

Most of our knowledge about hGH and IGF-1 comes from studying individuals with deficiencies. In children, hGH deficiency stunts growth and development. In adults, hGH deficiency (usually from disease, tumors, or surgery that destroys critical areas in the pituitary) causes weight gain, lipid abnormalities, cardiovascular disease, fatigue, poor immune response, and loss of muscle and bone mass. These individuals are also prone to depression and problems with sexual function. When they are injected with corrective amounts of the missing hormone, many of these problems are resolved.

Normally, hGH production peaks during puberty, then gradually declines after age 30—but the pituitary never completely ceases production. Decreased levels of hGH are thought to play a role in the decline of organ function and in the increase in fat and weight as we age.

Could supplementing with hGH prevent this wear, tear, and fat accumulation, and extend the quality and length of our lives? The scientific trials to date involve far too few people, for too short a time. Here is a quick recap of data from peer-reviewed journals:

In 1996, a double-blind study of hGH was published in the *Annals of Internal Medicine*. Fifty-two healthy men over age 69 were randomized to receive hGH or a placebo for six months. Those treated with hGH did not lose weight, but their fat content decreased and muscle mass increased. There was no corresponding increase in their muscle strength or cognitive abilities (intellectual skills and memory)—nor did they feel happier. Moreover, compared with the placebo group, they had more frequent side effects, such as swollen legs and pain in small and large joints; these were severe enough that a quarter of the hGH group had to have their dose reduced.

In 1998, *Science* carried a report on growth hormone research involving the Physicians' Health Study. Men who had naturally high levels of IGF-1 (the top quarter) were 4.3 times more likely to develop prostate cancer than men in the lowest quarter.

In 2001, the *Journal of Clinical Endocrinology and Metabolism* published a six-month, double-blind, placebo-controlled trial of hGH. Finally, this included forty-six healthy *women,* some taking HRT, as well as sixty-four men. The average age was 72 (the range was 65 to 88). It was found that neither growth hormone nor hormone replacement therapy—or hGH-plus-HRT—reduced abdominal fat in women, whereas hGH with and without testosterone reduced abdominal fat by 7 to 16 percent in men.

In 2002, another study, published in the *Journal of the American Medical Association,* examined the effect of six months of hGH, with and without hormone replacement therapy, on fifty-seven women (and seventy-four men), aged 65 to 88. The women treated with growth hormone averaged a 1-kg increase in their lean body (or muscle) mass, a 1.2-kg increase with HRT, and a 2.1-kg muscle benefit from combined hGH and HRT. But with or without HRT, hGH did not cause a statistically significant change in women's strength or cardiovascular endurance (as measured with a treadmill test). The men seemed to have a greater response to hGH, showing marginal improvements in muscle mass, strength, and endurance. However, this was equivalent to what they would have attained by exercising three times a week for six months. And as you saw in chapter 3, exercise provides additional life-prolonging benefits.

The most concerning aspect of this study was the high rate of side effects. Thirty-nine percent of women treated with hGH had edema (swelling), 46 percent had joint pain, and 38 percent had carpal tunnel symptoms. Diabetes and glucose intolerance developed more often after hGH treatment in men than in women.

In looking at the effects of added growth hormone, we should also review the lessons of nature. *Acromegaly* is a disease caused by excess pituitary production of hGH, which creates too much IGF-1—leading to serious overgrowth of every tissue it affects, and even death.

### Growth hormone and cancer?

In medical terms, IGF-1 is considered to be *mitogenic* and *anti-apoptotic*. That means it promotes proliferation of cells, and prevents them from dying—and this is exactly what happens to cancer cells. Are high levels of IGF-1 associated with the cancers we women are most concerned about, particularly breast cancer? We're not sure.

For example, 397 women from the Nurses' Health Study with diagnosed breast cancer were matched with 620 women who had not developed breast cancer, and their blood samples (collected almost ten years earlier) were compared. Among the premenopausal women, those with the highest IGF-1 concentrations had twice the rate of breast cancer as those with low concentrations. Among those younger than 50, the risk increased more than fourfold. There was no association found for postmenopausal women.

A 2002 article in *The Lancet* reviewed the fates of over 1,800 U.K. patients who had received human growth hormone in childhood or young adulthood (between 1959 and 1985—before synthetic growth hormone became available). They had a significantly higher risk of mortality from cancer, especially colorectal cancer and Hodgkin's disease. These patients received two or three injections a week; today's synthetic version is given daily. Critics argue that the higher hormone peaks created by less frequent injections might have encouraged abnormal cell growth, and that daily use could be safer. The researchers wisely suggested that we follow patients taking synthetic hormone over time to see what happens—but of course, those results won't be available for years.

To date, the FDA has approved the use of hGH for children with inadequate growth hormone production or growth-retarding diseases; in 2003, Humatrope (the most used synthetic hGH) was also approved to treat healthy but extremely short children. Since 1996, hGH use has been officially extended to include adults who have growth hormone deficiency due to pituitary or hypothalamic disease, surgery, injury, or radiation therapy. The prescribing information for Humatrope warns that safety and effectiveness have not been evaluated in people over age 65.

### What's the hGH bottom line?

Having given all of these caveats, I should mention that there's a burgeoning group of physicians and scientists who are hGH believers. They have formed a professional association called the Academy of Anti-Aging Medicine, which now has nearly twelve thousand members worldwide. In 2001, an estimated thirty thousand Americans were shooting up growth hormone. The yearly cost of such injections, depending on dose, ranges from $12,000 to $15,000.

After reviewing the data and perusing multiple Web sites with information that seems more commercial than scientific in tone, I personally veto hGH for most healthy-but-getting-older-and-heavier women. If you want to spend that kind of money, invest in research-supported paths to better health, good looks, and longevity: Hire a personal trainer and nutritionist, and buy prevention-oriented health insurance.

### Are there noninjectable growth hormone alternatives?

Human growth hormone is hard to synthesize; its large and complex molecular structure involves 191 amino acids. Since 1985, growth hormone has been made through recombinant DNA technology; bacterial or animal cells are given a gene that directs them to make human growth hormone. The cells are then grown in a tissue culture, which synthesizes a pure hormone identical to that produced by the human pituitary.

We can't copy this substance using the growth hormones of animals or plants, and molecules of this size can't be absorbed through skin or mucous membranes; in pill form, it would be deactivated by stomach acid and enzymes. So beware of marketing claims for products sold over the counter and on the Internet, stating that they provide "alternative" forms of human growth hormones or substances that will stimulate your pituitary to make more hGH. This hope in growth has created a billion-dollar-a-year market.

Human GH can only be manufactured by companies licensed by the FDA, prescribed and managed by a licensed physician, and administered via injection under the skin. It's legal for physicians to prescribe this or any approved drug off label (for nonapproved uses). Because injections are expensive, need strict supervision, and—according to the studies cited above—cause significant side effects, researchers have sought other ways to augment hGH:

*Secretagogues.* This word implies the stimulation of glands—in this case the pituitary—to secrete hormones. Recent research from Europe has found evidence that oral administration of certain secretagogues may help stimulate hGH release—but only for people who are hGH deficient. There is no good evidence that secretagogues can work as anti-aging products. There is also no evidence that "secretagogue" products available over the counter or Web contain any useful ingredients. Yet there are over one hundred secretagogue amino acid precursors or HGH spray products on the market. (In fact, the publisher of the *New England Journal of Medicine* has had to sue online hGH marketers that try to borrow the journal's credibility.)

## DHEA

From puberty, our adrenal glands flood our bodies with the hormone DHEA; production peaks in our late twenties, and it's downhill from there. DHEA levels fall by 50 percent in our forties, and are down to a trickle by our sixties and seventies. Should we shore up this dwindling supply?

DHEA is more than "just" a supplement. It is a hormone that can be converted into testosterone or estrogen. The FDA originally classified DHEA as a drug that was rarely approved for common use but could be prescribed by physicians. But in 1994, it was taken off drug status, and embarked on its maiden voyage into the uncharted sea of dietary supplements.

We don't even know what DHEA does on its own. No DHEA receptors have been isolated in our cells. We can only divine its powers by what is left unaccomplished when it's missing in individuals who have life-threatening adrenal insufficiency. A 1999 study of twenty-four women with adrenal insufficiency (due to either disease or surgery) showed that after four months of DHEA therapy, the women were less depressed and anxious, thought about sex more, and were more satisfied with their sexual experiences than before treatment. But all was not right in their added-DHEA world. Their levels of HDL cholesterol decreased, and most of the women developed male hormone side effects, including greasy skin, acne, and increased body hair.

What, if anything, should we do about DHEA levels naturally lowered by age? Once more, there is a dearth of proven worth (aside from the financial worth that is bestowed on DHEA manufacturers and marketers). Studies done on rats have shown that DHEA supplements prevent onset of cancer, atherosclerosis, viral infections, obesity, and diabetes, and make anxious rats calmer. Can we extrapolate these results to women? Rodents barely produce DHEA, so for them this is a foreign substance, given in supersized, never-to-be-found-in-nature quantities.

In the largest study of humans, blood levels of DHEA were measured in two thousand men and women between 1972 and 1974. More than twenty years later, the men who had previously "excelled" with above-average DHEA levels were 15 percent less likely to have died of heart disease than those who had lower levels. But the women with high DHEA levels had no heart disease benefits at all. Although this study did not show that higher levels protected women's hearts, it did demonstrate that this might help their mood. Out of nearly seven hundred nonestrogen-using women, there was an association between low DHEA levels and depressed mood. And a group of thirty-one women who had clinical depression had lower DHEA levels compared with those of ninety-three age-matched nondepressed women.

A French study of 280 healthy men and women between the ages of 60 and 75 showed that 50 mg of DHEA daily was associated with a small increase in bone mineral density in the women. But these women also had small increases in estrogen and testosterone levels, which could account for their bone improvement. Their libido scores also improved (however, the study did not provide partners).

There are several other studies frequently cited as scientific examples of positive effects of DHEA. They are woefully small and short-lived:

- Thirteen men and seventeen women, ages 40 to 70, reported that after a few weeks of 50 mg of DHEA daily, they had increased energy, better sleep, and improved mood. (The women also had a twofold increase in their male hormone level. Once more, this may have made them feel better.)
- Eleven postmenopausal women given 50 mg of DHEA had a twofold

increase in the destructive activity of their natural killer cells (hardly sufficient to prove that this will reverse the decline in our immune competence as we get older).

- A study of six patients with major depression and low DHEA levels showed that 30 to 90 mg of DHEA a day sparked improvement in some patients after four weeks.

There is evidence that DHEA supplements help one group of women: those who suffer from systemic lupus erythematosus. In studies that involved up to 120 women (finally, a number we can appreciate!), high doses of DHEA (200 mg) given daily for six months decreased episodes of disease symptoms and improved their overall sense of well-being. Some women on DHEA were able to lower the dose of other medications that they took to control their disease. As expected, however, they also had increased testosterone levels and acne.

Is DHEA the stuff that youth is made of? Sorry to disappoint you, but no. Our current body of research has not shown that it has any meaningful effect on our longevity or quality of life. That doesn't mean it can't help women with specific problems associated with a very low or absent DHEA production. These include:

- Women with documented adrenal insufficiency—from surgery, radiation, or disease
- Women who have chronic autoimmune diseases, especially if they take high-dose steroids that knock out their normal adrenal function (e.g., lupus and rheumatoid arthritis)
- Women with severe osteoporosis (but remember, there are a lot of other therapies that we know work)
- Women with both depression and low libido (this is really pushing the powers of DHEA to the limit, but in some cases it may help)

If you have medical conditions such as breast cancer or heart disease that make estrogen or testosterone therapy questionable—there's also no question that concerns about hormone therapy should apply to DHEA supplements.

One last warning: DHEA is unregulated, and there is no way of knowing exactly how much or what is in the pill. A recent report by ConsumerLabs.com found that three of seventeen DHEA products that they purchased had less than the claimed amount.

Most DHEA tablets (which you'll find prominently displayed on the counters of health food stores, drugstores, convenience stores, and even airport shops) are plain crystalline DHEA; when they are ingested, they are subject to "first bypass" in the liver, and a high rate of conversion to testosterone. This might give us an androgen punch, but if it's being taken for "pure" DHEA benefits, it's being pitched in the wrong hormone park. Micronized DHEA (minute pieces suspended in oil) will prevent some of this liver breakdown. This form of DHEA is made by compounding pharmacies and usually requires a prescription.

I reserve the right to alter the above negative statements if better, longer, and more convincing studies give us the wellspring of information we need to lend any credibility to this proclaimed and promoted fountain of youth. Meanwhile, let's get back to the more credible ways and means of preventing disease and maintaining our health.

## HERBS AND BOTANICALS

If you ever look at the package insert that comes with a prescription medicine, it's hard to avoid the feeling that you are putting an "unnatural" and possibly dangerous substance in your body. Something that's "natural"— especially when it doesn't involve an appointment with or stern admonitions from a physician—feels more comfortable, sort of like a loose housedress that requires no bra. And who knows your body better than you? Doctors freely admit that many of the medications they prescribe were first used by monks and wisewomen to heal disease. Why not go straight to the plants that were their source?

The word "natural" sounds so safe, but over the history of medicine, it took hundreds of years to figure out which parts of plants were medically active, and how to prepare and administer them without causing major complications or death. A good example is the heart drug digitalis, which originally was administered as leaves and seeds. Old textbooks showed forty different methods of processing the twelve varieties of plants, with potency and absorption differing from plant to plant, season to season, and plot to plot!

Even if therapeutic botanicals are farmed and processed, there is no guarantee that the resulting product isolates, concentrates, or gives standard doses of whatever substance is purported to have a beneficial effect. In fact, the therapeutic ingredient(s) often have not been identified, making standardization for many herbs virtually impossible. (An example: Ginkgo biloba extract makers try to achieve a concentration of 24 percent ginkgo-flavone glycosides—just because it's something they can measure.) You may be paying a lot of money for useless leaves and capsule fillers.

Finally, let me point out that not all of Mother Nature's plants are healing; consider hemlock, arsenic, and poison ivy. Some herbal "medicines" have been found to cause liver failure and even cancer. In a 1999 article published in the *Journal of the American Medical Association,* it was noted that "Assuming that 'natural' remedies must be safe, 60 million Americans spent $3.2 billion medicating themselves with herbals in 1996." (A 2001 estimate raised this to $4.2 billion.) The article went on to describe reports of over one hundred herb-related deaths, plus scores of serious complications requiring hospitalization and even organ transplants.

Some herbal therapies may be good for you; many are useless; a few are truly harmful. Moreover, herbs can interfere with prescribed medications, counteract OTCs such as anti-inflammatories, and increase the risks of anesthesia and surgery.

Here are the herbs most frequently used by women to help with hormonal imbalance or perimenopausal and menopausal symptoms; to diminish their risk of infection or disease; to improve memory and well-being; to lose weight; or to relieve physical and/or emotional distress.

## Herbs for Hormonal Imbalance?

> If menopause did not exist, dietary supplement manufacturers might well have invented it. It is hard to imagine a better target for their products—a natural process, but one accompanied by hot flashes, bone losses and other signs of aging, along with other changes that most women do not find pleasant, to say the least.
>
> —JANE BRODY AND DENISE GRADY,
> *THE NEW YORK TIMES GUIDE TO ALTERNATIVE HEALTH*

Before I begin this herbal saga, I have to voice my skepticism regarding some of the cited studies, as well as anecdotal proclamations of feeling better through herbs. Like depression, PMS and certain menopausal symptoms often improve during the initial phase of a trial in response to any treatment, including placebo. So the statement that "symptoms decreased by 30 to 40 percent in the first three months" or that "30 or 40 percent of

## How Do We Know What We Know?
## The German Commission E

An oft-quoted authority for herbal therapeutic claims is Germany's Commission E, a government health panel that has evaluated the effects of roughly four hundred botanicals. In Germany, about 30 percent of the drugs sold in pharmacies are herbal; the majority are prescribed by physicians and paid for by insurance companies.

While Commission E has been referred to as "the herbal FDA," its approval standards are far less stringent than those used by the American Food and Drug Administration (FDA) for pharmaceuticals: It only requires that there be "reasonable certainty" that the herbal product is safe and has evidence of therapeutic benefit. (Note: This sets up an unequal playing field. It's vastly less expensive for supplement makers to meet this "reasonable certainty" standard than it is for pharmaceutical manufacturers to make their case for approval to the FDA.)

So far, the commission has given the thumbs-up to over 250 botanicals, and thumbs-down to more than 125 that it has deemed unsafe and/or unefficacious. Some of the funding for the commission's research comes from industry (for example, the recent English translation of their monographs was paid for by forty-nine supplement companies). It has not acknowledged the deadly potential of nearly a dozen herbs, including ephedra.

The National Institutes of Health's Center for Complementary and Alternative Medicine (NCCAM), established by Congress in 1998, now provides us with an alternative source of herbal wisdom. The NCCAM funds preclinical (test tube and animal) and small clinical (human) studies, and selects herbs that show promise for randomized, controlled clinical trials. As these results come in, we'll be able to give much better advice on whether and how herbal remedies work, when they are safe to use, and when prescription medications are a better bet.

women responded to . . ." does not mean this product will continue to work for the long term, or indeed is significantly better than placebo.

## For PMS
The culprits behind the bloat, weight gain, mood swings, sleep disturbance, and other symptoms that can ruin one to two weeks of our lives every month are thought to range from nutritional deficiencies, to blood

sugar fluctuations, to inappropriate balance between estrogen and pro-gesterone—and their effect on nearly every cell in our bodies. Supple-ment makers reassure us that they have products that will "naturally" address one or all of these issues. Here is the bloated list of what's out there:

*Black cohosh.* This herb has become the nonprescription bête noire of menopausal hot flashes, which I'll discuss in greater detail under herbs used for those symptoms. Even though black cohosh has received the blessing of the German Commission E for the treatment of PMS and menstrual cramps, the studies don't support this.

*Chaste tree berry (Vitex agnus-castus).* There is only one placebo-controlled study of 178 women, lasting just three menstrual cycles. This showed a significant reduction in PMS symptoms (except bloating), with a dose of chasteberry dry extract ZE 440 three times a day. Other surveys have suggested chaste tree berry helps, but little science and many anec-dotes were involved.

*Dong quai.* This dried root, sometimes called "women's ginseng," is a common ingredient in traditional Asian herbal mixtures. Although it's been used for just about every gynecologic problem imaginable, it's hard to imagine why. While a number of flawed studies have sought to prove that dong quai helps with menstrual pain, they didn't. Nor does it seem to measure up beyond placebo when studied for PMS. Chinese healers, who have prescribed this for centuries, mix dong quai with other herbs; per-haps it works better blended rather than "straight up."

Contaminants (some toxic) have been found in dong quai prepara-tions—as well as pharmaceutical drugs not listed on the label, which could explain the anecdotal reports of their effects. Furthermore, if used with anticoagulants (including aspirin), dong quai can cause bleeding; it also increases skin sensitivity to the sun's rays.

*Evening primrose oil.* The seeds of this lovely-sounding plant produce an oil rich in fatty acids, especially gamma-linolenic acid (GLA). Because GLA causes the production of a certain prostaglandin that inhibits in-flammation, it was thought that this might be a remedy for conditions in-volving inflammation such as arthritis—and perhaps PMS and breast tenderness.

In small, three-month studies, breast tenderness did decrease, but only in those women who had neither large cysts nor benign lumps (fi-broadenomas). In other research, evening primrose oil's effect on joint pain was not sufficient to consider it as a replacement for NSAIDs such as aspirin. Finally, for PMS, only a few tiny, poorly controlled studies showed any benefit—certainly not enough to recommend it as therapy.

Don't forget, this is an oil—and like any oil, if you consume it in large quantities, you'll be getting extra, perhaps unwanted, calories. (The recommended dose is 3 grams daily.) Also, this fairly expensive product can cause nausea, headache, and soft stools.

## For perimenopausal and menopausal symptoms

*Soy products and the soy conundrum.* The joys of soy, as food or supplement, have been touted as a cure, treatment, or alleviator for disorders from breast cancer to heart disease, osteoporosis, and menopausal symptoms. The simple soybean is rich in protein, and also contains its famous phytoestrogens (plant estrogens) called *isoflavones*. These are further classified as genistein, diadzein, and equol. (Genistein is probably soy's most active isoflavone, and the one most often found in supplements.)

The molecules of all three look remarkably like estrogen; indeed, remember that natural progesterone capsules, as well as estradiol in many forms of HRT, originate and are concentrated from soy and yam plants. But isoflavones themselves are one hundred to one thousand times weaker than the estrogens used in hormone replacement therapy.

The functions of isoflavones are complex: On some estrogen receptors, isoflavones may promote estrogen activity; on others, they may block the receptors and prevent them from being stimulated by other, more potent self-created or administered forms of estrogen. This seemingly contradictory effect depends on the type of receptor, and the activity level and age of the cell in which the receptor is found.

Phytoestrogens may have a protective effect against DNA damage during active cell division in developing breast cells, during adolescence or young adulthood. But in older women, who have more stable breast cells, phytoestrogens may instead cause undesirable stimulation to the cells.

If you grow up eating a traditional Asian diet with up to 80 mg of isoflavones from soy products daily (perhaps together with vegetables, fish, and very little saturated fat), you are ultimately one-fourth less likely to develop breast cancer at a later age than your counterpart who consumed a typical Western, soy-devoid diet. But once your breast cells are no longer developing, suddenly dousing them with huge amounts of phytoestrogens may not decrease but actually increase the potential for breast cancer. Hence, our concern about suggesting large doses of phytoestrogens to women in midlife, or to women who've been diagnosed with breast cancer. Many soy supplement capsules and powders contain as much as 500 mg of isoflavones. A growing number of oncologists advise their patients not to take soy supplements, and either to avoid soy foods or to consume no more than 25 mg a day.

Women from Asian cultures—perhaps the most studied are the Japanese—are also far less likely to develop heart disease, osteoporosis, or menopausal symptoms than the typical American woman. (Or at least, they don't complain about the latter; there's some thought that this could be a cultural rather than physical phenomenon.) So, the question (in a soy-pod): Does soy in a supplement (a) help prevent these diseases and (b) relieve the miseries of menopause? Or could too much soy be dangerous?

*Heart disease.* The soy protein in food—not necessarily in supplements—in "doses" of 25 to 50 grams daily, have been found in over thirty studies to lower LDL cholesterol—especially when consumed in lieu of animal protein. There are phytoestrogens in three hundred plants, and it could be that these are among the dietary factors that give vegetarians their veg-upmanship against heart disease. However, we're not sure that simply taking a capsule or a powder, even if it's high in genistein, will do the same.

Soy products have also been shown to lower total cholesterol and raise HDL in female monkeys—and women—especially when given in doses as high as 80 grams. But at this level, there can be bloating or abdominal discomfort.

*Osteoporosis.* There is conflicting evidence here. One study found an increase in bone density when 40 grams of soy protein powder was ingested daily for six months. Another study, of five hundred women who took soy-derived supplements, did not show bone improvement.

*Hot flashes.* There is still no clear and definite statement on whether soy works for hot flashes. A 2002 review of eleven studies that pass some sort of muster (they were randomized and placebo controlled) on the effects of soy foods and/or isoflavone supplements for hot flashes gave somewhat disappointing results. Some of the short studies (less than six weeks) found significant benefits, but only three of the eight longer studies did; the longest, twenty-four weeks, found no benefits. What's more, the products varied in their contents and dosing, the scoring systems for hot flashes were inconsistent, and the patients varied in age and stages of menopause. Often, the placebo response was as good as the response to the active soy product (symptoms decreased as much as 60 percent!);

with time, the effects of both groups wore off. Even in the most favorable studies, soy isoflavone tablets had a very mild effect on symptoms, and none of them helped with other menopausal symptoms such as vaginal dryness or problems with short-term memory.

The best health results seem to have come from soy-containing foods rather than supplements. Not all soy protein concentrates and supplements are created equal; some may be missing many of the known (or unknown) healthful components found in soybeans. Those produced through alcohol extraction may be devoid of phytoestrogens altogether. Perhaps the biggest profood, antisupplement argument is safety: Soy foods have been a staple for Asian populations for thousands of years. Concentrated isoflavones are our own new invention and, in high doses, could be as potent as estrogen on the breast or the endometrial lining.

If you want to try to soy your way to better health, my advice is to start with food, but don't go overboard—no more than 30 to 40 mg a day (for comparison, 2 cups of soy milk or 6 ounces of tofu has 30 mg of soy protein).

If you try a supplement, and it works, I guess there's no need to argue about whether it has a placebo effect or not. But until we have more long-term studies, don't take huge doses, and make sure your doctor is aware of what you are taking.

## Black cohosh

A North American native, this plant has made a home in Europe as a treatment for symptoms of menopause. The German Commission E has approved this use, but for no longer than six months.

We're not sure how black cohosh works. It might affect estrogen receptors in some parts of the body, while having no effect in others—such as the vagina. (It hasn't been found to change the cells or decrease vaginal dryness.)

Most large studies have used a brand of black cohosh (Remifemin) produced by the pharmaceutical giant GlaxoSmithKline. Three of four randomized controlled trials found some hot-flash benefit, but these were short-term. The usual dose is one to two tablets twice daily. In studies, some women reported headaches, mild G.I. distress, dizziness, or weight gain.

Women who don't want to take estrogen, especially those who've had breast cancer, are searching for hot-flash remedies. Black cohosh may be one of them. However, long-term safety data are lacking on how black cohosh might affect women with breast cancer, or even whether it might promote endometrial cancer. There are also concerns that black cohosh could elevate liver enzymes.

### Flaxseed
This contains a form of phytoestrogen called *lignans*. Flaxseed's been popularized as a health food that may slow the growth of tumors, but evidence is way too skimpy to recommend this for all women. The German Commission E has authorized its use for G.I. problems such as constipation and abdominal pain. But there's no evidence that it helps with any menopausal symptom.

### Red clover
This plant is brimming with phytoestrogenic isoflavones and (no surprise) has been processed to produce a dietary supplement. The brand name is Promensil; each daily tablet contains 40 mg of isoflavones (supposedly four different ones). There are anecdotal reports that this helps hot flashes, but two small double-blind controlled studies did not find a benefit (even at 160 mg a day). We also don't have the safety assurance of previous consumption of red clover by women in any culture or time.

### St.-John's-wort
This "wort," which in Old English means "plant," has seasonal spots on its leaves that were felt to be symbolic of blood shed by Saint John. Because of its purported antidepressant properties (see page 219), it's been suggested for any condition associated with mood changes, including PMS, seasonal affective disorder, and menopause. To date, there are no good substantiating studies.

### The multiherbal solution (or pill)
If you peruse the shelves of herbal remedies, you'll find products labeled FOR MENOPAUSAL WOMEN that contain a hodgepodge of these herbs, and more. Obviously, if we don't know whether one herb works or is safe, there are no data as to what happens when you mix and match them.

## Other Popular Herbs: Do They Work?

### Cranberry extract
I'm writing this just before Thanksgiving. Cranberries certainly enhance the turkey, but does their extract enhance our health?

Yes, when it comes to bladder health. Cranberry juice decreases the ability of bacteria to adhere to and multiply on the bladder wall; small trials have found the same effect with cranberry extract in tablet form. If you tend to get recurrent bladder infections, you may lack an enzyme that limits this bacterial adhesion. Cranberry juice or extract may keep these bacteria from sticking around.

The recommended dose of cranberry extract tablets is 400 mg, two to four times a day. For cranberry juice, the dose is 4 ounces four times a day—which can be quite caloric.

## Echinacea

No part of this native American Midwest plant has been left unused by commercial herbal supplement companies, who have concocted capsules, drops, juice, and teas from the roots, leaves, and flowers. In Germany, where it's Commission E approved, more than three million echinacea prescriptions are written annually. In the States, we get it without prescription; it's over virtually every retail counter.

*Colds (acute upper respiratory tract infections).* A recent review of the research published in the *Journal of Family Practice* found that overall, echinacea can reduce the length and severity of a cold (cutting the average duration in one study from eight to four days). However, many of the trials were small, enrolled patients who may have contracted some other runny nose problem, and had varying criteria as to how bad the cold was or when it was really over. Some of the trials used placebos that patients could easily distinguish from the "real stuff." Finally, they used different products containing different plant varieties and plant parts.

The authors concluded that because we don't know which part of the plant works or how it works, bigger and better studies are needed before echinacea can be confidently recommended for use in early-cold therapy. I have to admit, I use it at the first sign that I'm probably coming down with a cold. And based on the evidence, if you take it as early as possible, there's a reasonable chance you might get better a bit faster.

Because echinacea products vary considerably, if one doesn't seem to help, next time try another. The dose varies, so read the instructions, and once you start, take it for seven to fourteen days. Note that there's little support for continued or long-term use to boost your immune system or prevent recurrent colds. (In fact, Commission E recommends that supplements not be taken for longer than eight weeks.) Goldenseal is frequently combined with echinacea in cold preparations, but there's no evidence that it adds to its benefit.

Wash your hands (the best known cold prevention) and *Gesundheit*.

## Garlic

Garlic is indispensable to great Italian cooking; unfortunately, the cooked kind doesn't seem to boost your health. Cloves have to be dried and processed into a powder or extract to obtain the active ingredient, allien.

*Heart health.* Garlic was originally thought to lower cholesterol. If it does, the effect is very limited: In some studies, it minimally reduced LDL cholesterol and triglycerides, but in many others it did not. Garlic may yet be heart-healthy through its antiplatelet action (it prevents platelets from sticking together and forming clots), and perhaps via a mild reduction in blood pressure.

*Colds.* Even though garlic makes you feel that nothing will ever again live in your mouth and nasal passages, once you have a cold, viruses do. Garlic is not a cold cure. However, a reasonable study suggests that if you catch cold frequently during the winter months, you might benefit from daily use of standardized garlic extract. The standard daily dose is 900 mg in a capsule or tablet, which should contain 1.3 percent allien. That's a lot of garlic, equivalent to an entire small garlic clove. Supplements can also give you stinky sweat and bad breath, although de-scented versions are sold. Garlic oil extract doesn't contain allien.

Due to its anticlotting effect, garlic can promote bleeding if taken with anticoagulants, aspirin, or even vitamin E. My recommendation is that if you're hypertensive and/or have abnormal lipids or coronary vascular disease, do not rely on garlic for heart protection.

## Ginkgo biloba

The ginkgo tree has its roots in the Mesozoic era, 150 million years ago. Its seeds and leaves have been used in Chinese medicine for centuries. Today, you can find pills with ginkgo leaf extract at your local grocery or pharmacy. Ginkgo is prescribed in some European countries for dementia, cerebral decline, peripheral artery insufficiency, and other disorders.

*Alzheimer's disease (and other dementias).* A number of small studies have suggested some benefit from ginkgo. Perhaps the best evidence comes from a yearlong double-blind, placebo-controlled study of three hundred people with dementia (mostly due to Alzheimer's). With a standard daily 120-mg dose, more of the ginkgo patients seemed to stabilize or show improvement on a commonly used test of memory and language.

Now, the caveats: Many patients dropped out before the end of the study. Family members and physicians did not report seeing significant differences between the ginkgo and placebo patients. Also, the improvement in test scores was less than with some currently available prescription treatments for Alzheimer's. I'd hesitate to recommend ginkgo over other options unless we see good results from the ongoing NIH trial (ending in 2006).

*Improved memory or concentration.* Many adults are popping ginkgo pills to improve their mental focus, or to remember where they put their keys; is there evidence that it works? An excellent 2002 study, published in the *Journal of the American Medical Association,* deflated these claims. When two hundred 60-plus adults were given fourteen different tests of learning, memory, attention, and concentration, there were no significant differences in the placebo and ginkgo group scores, or in the progress reports given by the subjects' relatives or friends. Looks like we're back to keeping lists to shore up our memories.

*Other diseases.* The NIH's Center for Complementary and Alternative Medicine is assessing whether ginkgo might have some effect on asthma, multiple sclerosis, and other conditions. Meanwhile, proceed with caution. Ginkgo can cause mild G.I. upset and headaches. Check with your doctor before using ginkgo if you have an illness involving blood circulation or clotting, or if you're taking anticoagulants (including aspirin).

## Ginseng (to adapt or not adapt)

"Adaptagen" is a fabulous term that I never heard mentioned in medical school; nor have I come across it in medical journals. But the Europeans and the Chinese embrace the concept. It refers to a substance or activity that helps your body adapt to psychological and physical stresses: emotional upset, sleep deprivation, temperature changes, toxic exposure, and even radiation. An adaptagen makes what's wrong right, but doesn't overcorrect. Oh, and it increases energy and overall well-being.

Ginseng (not to be confused with Siberian ginseng, which is altogether different) has been credited with all these qualities. Too good to be true? Not according to the makers of ginseng capsules, powders, liquids, extracts, teas, and soft drinks who are engaged in a tremendous commercial commitment to help us adapt to life's stresses.

Asian ginseng (*Panex* ginseng), used in Chinese herbal medicines, and American ginseng (*Panex quinquefolius*) are considered to have similar properties. It takes five years to grow and harvest the plant, so many ginseng products actually contain very little of the root—and what's marketed may be adulterated with caffeine (hence, you'll feel the energy) or other substances. There is also the concern that if it comes directly from Asia, distant root providers may cut it with toxic substances.

The scientific community does not know how ginseng works, or if it does. Here's a brief description of the more up-to-date, sort-of-controlled studies:

*Infections.* Most of the studies have been done on animals, but one done on a group of 227 human individuals showed that those who took a daily dose of 100 mg of Asian ginseng had fewer colds and flu after four to twelve weeks than those taking placebo.

*Brain "adaptation."* A twenty-two-month study that followed 112 middle-aged adults found that those who took ginseng had improved "abstract thinking ability," but there was no difference in reaction time, memory, or concentration between takers and abstainers. Another study of 120 adults apparently did show faster reaction time in ginseng users. I ponder slowly . . . could this be meaningful?

*Diabetes.* Some small studies concluded that Asian and American ginseng improved glucose control in type 2 diabetics.

*Athletic performance.* Two small studies of highly trained athletes found an increase in athletic endurance, but another short study of American university athletes did not. These possible benefits don't apply if you don't exercise.

*Sexual performance.* According to the Chinese, ginseng helps men exercise their tumescent abilities and achieve erection.

The usual daily dose—and as noted, it's hard to know if you're getting this—is 100 mg of extract standardized to contain 4 to 7 percent ginsenosides (in divided doses), or 1 gram of crude herb. The little bit of ginseng you get in other supplements, teas, or drinks probably doesn't compensate for the energy you'd expend earning money to pay for them.

There have been some reports of abnormal vaginal bleeding and breast tenderness with use of ginseng. Blood tests have shown no effects on a woman's estrogen levels. Right now, we don't know what you're getting, and we don't know how it works. I would not suggest ginseng-ing. For long life and well-being, try a known "adaptagen": exercise.

### Goldenseal

Often patients say that they take goldenseal as their "natural antibiotic." But there's no good evidence that it strengthens the immune system in humans. Some studies show it improves the symptoms of diarrhea, but there are so many other ways to do this that I would not suggest this herb as a first-line diarrhea defense. High doses of goldenseal have been shown to elevate blood pressure and cause nausea and vomiting and even convulsions. It can also interfere with the anticoagulant heparin.

### Kava

Coming to us from the Pacific Islands, where it was used in beverages on relaxing social and ceremonial occasions, kava is a root that has been dried and ground into a powder for pills, capsules, extracts, and drinks. And although not specifically marketed as an anti-anxiety medication (because it has not been approved as such by the FDA), it has become a popular New Age "root" to calm and inner peace.

One kava study from Germany that looks quite convincing was done on 101 outpatients with clinically defined anxiety disorders. The treated group showed significant reduction in symptoms (compared with the placebo group) beginning at eight weeks, and continued to improve throughout the six-month study. Other studies have found a more rapid anti-anxiety effect. Kava seems to work by increasing the number of GABA receptors in the brain (see chapter 8).

The recommended dose of kava extract is no more than 300 mg a day, and German experts do not recommend its use for more than three months (although they found no evidence that it was addictive). Long-term use can cause a skin rash, and kava has been implicated in cases of liver failure. (As of this writing, at least eleven kava users have required liver transplants, leading several countries to restrict its use. The FDA has issued a consumer advisory.) It's not known whether the products sold in the United States have the same properties as those tested in Germany. And kava can be mind altering; there have been cases in the United States where motorists arrested for drunk driving were intoxicated on kava beverages, not alcohol.

### Red yeast rice

This yeast is fermented on rice, and contains substances that are present in statins—the drug of choice to lower "bad" cholesterol and decrease the risk of atherosclerosis and coronary vascular disease. A red yeast rice product marketed under the name Cholestin has been the focus of legal debate. The FDA said it was a drug and sought to regulate its use; the company that sold it protested, saying it was a "functional food." In 1999, a judge ordered the FDA to lift its ban on importing red yeast rice powder to produce this product.

The medicinal properties of this supplement have been given scientific credence: A study published in the *American Journal of Clinical Nutrition* found that red yeast rice lowered cholesterol 18 percent after eight weeks—but noted that it was not as effective as statin drugs. The dose that lowered LDL and triglycerides in past studies is 1.2 to 2.4 grams of powder daily.

The original Cholestin has been taken off the market and has now been replaced with—you guessed it—New Cholestin. Don't try this at home without monitoring your cholesterol levels and liver function. If your cholesterol profile remains abnormal after twelve weeks, stop supplementing around and get a prescription-strength statin—and certainly don't mix the two.

## St.-John's-wort (hypericum)

As an herbal remedy, St.-John's-wort is found everywhere these days, even in some juice drinks. It is the most commonly used antidepressant in Germany. A review of existing studies shows that this herb probably works better than a placebo for mild to moderate depression. (The American College of Physicians/American Society of Internal Medicine states that St.-John's-wort may be considered for short-term treatment of mild acute depression, as long as patients are cautioned that this treatment is not approved by the FDA.) However, a 2002 study published in *JAMA* found it completely ineffective for moderately severe depression.

One problem is that since the active ingredients in St.-John's-wort are still unknown, you can't be assured of an optimal dose. We do know that this herb affects an important metabolic pathway used by many common prescription drugs—including life-sustaining antirejection drugs taken by organ transplant recipients, and cancer chemotherapy drugs. Drugs for heart disease, seizures, and depression can also be affected. For these reasons, the FDA issued a consumer advisory on St.-John's-wort in 2000, and I'm issuing my own warning not to take St.-John's-wort casually, without medical supervision. (See chapter 8 for information on FDA-approved antidepressants.)

## Valerian

Can a traditional European herb provide better living through better sleeping? According to those who market valerian, it might be the answer to your dreams. There are more than two hundred plant species. The one that works is malodorous; it's called *Valeriana officinalis,* and is dried and processed as capsules, liquid extract, or tea.

Valerian does seem to create drowsiness; it's used in some European nonprescription sleep preparations. In small trials, subjects given valerian said they slept better with the herb than they did on placebo. But since this was not a "nose blind" study, they may have smelled the difference between the two. Another study showed that for patients with a history of insomnia, taking valerian nightly helped, but only after twenty-eight nights. We're not sure how valerian works, or if it's best to use it for occasional sleepless nights or more regularly to improve sleep. Unlike many prescription sleep aids, valerian has not been linked to any overdose deaths, seldom causes morning grogginess, and does not seem to create dependence (unless you fear you won't be able to sleep without it). The FDA put valerian on its "generally recognized as safe" (GRAS) list—but as a food. (I doubt this smelly root will become a popular salad ingredient.)

The usual dose for insomnia is 270 to 450 mg of valerian extract in solution, or a 600-mg capsule, taken thirty to sixty minutes before bedtime. Alcohol may compound valerian-induced drowsiness. Don't take valerian before you drive. (And—as noted with so many other meds—don't operate heavy machinery. I'm never quite sure what this means!)

## Yohimbe

There is a prescription drug called yohimbine that contains the bark of the yohimbe tree. It's been used, with questionable results, to treat erectile dysfunction in men but has now been overshadowed by the more potent Viagra and Levitra. Over-the-counter herbal yohimbe preparations often contain just trace amounts or no bark at all. When it comes to our female equivalent of erectile dysfunction—lack of arousal and lubrication—one small trial suggests that combining yohimbe and the amino acid arginine might help. But because the suggested dose can cause anxiety, insomnia, nausea, hypertension, and urinary frequency, I don't recommend it. There are prescription medications that are safer and work better (see chapter 2).

## Ephedra (ma huang)

Despite its long history as a Chinese medicine, this herb's bad press is well deserved. Ephedra has been widely marketed in this country for weight loss, energy boosting, and improved athletic performance. It contains amphetaminelike chemicals that powerfully stimulate the heart and nervous system and can cause irregular heartbeats, strokes, seizures, acute psychosis, heart attack, and death. More than 1,500 serious reactions related to ephedra have been reported to the FDA. A government-sponsored study by the RAND Corporation reviewed another fifteen thousand reports submitted by Metabolife in the summer of 2002, which included two deaths, four heart attacks, and nine strokes attributed solely to ephedra use. The 2003 death of Baltimore Orioles pitcher Steve Bechler, from multiple organ failure linked to his use of an ephedra weight-loss product, increased public awareness of the danger. Ephedra was banned in Canada, and finally after ongoing efforts at the state and federal levels (supported by the FDA and the American Medical Association) it has been banned in the United States.

## *Chinese Herbal Mixtures*

Most Chinese "natural" remedies contain at least several Asian herbs purported to work in sync to improve your health. A scientific look at even a handful of the thousands of combinations is beyond the scope of this book (and of my knowledge). But caution's in order before you purchase an imported compound or one locally made up by a Chinese herbal practitioner. A review by the British research group Bandolier of 2,600 herbal medicines sold in Taiwan found that 24 percent were adulterated with at least one synthetic medicine, including steroids, NSAIDs, anticonvulsants, and anti-anxiety and glucose-lowering medications. The California Department of Health reported that 32 percent of Asian patent medicines sold in the state contained heavy metals (lead, mercury, arsenic) or undeclared pharmaceuticals (Viagra, adrenal steroids, Xanax, fenfluramine, or the cancer-causing painkiller phenacetin).

This adulteration with the "real" stuff may be the reason that some of these preparations work. Because you don't know what your mixture might contain, you risk serious side effects from the product, especially when you add other drugs or medical conditions to that mix. (For example, deaths were reported in 2002 from Chinese herbal weight-loss

# Before Surgery

Where hat you, your surgeon, and your anesthesiologist should know:
Herbal supplements should be taken as seriously as prescription medications in terms of their side effects. Always let your doctor know what supplements you take, especially when you may have to undergo surgery. Many supplements—including garlic, ginseng, ginkgo, feverfew, fish oils, fenugreek, and licorice—can affect your risk of bleeding, leading to complications or the need for blood transfusions. When in doubt, it's safest to stop taking supplements two weeks before surgery. Here is specific information on some of the more popular herbal supplements:

| Herb | Possible side effects | Stop before surgery? |
|---|---|---|
| Echinacea | Suppressed immune system, delayed wound healing | Not known, but stop ASAP if facing organ transplant surgery or surgery that will affect liver function |
| Ephedra | Heart attack and stroke, hypertension, irregular heart rhythm, shock | At least 24 hours (remember, it's illegal!) |
| Garlic | Increased risk of bleeding, esp. if combined with anticoagulants | At least 7 days |
| Ginkgo | Increased risk of bleeding, esp. if combined with anticoagulants | At least 36 hours |
| Ginseng (Asian and American) | Low blood sugar, increased risk of bleeding, decreased effect of heparin | At least 7 days |
| Glucosamine and chondroitin | None known | Probably okay to continue |
| Kava | Oversedation | At least 24 hours |

| St.-John's-wort | Faster breakdown of other drugs, including heparin, steroids, tranquilizers, antihypertensives (calcium channel blockers), digoxin, and antirejection drugs (cyclosporine) | At least 5 days |
| Valerian | Oversedation; acute withdrawal symptoms if stopped suddenly; long-term use may increase required dose of anesthetic | No data; best if tapered slowly over several weeks |

(Adapted from M. Ang-Lee et al., *JAMA,* 11 July 2001.)

capsules containing fenfluramine.) Even if you tell your doctor the name on the bottle, you'll both just end up playing "guess what I'm taking"—a game that is unlikely to improve your health or medical care.

## "All Natural" Dangers

Since the 1994 Dietary Supplement Health and Education Act, we trust in God, country, and the supplement maker, who we assume sells a safe product and does not make misleading claims. Unless the product contains a new dietary ingredient, the manufacturer need not give notice to the Food and Drug Administration before putting it on store shelves. Once it's there, the burden is on the FDA to prove that this supplement is unsafe, before it can be restricted or banned. We need better regulations, but until then we consumers and doctors need to report supplement-related adverse effects to the FDA's Medwatch Program at 800-332-1088, or online at www.fda.gov/medwatch. Here are a few of the herbs that have been found unsafe (for everyone or for certain conditions):

| Herb | Purported uses | Dangers |
|------|----------------|---------|
| Belladonna | Digestive problems, asthma, muscle pain | Contains 3 toxic alkaloids; can cause death |
| Broom, foxglove, and other herbs containing digoxinlike substances | Low blood pressure, heart ailments | Heart damage, miscarriage; an overdose can kill |
| Comfrey | Bruises, cuts, indigestion, ulcers | Contains toxins linked to liver disease, cancer; death |
| Ephedra | Weight loss, boosting energy | Heart attack, stroke, unconsciousness, death |
| Garlic | Cholesterol reduction | Side effects in persons taking HIV drugs |
| Kava | Anxiety | Liver failure requiring organ transplant |
| Kombucha tea | AIDS, insomnia, acne | Liver damage, intestinal problems, death |
| Lobelia | Asthma; induce vomiting | Even 0.6 gram can cause irregular heartbeat, breathing problems; 4 grams is fatal |
| Pennyroyal | Indigestion; liver and gallbladder problems | Causes liver damage, miscarriage (even 1 tsp. of oil can cause paralysis; more can kill) |
| Sassafras | Stimulant | Contains a carcinogen banned from use in food |
| Skullcap | Tranquilizer | Can cause liver damage |
| St.-John's-wort | Depression | Organ rejection after transplant |

## A Final Word

When it comes to herbs, there are several things we as consumers want to know: Does this work? What's in it? Could it be harmful to my health? Can it be safely taken with medications? It takes a lot of experience, analysis, research, and testing before we can get those assurances. In the meantime, try not to be fooled by false advertising promises. The clerk at the health food store does *not* know how to guide your herbal or supplement choices, but she does know how to ring up the sale. Don't bet your money or health on her or his advice.

# 6

## *Disease Prevention and Detection for Longer, Better Life*

Nicole obsessed about her weight. She aggressively dieted and exercised from her teens through her forties. She thought dairy products would make her fat, and high-fiber foods caused bloat. I worried that Nicole had osteoporosis, but her bone density scan showed only mild bone loss. (The exercise must have helped.) Her greatest fear was breast cancer; her breasts had no subcutaneous fat, so she could feel every gland. She religiously scheduled an annual mammogram, demanding an ultrasound for every palpable lump.

When Nicole turned 50, I suggested she get her first colonoscopy. For the next seven years, she put it off. She even refused a take-home test to check for occult blood in the stool: "I'm not going to wipe feces on a card; how disgusting!"

At 57, she relented and had the colonoscopy. A four-inch cancerous tumor was found in her large bowel (colon). Miraculously, her lymph nodes were negative, and there were no signs that the cancer had metastasized. A portion of her colon was removed, and she was given a short course of chemotherapy.

Two years later, Nicole is clear of any recurrence. She comes to see me every few months, "Just to make sure everything else is okay." As she sits in my waiting room, Nicole preaches to all present on the importance of colonoscopy, and how she should have had one earlier. Her story has converted many of my more reluctant patients into colonoscopy believers.

At 42, Leah received the frightening diagnosis: stage I invasive breast cancer. She was treated with lumpectomy, radiation, and five years of tamoxifen therapy. She became my patient in her late forties, and diligently had repeat mammograms and physical exams.

Leah was of Ashkenazi (eastern European) Jewish descent. Her paternal aunt had succumbed to ovarian cancer, and her father had been diagnosed with prostate cancer. We discussed genetic testing, but she wasn't ready. After a friend died from breast cancer, Leah decided to be tested "just" for the three BRCA gene mutations more commonly found in Ashkenazi Jews. She tested positive for a BRCA 1 mutation.

I removed both of Leah's ovaries via laparascopic surgery; she went on to have a bilateral mastectomy and breast reconstruction. An early cancer was found in her "healthy" breast.

Shailaugh was 51 years old. She exercised, kept her weight down, didn't smoke. She hated doctors, and didn't believe she needed checkups except for the very occasional Pap smear and mammogram. Her mother had died of a stroke in her early sixties; her father, who smoked, drank heavily, and was overweight, died suddenly at the age of 45 from a heart attack.

Shailaugh reluctantly made an appointment to see me to discuss her bothersome hot flashes, and to get a long-overdue Pap smear. She was my first patient that morning, and she hadn't had breakfast. So, I persuaded her to let me draw her blood to check her cholesterol levels, CRP (C-reactive protein), fasting blood sugar, and TSH (thyroid stimulating hormone). Her cholesterol was over 300, with very high LDL and triglyceride levels. Her CRP was elevated. I referred her to a cardiologist, who not only started her on cholesterol-lowering statins, but performed an echo stress test (which Shailaugh failed), a thallium stress test (results abnormal), and subsequently an angiogram and angioplasty (coronary artery repair).

Shailaugh's Pap smear was normal, and I didn't give her hormone replacement therapy. But those hot flashes probably saved her life.

• • •

I could fill this chapter with patient stories such as these. Every time I see a woman whose quality and years of life have been changed because she paid attention to her risks and sought the right diagnostic test, I silently thank the thousands of physicians, scientists, and statisticians who conducted the myriad studies and published the reports that have built our medical safety net.

Most of us don't have the time, interest, or insurance coverage to run from specialist to specialist to check for every possible disorder. However, there are basic tests that every one of us should have, starting in our teens. You have to understand their purpose and how to prioritize them, based on which disease is most likely to speed your clock forward and shorten your life.

## WHAT WE DIE FROM

At the start of this century, the average life expectancy for American women at birth was 79.5 years. According to the most recent National Vital Statistics Report from the Centers for Disease Control, the leading causes of death for American women are:

- Diseases of the heart: 30 percent of deaths
- All cancers: 22 percent
- Stroke (cerebrovascular diseases): 8 percent
- Chronic lower respiratory diseases (not including lung cancer): 5 percent
- Diabetes; flu and pneumonia; Alzheimer's disease; and accidents: about 3 percent each

The overall statistics are interesting, but it's more compelling to find out what conditions might cause you, or other women in your age group, to die within the next decade:

## DEATHS PER THOUSAND AMERICAN WOMEN, BY AGE (NEVER-SMOKERS)

| Age | Heart attack | Stroke | Lung cancer | Breast cancer | Colon cancer | Cancer, ovaries | Cancer, cervix | Pneumonia | AIDS | Accidents |
|---|---|---|---|---|---|---|---|---|---|---|
| 40 | 1 | 1 | — | 2 | 1 | — | — | — | 2 | 2 |
| 45 | 2 | 1 | 1 | 4 | 1 | 1 | 1 | — | 1 | 2 |
| 50 | 4 | 2 | 2 | 5 | 2 | 1 | 1 | 1 | 1 | 2 |
| 55 | 7 | 2 | 3 | 6 | 3 | 2 | 1 | 1 | 1 | 2 |
| 60 | 14 | 4 | 5 | 7 | 4 | 3 | 1 | 2 | — | 2 |
| 65 | 30 | 10 | 7 | 9 | 6 | 3 | 1 | 4 | — | 3 |
| 70 | 52 | 19 | 10 | 10 | 8 | 4 | 1 | 7 | — | 5 |
| 75 | 90 | 36 | 11 | 11 | 11 | 4 | 1 | 15 | — | 7 |
| 80 | 153 | 62 | 11 | 12 | 14 | 4 | 1 | 30 | — | 11 |

(Adapted from Woloshin, Schwartz, and Welch, *Journal of the National Cancer Institute*, June 5, 2002.)

Wherever you are on this age spectrum, your odds of dying in the next ten years are greater if you smoke cigarettes. Among women who smoke, lung cancer is the leading cause of death from age 40 to age 75; after that, heart attack tops the list.

## WHAT DISABLES US

When we're talking about slowing down the clock, it's not just the amount of time we live but our quality of living. The chronic conditions that most limit activity for Americans include:

| Condition | Percent of all disabilities |
|---|---|
| Arthritis or rheumatism | 17 |
| Back or spine problems | 13.5 |
| Heart disease | 11 |
| Lung or respiratory problems | 7 |
| Hypertension | 5 |
| Diabetes | 4 |
| Stroke | 2.5 |

Contrary to general belief, cancer falls near the bottom of the list of disabling illnesses. As you'll see, many of these illnesses share common and *preventable* risk factors.

## OUR DISEASES: WHAT WE SHOULD KNOW

### Our Vulnerable Hearts

Most of us know what to do if a male over 40 has crushing chest pain that radiates to his left arm, or if he just clutches his chest and says, "Something's not right": We call the doctor, the paramedics, or drive straight to the emergency room. (The one time I did the latter for my husband, he was—thankfully—diagnosed with heartburn.) As we care for the men in our lives, we maintain a personal cardiac complacency; after all, we have ovarian estrogen that protects us in our forties. Men have heart attacks, and die from them, seven to ten years earlier than we do.

It's true that men develop heart disease at a younger age than women.

But we play rapid catch-up, and some of us with risk factors don't require any extra time to establish equality as cardiac casualties. Our female hearts are smaller and beat faster than those of men. The blood vessels feeding the heart, called *coronary arteries,* are also somewhat smaller. Small doesn't mean less competent, and for most of us this crucial organ works phenomenally throughout our reproductive lives.

As the beat goes on, our clocks advance and our ovarian follicles get used up; heart disease becomes our leading cause of death and illness. While the number of cardiovascular deaths in men has declined, the number in women is still rising.

Here are the disheartening statistics:

- More than 400,000 American women will suffer a heart attack this year.
- 35 percent of these heart attacks go unrecognized.
- 42 percent of women die within one year of a recognized heart attack, which is double the rate of men.
- One-third of women who've had a heart attack will have another within six years (versus one-fifth of men).
- The death rate from coronary vascular disease (CVD) in African-American women is 69 percent higher than in Caucasian American women.

To add injustice to injury, we women are less likely than men to receive timely, lifesaving diagnosis and therapy, including EKGs (electrocardiograms), stress testing, coronary catheterization (angiograms), angioplasty, clot-busting drug therapy, and bypass surgery. We are also less likely to be given medications that prevent a second heart attack, or to be referred to or complete a program of cardiac rehabilitation. Both patients and caregivers need to be aware of these stats, and not let old men's tales about our cardiac health impede our appropriate care.

Younger women *do* have heart attacks, and the younger they are, the worse the outcome. Women under the age of 65 are 50 percent more likely to die from a heart attack than men in the same age group. It's thought that a sudden spasm of a coronary vessel, the formation of a vessel-blocking clot, or an erosion (shearing off) of a piece of plaque is to blame—in contrast to the generalized narrowing of vessels we see in older heart attack victims.

While heart disease is the major killer of women, it is too often ignored. So I am expanding this section in protest. We have a lot of work to do, so let's put our hearts to it.

## Evaluating Your Risk of a "Broken" Heart

It's not hard to figure out if you are at risk. Look to your ancestors, your past and present uses and abuses of your body, and your weight and exercise level. Then, have your blood pressure checked, and have a prebreakfast blood sample drawn (see the list of tests below). Together, these will give you a very accurate picture of your cardiac risk—even before more specialized testing is done.

There are nearly three hundred risk factors for coronary heart disease, but the ones listed in the table below account for at least 80 percent of your risk prediction:

| Factor | Increased risk |
|---|---|
| Family history of early heart attack (earlier than age 55 in men, age 65 in women) | Six to seven times |
| Smoking | Five to six times. Even just 1 to 14 cigarettes a day triples your risk of a coronary event. This is twice the effect seen in men who smoke |
| Diabetes | Four times; twice that of men with diabetes |
| Inflammatory markers Elevated CRP (C-reactive protein) | At least four times, if elevated over 0.85 mg/dl |
| Elevated homocysteine (an amino acid) | Two times, if greater than 15.7 |
| Abnormal lipids/high cholesterol (low HDL, high LDL, or high triglycerides; 45 percent of women over 55 have abnormal lipid profiles) | |
| Total cholesterol | 2.4 times greater if over 267 |
| LDL | 2.4 times if greater than 156 mg/dl |
| Ratio of total cholesterol to HDL | 3.4 times if greater than 6.3 |
| Obesity Gaining 45 pounds between ages 25 and 50 | Three times greater |

| | |
|---|---|
| *Untreated hypertension* (One-third of white women and nearly half of black women in their fifties have high blood pressure.) | Two to three times greater, even if "just" 130/90. The risk goes up in direct correlation to the elevation of either *systolic* or *diastolic* pressure |
| *A sedentary lifestyle* (lack of exercise) | Two times greater |

To fine-tune your risk assessment, your doctor may run additional blood tests (half of all heart attacks occur in women who have normal cholesterol levels). These include a test for lipoprotein (a), which when elevated (greater than 329 mg/dl), increases risk by 30 percent. (Note: In the HERS I study, women with heart disease who had high lipoprotein (a) levels lowered this substance and their risk of heart attack when they took estrogen; see page 54.)

Most of us will find that we have at least one of these risk factors, and that the organ we so take for granted might indeed not grant our wish for longevity. But now that the cardiac research gender gap has been recognized, there have been huge advances in our cardiac care. The good news is that we have a battery of specific tests (listed in the following section) that can accurately diagnose coronary vascular disease. The bad news is that too few women get them.

**Specific cardiac testing**
If you are over 40 and have a male partner, and you both go to the same family physician or internist, your partner's "routine checkup" will invariably include an EKG (electrocardiogram) and a stress test (on a treadmill)—whereas you, the woman, will probably have neither, or at most a resting EKG. Lying down and having those electrodes put on your chest will allow your doctor to evaluate the electrical conduction of your heartbeat, but this may not be adequate to detect developing heart vessel blockage or heart attack.

A treadmill test would seem the logical next step, but it is falsely abnormal (a "false positive" result) in as many as half of the women who take it. For a more accurate assessment of your coronary arteries, your heart should be viewed before and after exercise with a cardiac ultrasound.

The most accurate assessment, particularly for those of us at high risk, is a *thallium exercise stress test,* in which blood flow to the heart is imaged with radio tracers injected into a vein. This requires a specialized medical team (often hospital based) and can be expensive. You'll probably need a

## Pay-per-Cardiac-View: EBCT

There is one more test whose popularity has been boosted by direct-to-the-heart consumer advertising: the electron-beam computerized tomography (EBCT), commonly called a "heart scan" or "coronary calcium scan." A rapid series of X rays of your heart are amassed on a computer, and a picture is built that shows whether, and to what extent, calcium (present in plaque) has been deposited in the arteries. It's quick, effortless (you don't even have to undress), and gives immediate visual results. You'll receive a picture showing the bad white stuff and a score grading it.

The EBCT is an out-of-pocket test that will set you back about $400. For the radiologists, it's a high-cash-flow (and no insurance woe) business, and scanning centers have proliferated at an astounding speed.

However, a cardiologist may point out that it's not just the presence of plaque that raises concern, it's the stability. Unstable plaque may shed pieces that travel to smaller vessels, where they can cause complete obstruction. Since heart attacks, especially in women, are often due to vessel spasm, sudden clot formation, local inflammation, or rupture of small, unstable plaques that have little or no calcification, the absence of calcium deposits is not a guarantee of future heart health. Even if your calcium score is low, you and your doctor should evaluate your other risk factors. So, if your score is high, don't panic; the plaque may be stable, but lipid and inflammatory marker testing is called for, and perhaps an echo or thallium stress test.

referral from a cardiologist to get this scheduled, *and* paid for by your insurance company (it can cost more than $1,000).

If abnormalities are found, you should be referred for an *angiogram,* in which dye is injected via a catheter inserted into a femoral (leg) vein, and threaded into the coronary vessels. This accurately measures obstruction, scarring, and the ability of vessels to feed the heart muscle with blood.

This test will be the final determinant of whether you need *angioplasty:* reopening and widening a narrowed vessel by inserting a catheter and inflating a tiny balloon. Once opened, a fine-mesh medicated tube (*stent*) may be inserted to keep it open. If this is not an option (or it fails), you may have to undergo open-heart surgery and a *coronary artery bypass graft* (CABG) to replace the diseased vessel with a healthy vein from another part of your body.

## Anything else? More facts about heart attack risk in women

If you've been diagnosed with polycystic ovarian syndrome, or have what's now called Syndrome X (or metabolic syndrome) with insulin resistance, abdominal obesity, hypertension, high blood sugar, and abnormal lipids—you are especially prone to coronary vascular disease. Overproduction of insulin resistance harms the lining of the blood vessels so they can't produce the nitric acid they need to expand and allow proper blood flow. One-third of all women develop insulin resistance, which frequently accompanies weight gain (see chapter 4).

How often have we heard the expression "This [add source of stress] will give me a heart attack"? Studies show that particular stresses do increase our heart attack risk. Women who feel they have little control over their work environment or who experience relationship problems at home are more likely to suffer a heart attack than their calmer sisters.

Incidentally one more test can demonstrate your personal risk for heart disease: a mammogram. Calcifications of the milk ducts (seen in at least 2 percent of women) seem to predict a nearly twofold increase in subsequent coronary heart disease. These are probably a sign of chronic inflammation—not just in the ducts, but also in vital heart vessels.

If you experience the symptoms of a heart attack (see below), you should get rapid medical attention; in fact, the American Heart Association (AHA) recommends calling the paramedics right away. Perhaps you've seen ads that claim you can save your life if you have symptoms of a heart attack and take an aspirin on the way to the hospital. (Actually, you should chew it for faster absorption.) The AHA recommends that you wait for directions from emergency personnel before taking an aspirin, as you might have an allergic reaction or a health problem that makes aspirin dangerous—or aspirin could interfere with other drugs

### Is This Indigestion, or a Heart Attack?

Our symptoms differ from the classic chest pains that signal a heart attack in men. They include:

Pain or pressure anywhere above the waist (chest, jaw, neck, shoulder) that occurs during exercise or even at rest. It need only last a few minutes, and often recurs.

At the same time, there may be:

Nausea, vomiting, fatigue, shortness of breath, and/or lightheadedness.

you're taking or might be given. Many cardiologists, however, disagree. An estimated five to ten thousand lives would be saved yearly if everyone chewed aspirin at the first sign of a heart attack. There is little to lose (except our hearts) and I go on record here: Chew two low-dose "baby" aspirin, or half of a regular aspirin, if you think you're having a heart attack.

Know that you or your family may have to demand your heart care. Emergency-room "door to needle" time for treatment of a heart attack in women has historically been longer than for men. There is a crucial sixty-minute window in which clot-busting medications and other treatments are most effective. Don't leave the E.R. or doctor's office without getting basic heart tests, such as an electrocardiogram (which shows similar changes in men and women during an acute or active heart attack) and blood tests for substances released when the heart is damaged.

## How to "Take Heart": Preventing Coronary Vascular Disease

It begins with your behavior. I can think of no other major disease where what you *do* can make such a positive difference in the outcome.

I hadn't seen Amy for ten years, since delivering her last child. She had gained 50 pounds and was smoking, and her only exercise was turning the steering wheel of her car. She greeted me with a guilty smile. "I haven't had time for checkups, but I'm finally here. So run all your tests, and make sure I'm all right."

She wasn't. Her cholesterol, inflammatory markers, and blood pressure were all high. Amy's response? She "might cut down" on her smoking, but eating was one of her "joys in life." And she was much too busy with her job and family to exercise.

Exasperated, I referred Amy to our hospital weight loss program and strongly suggested she see an internist who would do cardiac testing (including an echo stress test) and prescribe appropriate medications. It's been a year; so far, she hasn't come back. Unless Amy changes her behavior, she may become a "30% female mortality from heart disease" statistic.

So many of my patients tell me they know what they should do, but just can't commit to doing it. They are somehow unwilling to make or sustain changes. "Medical enforcement" is not constitutional, and there's no law against committing self-body wrecking. "I told you so" gives doctors no satisfaction, and hearing "If only I had . . ." leaves only sadness. So please, take the time to extend your time and become responsible for your heart. Let's keep "Achy-Breaky Heart" the title of a song, and not an epitaph. . . .

### Things you can do on your own

Here's how you can get an "A" for effort:

*Stop smoking.* This may be the single most important thing you can do for your heart. The thousands (yes, thousands) of chemicals in cigarette smoke diminish the oxygen content in your blood, damage the lining of blood vessels, make blood platelets stickier, increase clotting and inflammatory factors, and raise LDL and lower HDL. (Note: When this affects your heart, it's called cardiovascular disease. When it affects your brain, it leads to cerebrovascular accident [CVA], or stroke.)

Just one to four cigarettes a day doubles your risk of coronary artery disease. For women under 50, most coronary heart disease can be traced to smoking alone. A cigarette may look elegantly white and slim, but it makes your arteries thick, yellow, and blocked.

It's never too late to quit. The benefit to your heart is immediate, and you can reduce your risk of heart attack to nearly that of a nonsmoker in five years. For thoughts on how to quit for good (in both senses of that word), see page 256.

*Exercise.* The latest recommendations from the Institute of Medicine call for an hour of exercise a day, but don't feel that it's this or nothing. Thirty minutes a day of brisk walking has been shown to dramatically decrease heart attacks in women. If you want a measure of success, other than your watch or the treadmill timer, here's another worthy statistic: Walking just ten blocks a day will decrease your risk of a heart attack by one-third!

*Control your weight.* Losing just 10 percent of your body weight can have a much more weighty effect on your blood pressure, lipid levels, insulin levels, heart load, and risk of developing heart disease. (See chapter 4 for more on weight loss.)

*Eat right (or at least better).* Lower your intake of total fat to between 10 and 30 percent. (There are huge debates over this figure. I generally tell moderately high-risk patients to aim for 25 percent.) It's probably more important to change the *type* of fat than the total amount. Limit saturated fat from meat and dairy products. Avoid trans fats (partially hydrogenated fats), often found in commercial baked goods and in solid margarines. Go for the good, unsaturated fats found in cold-water fish (such as tuna and salmon), olive oil, canola oil, nuts, and avocados. Make fruits, vegetables, and whole grains the major source of your calories. A recent Canadian study found that a high-fiber vegetarian diet heavy in soy, almonds, oats, barley, legumes, eggplant, and okra dramatically reduced cholesterol levels. Simple starches (the white stuff: breads, cookies, cake, potatoes, white rice) should no longer be the mainstay of your diet.

## A Joint Venture: Things You Can Do with Your Doctor's Help

### Cholesterol-lowering medications

*Statins (Lescor, Lipitor, Mevacor, Pravachol, Zocor).* Statins inhibit the last step in the production of cholesterol, and can lower total cholesterol, raise HDL, and lower LDL and triglycerides. They also decrease some inflammatory markers and act as plaque stabilizers, preventing the dislodging of plaque as well as additional plaque formation. These medications can lower your risk of heart attack and stroke by 30 to 40 percent. Statin therapy is recommended if:

- You have had a heart attack or have documented coronary vascular disease—even if your cholesterol levels are normal. (The aim is to lower your LDL to below 100 mg/dl.)
- You have diabetes or other serious risk factors for coronary vascular disease, and your LDL is greater than 130 mg/dl, HDL is less than 45 mg/dl, or triglycerides are over 150 mg/dl.
- You don't yet have known coronary vascular disease (CVD), but your lipid levels are abnormal and did not improve after three to six months of diet and exercise. Begin statin therapy if your LDL is greater than 130 mg/dl (even if your HDL is normal). In the past, we thought that as long as your HDL was good (greater than 60 mg/dl), we didn't have to worry about the LDL. But as you get older, or if you have risk factors, it is now recommended that LDL be brought down with statins.
- Your triglycerides are greater than 200 mg/dl. In women, high triglycerides are considered an independent risk for CVD, increasing risk of a heart attack by 37 percent compared with just 14 percent in men.

When Miranda, a 58-year-old patient with a strong family history of heart disease, was informed that her high LDL and low HDL needed to be treated with a statin, she balked. "It will damage my liver!" I had to use all my powers of persuasion to assure her that we would not sacrifice her liver for her heart. Liver damage occurs in less than 1 percent of patients taking a statin, is usually mild, and goes away quickly once the medication is discontinued. Lipid management may save more lives than angioplasties and coronary bypass surgery—and with a lot less pain and effort.

Statins can also cause pain and inflammation in muscles. Once you begin therapy, liver function and muscle enzyme levels should be checked within three to six months, and repeated every six to twelve months thereafter. If you do develop generalized muscle pain, report this to your doctor.

The cost of the medication may also cause you to skip a beat. This, too, should be discussed with your physician. Some statins will be more readily covered by your insurance company, and some pharmaceutical companies have reduced-cost programs for patients who lack drug coverage.

*Fibrates (Gemfibrozil).* This potent triglyceride-lowering medication may be added to your therapy if you have CVD and statins have not sufficiently lowered your triglycerides, or if you have a genetic disorder causing very high triglyceride levels (over 400 mg/dl).

*Nicotinic acid (niacin).* This type of vitamin B can lower total cholesterol, LDL, and triglycerides, and raise HDL, but is hard to take long-term due to side effects such as flushing (not welcome if you're having menopausal symptoms!), itching, and nausea; the long-acting forms may be more tolerable. Nicotinic acid is often added to a statin or fibrates if they don't sufficiently lower triglycerides or raise HDL. Even though nicotinic acid is available without a prescription, it's definitely not wise to self-prescribe off-the-shelf doses. Use this *only* under a doctor's supervision.

*Antihypertensive medications* (also see page 243). You and your doctor should aim low—at or under a blood pressure of 120/80—and use whatever meds will get you there, beginning with *diuretics* (which, in women over 60, can reduce chances of dying from CVD by 25 percent) and proceeding to *beta blockers* (Tenormin, Toprol, Inderal), and *ACE inhibitors* (Lotensin, Capoten, Vasotec, Monopril, Prinivil, Zestril, Univasc, Accupril, Altace). This last group of medications not only do an excellent job in helping blood vessels relax and dilate, but also seem to save more lives from CVD than expected solely from their blood-pressure-lowering capability.

*Blood-sugar-lowering medications.* Oral medications that lower glucose output by the liver and increase insulin sensitivity (so that your body doesn't need to produce large amounts of insulin in order to control blood sugar levels) may also improve your lipid profile, and prevent plaque formation and CVD. These include Glucophage, Avandia, and Actos.

Too little insulin causes glucose levels to become high, so we develop diabetes; too much insulin causes triglycerides and LDL to increase and reduces the production of nitric acid (which helps vessels relax and fights inflammation). With age, insulin insensitivity—usually linked to or caused by obesity—occurs in up to 33 percent of women and ultimately may lead to type 2 or late-onset diabetes, but even if that doesn't occur, years of insulin insult contribute to CVD.

Lowering insulin is good for the heart, but if you develop type 2 diabetes (see page 249), you may need to take insulin. In that case, maintaining normal glucose levels will help prevent blood vessel damage in all your tissues, including your heart.

### No doctor's prescription needed

*Vitamin E.* There was some initial hope, based on the Harvard Nurses' Health Study, that vitamin E (over 100 IU daily) would reduce the risk of cardiovascular disease by soaking up the marauding free radical molecules that form as your body metabolizes oxygen. These radicals' goal is to take back electrons lost during oxidation; in so doing, they oxidize LDL and promote atherosclerosis. But other large observational studies have not shown substantial benefit, other than that eating foods (such as nuts, vegetable oils, and leafy greens) with high levels of antioxidants is better than not eating them. Also, since vitamin E increases bleeding risk, I don't recommend a dose higher than that found in a multivitamin for women who are hypertensive and at risk for stroke.

*Folic acid.* This will bring down homocysteine levels. Unless your levels are higher than normal, the 400 mcg found in most multivitamins should suffice. Your multivitamin should also contain $B_6$, which appears to work in concert with folic acid to reduce homocysteine levels. If you're homocysteine challenged, you may need doses of 1 mg or more, but this should be initiated by your doctor.

*Aspirin.* A famous 1983 Harvard study of physicians showed that men could decrease future risk of heart attack by as much as 44 percent with use of aspirin (a standard dose of 325 mg every other day). Our own study (of nurses) found that taking one to seven aspirin tablets a week decreased the risk of heart attack by 32 percent. Aspirin decreases the stickiness of platelets, so clots can't begin to form.

The American College of Chest Physicians has recommended that all women over 50 who have one or more cardiovascular risk factors take one low-dose or "baby" aspirin per day. The FDA recommends this only if you've had a previous heart attack angina, or have undergone coronary vessel surgery (angioplasty or bypass). If you've had a history of ulcers or bleeding problems, or are taking anticoagulation therapy, or have an aspirin allergy, you probably are not a candidate for preventive aspirin therapy.

## Hypertension: What's Pressing About Blood Pressure?

When that cuff is inflated on your arm, it's measuring two blood pressures. The first one (*systolic*) is created as blood is actively pumped through the artery by your heart; the second, or lower, number (*diastolic*) represents the resting pressure in the artery, between heartbeats. Your optimal blood pressure will be less than 120/80 mm Hg. You are "prehypertensive" if you are between 120 and 139 and 80 and 89, and "hypertensive" once pressure climbs to 140/90 and above.

Blood pressure readings represent the rigidity of your vessels. Their ability to allow free and easy blood flow diminishes when narrowed by plaque (atherosclerosis) or with generalized thickening and loss of elasticity (arteriosclerosis)—meaning your heart has to pump harder to force blood out to your body. This "excessive use of force" can damage the arterial walls, causing them to rupture. In the brain, that's a stroke; in a major vessel such as the aorta, a ruptured aneurysm. Either can be fatal.

Narrowed, uneven vessels also create turbulent blood flow that bruises blood cells, which then tend to clump together and form clots.

As the heart tries harder to pump blood through unyielding, narrow vessels, its pumping chamber (left ventricle) often thickens (*hypertrophy*). Extra pounds create an even greater demand for blood. It's easy to see why this can lead to heart failure, causing fluids to back up into the lungs and other tissues. Add cigarette smoke, which promotes vessel spasm and plaque buildup, and it's a wonder that blood gets to where it should be at all.

Nine out of ten women in their midfifties already have, or will develop, high blood pressure. A third of them don't know they are hypertensive; there are few, if any, symptoms until an organ fails. (If your blood pressure's not measured yearly, you'll lose valuable time in which to battle the consequences of this silent disorder.) Only a fifth of women get adequate treatment—"adequate" being defined as bringing blood pressure below 140/90, or 130/80 with diabetes or kidney disease.

## De-pressing the Pressure

There is a myth that a high systolic number represents "stress," whereas a high diastolic value measures "disease." We now know that an increase in systolic pressure can represent *more* future damage than an increase in diastolic levels, and should be closely monitored and treated, especially in older women. Today, when doctors treat hypertension, we gear the therapy toward reducing the systolic pressure, knowing that the diastolic will follow.

Most of us are destined to become hypertensive. But you are twice as likely to reach this destiny if you are prehypertensive. You can make lifestyle changes before those numbers go up, and cut your risk of sickness and death:

- *Stop smoking.*
- *Get regular exercise* that increases your heart rate. The ideal is to work up to a thirty- to forty-five-minute session on most days of the week. Start slowly (walk ten minutes a day) and monitor your pressure with a home blood pressure cuff (available at your local pharmacy) and at the doctor's office. (See chapter 3 for more.) Avoid weight-resistance exercises (such as lifting weights) until your blood pressure is under control.
- *Lose weight* if you're overweight. For every 22 pounds of weight lost, you can reduce your systolic pressure by as much as 20 mm Hg.
- *Reduce your salt intake.* Some of us (especially those of African heritage) are particularly salt sensitive; just cutting back on salt will lower blood pressure in one-third of women with hypertension. The recommendation is to consume no more than 2.4 grams of sodium or 6 grams of salt per day; labels on food packages should list the sodium content.
- *Eat right.* The low-sodium DASH diet—Dietary Approaches to Stop Hypertension—may be right for you. It's rich in fruit, vegetables, and low-fat dairy products, with reduced saturated fat and total fat. DASH can reduce systolic blood pressure by 8 to 14 mm Hg, which is equivalent to the effect of most single forms of drug therapy. (There is a very

clear and useful brochure about DASH-ing at the National Heart, Lung, and Blood Institute Web site, http://www.nhlbi.nih.gov.)

- *Limit alcohol* . . . no more than one drink per day. Why? Alcohol can cause blood vessels to constrict.
- *Take prescribed medications faithfully.* Hypertension does not respond to a short-term fix; you will probably need to take your medication for the rest of your life. Antihypertensive therapy, when given in correct amounts and combinations that lower your blood pressure to less than 140/90, will reduce your risk of stroke by as much as 40 percent, of heart attack by 25 percent, and of heart failure by more than 50 percent. It's likely you will need at least two antihypertensive medications to reach your blood pressure goal.

Your doctor may prescribe one or more of the following for you:

*Diuretics.* These work by reducing the volume of fluid your heart has to pump, and can decrease heart attacks in older women by 25 percent. A landmark 2002 study found that inexpensive diuretics work just as well as ACE inhibitors and calcium channel blockers (see below) to prevent heart attacks, with added protection against heart failure and strokes—and minimal side effects.

*Beta blockers.* If you have CVD, beta blockers will slow your heart and increase the force of its contractions. When combined with a diuretic, they help prevent strokes and, to a lesser extent, heart attacks.

*ACE inhibitors (angiotensin converting enzyme).* If you have diabetes, high systolic pressure, and/or CVD, this type of drug may be most effective. ACE inhibitors work by reducing your kidneys' production of angiotensin, a hormone that constricts arteries.

*ARBs (angiotensin receptor blockers).* These are an alternative to ACE inhibitors for those who have problems with side effects such as a cough or rash. ARBs have been shown to help prevent strokes.

*Calcium channel blockers.* These relax blood vessels and decrease risk of stroke, but may increase the risk of heart failure. (I'm sorry that this is so complicated; this is why God created cardiac specialists.)

- *Measure for yourself.* Get a home blood pressure monitor (it can be the digital kind but should have an arm cuff). Check your blood pressure at rest and after physical or stressful activities, and note your blood pressure variations throughout the day, to help you and your doctor monitor your response to therapy. If your average BP at home is 135/85, you are considered hypertensive.

- *Reduce your stress level.* Relax, relax, relax. . . . Try yoga or meditation. For many of us, a warm bath accompanied by soothing music and candlelight is a wonderful de-stressing ritual.

## Stroke

After heart disease and cancer, stroke is the most common cause of death for American women. Most strokes (80 percent) are caused by blocked blood flow to the brain, subsequent lack of oxygen (*ischemia*), and irreversible damage to brain tissue. The other 20 percent of what we call CVAs (*cerebrovascular accidents*) are caused by bleeding (*hemorrhage*) in the brain, due to a leaking or ruptured vessel.

### When time runs out for your brain

Our brains are sometimes smarter than we are, and issue warning signs before a disabling or deadly stroke occurs. Temporary episodes of diminished blood flow to the brain (called *transient ischemic attacks,* or TIAs) cause the following symptoms that come and go:

- A sudden feeling of numbness or tingling
- Muscle weakness or paralysis
- Difficulty finding the right words or pronouncing them
- Disorientation or confusion
- Sudden memory loss
- Double vision or gaps in vision
- Lack of coordination or feeling unsteady on your feet

The fact that these go away is false comfort, you must seek immediate medical attention. Even small brain accidents can cause permanent memory deficits. Your life depends on where and how much of your brain is damaged. Rapid recognition and treatment of prestroke and stroke symptoms can limit this damage. Your health and independence are also at stake. A stroke can affect your ability to remember, speak, read, or understand what people are saying; to move your arms or legs; and to feel and express emotions. This is no time to "wait and see"; clot-busting medication works best if given within three hours of the onset of a stroke. Procrastination can be disabling or deadly.

## Preventing "brain attacks"

The same "insults" that cause CVD (coronary vascular disease) also cause CVAs. Treating and/or eliminating these can reduce your risk of stroke:

- *Smoking.* If you quit now, within five years your extra risk is gone.
- *Hypertension.* Controlling your blood pressure can cut stroke risk in half.
- *Lipid abnormalities.* Studies suggest that cholesterol-lowering drugs can reduce the risk of stroke by one-third.
- *Diabetes.* Treating prediabetes and insulin resistance (see page 246 ) may decrease stroke risk. (Once you have overt diabetes, we're not sure if controlling blood sugar reduces your risk.) .
- *Obesity.* Losing weight lowers your blood pressure, which decreases your stroke risk.
- *Atrial fibrillation.* This very common form of irregular, rapid heartbeat (cardiac arrhythmia) causes the heart valves to quiver, which promotes clot formation. These solidified pieces can travel to the brain, where they clog small vessels. The symptoms of atrial fibrillation include palpitations (they feel like hiccups in your chest), dizziness, chest discomfort, shortness of breath, and/or fatigue. Your pulse may feel fast and irregular. This condition causes a sixfold increase in your risk of stroke, and accounts for a third of all strokes in women over age 80. If heart medications can't control the fibrillation, an anticoagulant or blood-thinning drug (usually Coumadin) should be prescribed; this decreases stroke risk from this disorder by two-thirds.
- *Carotid atherosclerosis (carotid artery blockage).* If plaque blocks more than 60 percent of the major vessel supplying blood to your brain, there is a significant risk that the resulting turbulent blood flow will create clots and strokes. This uneven flow can be heard through a stethoscope placed on your neck, and is known as a *carotid bruit.* (After age 50, during your annual physical, your doctor should be listening to your neck as well as your heart.) If your neck sounds suspicious, an ultrasound exam can reveal the degree of blockage. You may be a candidate for a plaque-removing surgical procedure called *carotid endartrectomy,* which can cut your risk of future stroke in half.
- *Heart attack.* This is the ultimate sign of clogged arteries. The risk of stroke is greatest during or immediately after a heart attack. Anticoagulant drugs given to treat the heart attack can prevent an added "brain attack."

In sum, all of the behavioral changes I listed for prevention of heart attack will help prevent stroke. If you've had TIAs (and don't take other anticoagulants or have bleeding tendencies), it's a good idea to take a daily low-dose aspirin.

## Insulin Resistance (Prediabetes)

One in three women has a condition that predisposes her to develop diabetes, heart attack, and stroke, but most have never even heard of it. Our twenty-first-century fat epidemic is creating an epidemic of *insulin resistance*. There is much you can do to stave off the initial disorder and the subsequent complications—but you and your doctor must become insulin-excess vigilantes, so that the diagnosis can be made and therapy initiated as early as possible.

### What is insulin resistance?

This condition happens when tissues stop responding as they should to insulin produced by the pancreas. For your body—especially your brain—to function normally, blood levels of glucose (sugar) must be kept fairly constant. As your glucose level rises after you eat, insulin is secreted to promote cell uptake of this "fuel." If blood glucose falls too low, other hormones help your body produce and release glucose to the bloodstream. Plummeting glucose levels can cause seizures, coma, or even death.

On the other hand, if blood sugar levels are too high, your body copes by making you thirsty; drinking fluids dilutes the sugar and helps your kidneys remove it through urination. High blood sugar promotes frequent yeast and bladder infections, and over time, can cause blindness, kidney failure, arteriosclerosis, heart disease, stroke, and nerve damage. Clearly, your body requires a critically tight glucose framework.

Here is how insulin resistance promotes disease. As tissues become less sensitive to insulin, your pancreas churns out extra insulin to take care of excess blood sugar. As long as this tactic works, you will not become diabetic. But eventually the overworked pancreas gives out and stops producing enough insulin to keep blood sugar down. Levels rise and stay up. You have developed type 2 diabetes.

This transition from insulin resistance to type 2 diabetes may take a decade, but during this "prediabetic" span of time, your body is already suffering damage from insulin overload. Excess insulin causes increased production of triglycerides (an especially dangerous risk factor for heart disease in women), and encourages abdominal fat accumulation, which in turn promotes insulin resistance, creating a vicious cycle. Insulin also promotes oxidation, inflammatory changes, and damage inside blood vessels, so that plaque is deposited and atherosclerosis develops. Even worse, insulin resistance and obesity often occur together with hypertension, culminating in extraordinary risk for heart attack and stroke. This combination has rated an equally hard-core name: Syndrome X (or metabolic syndrome).

**Are you becoming resistant?**
The more of these factors you have, the greater your risk for insulin resistance:

- You are overweight, i.e., your body mass index (BMI) is 25 or greater, your waist measures over 35 inches, or you developed obesity in childhood or adolescence.
- You are sedentary.
- You are over age 40.
- You are non-Caucasian (Latino/Hispanic, African American, Native American, Asian, Pacific Islander).
- You have a family history of type 2 diabetes, hypertension, or heart disease.
- You have a history of gestational diabetes or gave birth to a baby weighing more than 9 pounds.
- You have been diagnosed with hypertension, high triglycerides/low HDL, or coronary vascular disease.
- You've had polycystic ovarian syndrome (see page 9).

While genetics play a role here, there is no question that becoming overweight or obese is correlated with insulin insensitivity—and probably causes it. Presenting the body with too much food, especially the quick-release glucose from carbohydrates, causes insulin highs and subsequent lows that make tissues less sensitive to the effect of insulin.

**How is the diagnosis made?**
Your doctor should inquire about your family history of disease and obesity, and your personal medical history (including irregular periods, weight gain, infertility, pregnancies, and related issues). She or he should

perform a thorough physical exam, and order blood tests. Insulin testing is not routine and requires special labs, but other tests can help your doctor determine if this syndrome is present. These include a *fasting blood glucose test* (no food for twelve hours beforehand), and an *oral glucose tolerance test* (OGTT), where blood is drawn two hours after ingesting a special sugar drink containing 75 grams of glucose. The tests indicate insulin resistance if:

- Fasting glucose is 110 to 125 milligrams/dl
- Blood glucose is 140 to 199 mg/dl two hours post–sugar drink

Additional tests, which help confirm the diagnosis, include:

- High triglyceride level: greater than 150 milligrams/dl
- Low HDL: lower than 50 milligrams/dl
- High blood pressure: greater than 130/80

If your doctor simply says you have "borderline diabetes," ask for your exact blood sugar and lipid level results. (In the past, insulin resistance was seen as no big deal, or even considered normal, and not all doctors are aware of the latest research and treatment guidelines.) If you have or are at risk for insulin resistance syndrome, you should have your glucose levels retested every year.

## Can insulin resistance be treated?

Yes! You can vastly improve insulin sensitivity by *losing just 7 percent of your body weight*. A recent study of high-risk patients found that thirty minutes a day of walking and a loss of 10 to 15 pounds reduced their odds of developing diabetes by nearly 60 percent.

You should also limit foods that have a high glycemic index. This index is derived by comparing the amounts of glucose released to the bloodstream by various foods with the effects of eating pure glucose or sugar. (Note that it won't precisely predict the amount of glucose released during a particular meal; this varies depending on what foods are eaten together and how much of a food you eat.)

My rule of thumb (or sugar) is that the more processed the food, the whiter it is, and the more sugar it contains, the worse it is for insulin levels. So, cut way back on the white bread, white rice, sugar, and potatoes. Go for the complex starches and carbohydrates: whole grains (oatmeal, stone-ground breads), fruits, and vegetables—and control portion size and calories to lose weight.

Adding nuts and/or peanut butter to your diet may also help prevent the transition from insulin resistance to type 2 diabetes. Since nuts are calorie-dense foods, you should make calorie room for them by cutting down on saturated fats and sugary carbs.

Third, *add exercise to your schedule.* It burns calories, lowers insulin levels and blood pressure, and raises HDL cholesterol levels.

Finally, some women will benefit from *medications* that lower glucose output by the liver and intestine, and enhance the action of insulin. These include Glucophage (metformin), Avandia and Actos (glitazones), and Xenical.

However, to prevent the near-inevitable development of cardiovascular disease, you must go on to treat the other components of metabolic syndrome: the high triglycerides with lipid-lowering drugs (statins), and the high blood pressure with antihypertension medications. Evidence suggests that coronary vascular disease develops early with insulin resistance, so you should also have a stress echocardiogram and/or a thallium stress test to assess your heart.

## TYPE 2 DIABETES: THE FINAL EPISODE

### Sheila's Story

Sheila sat on my exam table wearing the standard cotton gown, which she could not manage to close. She greeted me with a sigh: "It finally happened. I'm diabetic."

Sheila was 50 years old and the comptroller for a clothing manufacturer. She noticed that her attention was flagging during business meetings, and that she felt more tired and irritable than usual. She assumed all this was due to perimenopause, but when her internist checked her blood sugar, it was 140 mg/dl before breakfast and rose to 260 after eating.

Sheila weighed 210 pounds, and her BMI was 38. She began her rise toward obesity in her teens. She tried fad diets, but neither they nor exercise fit into her lifestyle, and she surrendered to creeping weight gain. The diagnosis of type 2 diabetes did what years of physician coaxing had failed to do. She was ready to take her weight and risk factors seriously. Sheila started an exercise program, a diabetic diet, and an oral hypoglycemic medication. Since her lipids were abnormal, she began taking a statin. Her mildly elevated blood pressure, which she'd ignored in the past ("Oh, it's just stress"), was treated with a diuretic. She was also given Xenical to help her lose weight.

Her blood sugar is now below 120 throughout the day, and so far her echo stress test looks fine. She sees her internist every few months to monitor her condition.

### The arrival of type 2 diabetes

After years, if not decades, of insulin resistance, "late onset" diabetes finally appears as the pancreas exhausts its ability to keep up with the body's incessant, growing (literally, as weight increases) demand for insulin. Type 2 diabetes need not be heralded by a sudden change in symptoms; the decline can happen gradually. Look out for:

- frequent need to urinate
- unusual thirst or hunger
- unexplained fatigue or weight loss
- irritability
- blurry vision
- tingling or numbness in your hands or feet
- bouts of bladder, gum, vaginal, or skin infections, or
- wounds that won't heal

You officially have type 2 diabetes if your fasting blood glucose is greater than 125 mg/dl (or if your blood glucose measures 200 mg/dl or higher with an oral glucose tolerance test).

### Managing Diabetes

The only way to prevent or reverse some of the direct outcomes of diabetes is by aggressively controlling blood glucose, keeping it between 90 and 130 mg/dl when fasting, and making sure that levels never go higher than 180 mg/dl after eating. Avoid "instant" glucose foods that have a high glycemic index, and embrace the healthy complex carbs found in vegetables, fruits, and whole grains. (I was amazed to learn that the average adult American consumes 158 pounds of refined sugar a year, and

## Diabetes Statistics That Aren't Sweet

- Nearly one in five adult Americans will develop type 2 diabetes.
- Typically, there's a four- to seven-year delay between onset of the disease and its diagnosis.
- Once the diagnosis is made, 20 percent of people already show evidence of damage to their vascular and nervous systems.
- Type 2 diabetes is the primary cause of kidney failure, limb amputation, and new-onset blindness, and it is a major cause of heart disease and stroke. Diabetic women are more likely to develop heart disease and die of diabetes-related heart attacks than diabetic men: 70 percent of women with type 2 diabetes will die of cardiovascular disease.
- These complications make diabetes the fourth most common cause of death.

that sugar intake increased by 25 percent over the last three decades!) In fact, a diabetic meal plan is not so different from what I propose to keep bodies healthy and slow our clocks down (see chapter 4).

### Managing diabetes with medications

With weight loss, careful eating, and regular exercise, it may be possible to manage your diabetes without medication. If not, there are four types of oral medications that can be used separately, together, or with insulin.

*Metformin, or biguanide* (Glucophage, Glucophage XR, Glucovance). These drugs suppress liver production and release of glucose, lower blood fat levels, and may help curb appetite. Their effectiveness often wears off within five years, after which most women either need to change to a different medication or add new ones.

*Sulfonylureas* (Glucotrol, Diabeta, Amaryl). These older medications increase insulin secretion, which helps lower blood sugar. However, higher levels of insulin can cause weight gain.

*Alpha-glucosidase inhibitors* (Precose, Glyset). These "starch blockers" slow down carbohydrate digestion in the small intestine, moderating glucose entry into the bloodstream, so there's less need for insulin. They are often used to support the work of other diabetic medications.

*Glitazones or thiazolidinediones* (Avandia, Actos). These improve tissue sensitivity to insulin, increase the uptake of glucose by muscle and fat cells, and lower production and release of glucose from the liver. Again, these are most often used in combination with other drugs (Avandamet handily combines metformin and Avandia into one dual-action pill). As the glucose is picked up and used by your tissues, weight gain can occur.

### The next step: Insulin injections

This is the ultimate "replace what's missing" medication. The higher the dose, the more it forces blood glucose levels down. Since insulin "feeds" glucose to the tissues and increases fat production, it can cause weight gain, but a reduced dose won't adequately control the effects of this disease. Too much insulin causes dangerously low glucose levels (*hypoglycemia*). Constant vigilance is therefore required to balance food, physical activity, state of health, insulin injections, and glucose monitoring. Many diabetics require combinations of rapid, intermediate, and long-acting insulin. Some of my patients have successfully maintained tight glucose control with an insulin pump. The size of a pack of cards or a pager, the pump contains a supply of insulin that enters the body through thin tubing connected to a disposable device attached to the skin. This painlessly injects very small measured amounts of insulin according to programmed instructions.

## CANCER

Our mothers and grandmothers whispered the "C" word with fear and even shame. We're no longer lowering our voices; we're shouting for improved detection and treatment of women's cancers! The latest estimates are that nearly 650,000 American women will be diagnosed with invasive cancer in the next year, and close to 270,000 will die from it. Our overall probability of developing cancer (38.3 percent) is lower than that of men (43.5 percent); however, we're more likely than men to receive this diagnosis before the age of 60.

Like most women, when you hear the word "cancer" you probably think "breast." While this is our most *common* cancer, diagnosed in over 200,000 women per year, it will kill fewer women (40,000) than will lung cancer (over 67,000). In the following sections, I'll cover the most prevalent malignancies, and the ways you can help prevent these cancers—or detect them early enough so they're less likely to steal years from your life.

Space, time, and the limitations of my own expertise (I'm not an oncologist) preclude an in-depth look at the very complicated development and progression of each type of cancer. There are many new therapies that can slow or counteract malignancies. If you receive a cancer diagnosis, immediately consult a qualified, specialized physician and get information from reputable cancer institutes. Millions of women have been able to live long, healthy lives despite this disease.

## Numbers Speak Louder Than Fears

The most common cancers aren't necessarily the most deadly ones. Here are figures from the American Cancer Society:

### ESTIMATED NEW CASES OF CANCER IN WOMEN (2002)

| Type of cancer | New cases (incidence) | Deaths (as a percentage of all cancers) |
|---|---|---|
| Breast | 31 percent | 15 percent |
| Lung and bronchus | 12 percent | 25 percent |
| Colon and rectum | 12 percent | 11 percent |
| Uterus (endometrial) | 6 percent | 2 percent |
| Non-Hodgkin's lymphoma | 4 percent | 4 percent |
| Melanoma (skin) | 4 percent | — |
| Ovary | 4 percent | 5 percent |
| Pancreas | 2 percent | 6 percent |
| Thyroid | 2 percent | — |
| Urinary bladder | 2 percent | — |
| Leukemia | — | 4 percent |
| Brain | — | 2 percent |
| Multiple myeloma | — | 2 percent |
| **All other sites** | 20 percent | 23 percent |

A blank denotes less than 1 percent of all cancers; percentages do not total 100 due to rounding.

## Carrie's Story

At 21, Carrie was wonderfully quirky, funny, and sensitive, and making a name for herself as a musician. She was also a heavy smoker, since her early teens. With each visit, we assumed our respective doctor and patient roles: "It's time to stop smoking." "I'll try." This went on for the next sixteen years. She was diagnosed with metastatic lung cancer at 37, and died nine months later. Countless friends left the memorial service weeping—and lighting up.

## Lung Cancer: Women's Cancer Enemy Number One

Cancer of the respiratory system, which includes the larynx (voice box), lungs, and bronchi (lung branches), kills more women than breast, colon, or any gynecologic cancer. This year, lung cancer will kill over 67,000 American women, and more than 100,000 of us will receive this diagnosis—usually once the cancer has spread. At least 85 percent of lung cancers are due to smoking. Lung cancer deaths in women have escalated 150 percent over the last two decades, while deaths in men have actually decreased. We've come a long way . . . and died along the way, baby!

### Follow the cigarette smoke

The number of chemicals in cigarette smoke is mind numbing: researchers have counted four thousand. They damage the DNA in cells, leading to mutations that can become cancerous in every part of your body: starting from where you suck it in (mouth and throat), on to its first locale (bronchi and lungs), through gastrointestinal absorption (esophagus, stomach, small intestine, and pancreas), to where you metabolize the chemicals (the liver) and collect their byproducts (the lymph nodes). Eventually, the chemical products spread to your reproductive organs (ovaries, cervix, and vagina), and finally are excreted (by way of your kidneys, bladder, and colon).

We are gender-challenged when it comes to processing these inhaled carcinogens. Women who smoke are 50 percent more likely to develop cancer than male smokers. And the younger you are when you start, the more extensive the DNA damage to respiratory tract cells, and the less likely this damage can be repaired. Even fifteen years after quitting, the residual devastation from smoking can double your risk of lung cancer.

But this beats the twentyfold greater risk for women who continue to smoke! Black women seem to have an even higher risk of tobacco-caused lung cancer.

And now a plug for smoke-free laws: Secondhand smoke increases your risk for lung cancer by 20 percent. Sidestream smoke has an extremely high concentration of carcinogens, and does disproportionate harm to nonsmokers' virgin lungs. If you are married to a smoker, your risk of getting *any* cancer is increased by 50 percent.

*Aren't there other risk factors for lung cancer?* Lung cancer was uncommon in women until tobacco came along. Serious exposure to industrial chemicals (asbestos, radon, gas, or diesel exhaust) can increase our risk, but their contribution pales compared with smoking. Occasionally, a seemingly healthy person develops lung cancer without a clear cause.

## Lung cancer detection: Won't a chest X ray do it?

No. There's no simple test for lung cancer. Neither yearly chest X rays nor sputum (phlegm) screening reduces deaths from this disease. Only 16 percent of women are diagnosed with lung cancer at an early stage, before it has spread. (*If* cancer hasn't spread to the lymph nodes, the five-year survival rate is 50 percent.)

Media reports and screening centers have promoted the new spiral CT scans (spiral computerized tomography) as the best option for early lung cancer detection. This quick computer-controlled scan of your chest cavity produces a 3-D model of your lungs. National Cancer Institute research on the value of this scan for smokers is under way. The problem is that the small abnormalities frequently found may represent old scars from previous (or even current) infections, and smokers get a lot of infections. So, if you undergo this scan, be prepared for the possibility (and associated major anxiety) that the scan finds something, and you now have to wait three months to make sure there's no change and that it's not cancer. You may require more extensive tests, including PET scans (positron emission tomography), or even surgery, to rule out that this "something" is not cancer. Most insurance plans will not cover the cost of a spiral CT scan (which is five times that of a chest X ray). The price of smoking is much greater than the rising cost of a pack of cigarettes.

## "If I breathe okay, are my lungs okay?"

No. Early lung cancer generally has no symptoms; it's sometimes found by chance during a medical checkup. More advanced cancer can have symptoms such as hoarseness, a chronic cough, coughing up blood, short-ness of breath or wheezing, chest pain, and recurrent pneumonia or bron-chitis. Unfortunately, by then, therapy may be too late.

**Preventing lung cancer**
Don't smoke, or stop. The greater the dose (packs per day, years of smok-ing), the greater your risk. (And low-tar cigarettes don't diminish the risk; studies show that people tend to suck in harder to soothe their nicotine craving.) If you quit before a cancer develops, your lungs can gradually heal; ten years later, your risk will be just one-third of what it was when you smoked. As for secondhand smoke, aside from wearing a gas mask around other smokers or in venues where smoking is permitted, there is no known protection.

Chugging vitamins won't help; in fact, high doses of beta-carotene supplements have been shown to actually *increase* the risk of death in male smokers. (Eating fruits and vegetables that contain beta-carotene won't have this scary effect.)

**Don't quit on yourself: You *can* quit smoking**
When I see a new patient who smokes, I ask, "Has one of your doctors encouraged you to quit, or offered to prescribe medication to help you do it?" I'm always amazed at how many patients say their doctor has done neither. And when a woman comes in sporting those telltale wrinkles around her lips and eyes, I'll ask how much she smokes. Some patients are startled. "How did you know?"

"Oh," I respond, "I can tell by your face."

I know smoking is also aging my patient internally, eroding her bones and clogging her vessels. No behavior hastens aging more than smoking. Women who die of smoking-related illness lose an average of fourteen years of potential life. (In the United States alone, this totals an annual loss of over two million woman-years of life. What a waste!) But given that 46 percent of women have smoked at some point in their lives, there are clearly many successful quitters out there.

*Judy's Story*

My nurse, Judy, was a secret smoker. She started during her nursing train-ing in the army. How could she tell me that she smoked while working in my office? I would have killed her before the cigarettes did! (She was good—must have spent a fortune on mints and gum.) Judy had tried to quit many times. She had three young children and was determined that they would not smoke.

When she saw that many of my patients successfully quit with Zyban and the nicotine patch, she quietly raided my sample supply closet and started to use them herself. One year later, she proudly announced that she was smoke free.

Six years later, Judy is the first to "tell" on patients: "I smell smoke on her breath/her clothes." Before I get a chance to expound on the medical consequences of smoking, she's offering advice on why and how to quit. "I did it; you can, too!" As an ex-smoker, she is more convincing than I (a never-smoker) can be.

Women respond differently to nicotine (and to withdrawal from this drug) than men, and their treatment needs to take that into account. For example, cravings may change with the hormonal fluctuations of the menstrual cycle. And women are more likely to use nicotine to manage stress and moodiness. The standard recommendations are to use patches, lozenges, or gum for eight to twelve weeks, and inhalers and sprays for three to six months. Zyban is prescribed for seven to twelve weeks, or up to six months if needed to maintain abstinence. This is enough for many smokers to change their habits and wean themselves slowly from nicotine.

What if you can't keep away from cigarettes unless you keep on medication? A recent report concluded that, despite the lack of long-term studies, you're almost certainly better off taking the medication than inhaling known poisons.

Another potential plus: There is evidence that using Zyban or nicotine replacement helps limit weight gain. While a lot of women are concerned about gaining weight if they quit smoking, research shows that large weight changes are unusual. Adding a few (perhaps temporary) pounds seems a tiny price for adding years to your life. If you increase your physical activity, you can maintain a healthy weight. Burn those calories, tone those muscles, get your heart rate up, and use those lungs to bring in the oxygen—not smoke!

### Counseling and mental preparation

Counseling makes all of these methods work better. The American Cancer Society website (www.cancer.org) can link you to smoking cessation resources in your community. There is also excellent information available on the Web on ways to prepare for quitting, and how to handle those

## Medications That Can Help You Quit for Good

Nicotine addiction is a chronic health problem, and should be treated as seriously as high blood pressure or high cholesterol. While some women do quit cold turkey, many do better with pharmaceutical support. Here are options to consider:

### Nicotine Replacements

These products supply your nicotine "fix" in a far less dangerous way, so you can focus on changing the many daily routines you've created around smoking. From your heart's perspective, nicotine replacement therapy is preferable to smoking. It is generally safe to use if you have cardiovascular disease, including stable angina—while cigarettes definitely are not. But if you have heart or blood vessel disease, consult your doctor before you try nicotine replacement.

### Patches

These work by gradually releasing nicotine through your skin into your bloodstream, maintaining a low, even dose. They come in various shapes and strengths.

*Types:* NicoDerm, Habitrol, and ProStep are usually worn twenty-four hours a day; Nicotrol is put on in the morning and taken off at bedtime.

*Starting dose:* Probably the 21-mg patch. If you weigh less than 100 pounds, or smoke fewer than ten cigarettes per day, start with the 14-mg patch.

### Gum (Nicorette)

Gum handles those sudden urges to smoke.

*Starting dose:* If you smoke fewer than twenty-five cigarettes per day, buy the 2-mg gum; if more, buy the 4-mg gum. Chew when the craving hits, every hour or so—not more than twenty-four pieces per day. For best results, chew slowly until you get a distinctive taste (the nicotine); then tuck the wad between your cheek and gum so the nicotine can be absorbed into your bloodstream. Keep it there until that taste is gone.

### Lozenges (Commit)

This newest form of nicotine replacement comes in 2-mg and 4-mg strengths. If you usually light up within thirty minutes of waking, the higher dose is recommended. Pop a lozenge every hour or two for the first six weeks, then gradually space them farther apart. To get the full dose, you must hold the lozenge in your mouth until it completely dissolves (twenty or thirty minutes)—no chewing allowed.

### Vapor inhaler (by prescription; Nicotrol Inhaler)

The nicotine is delivered through a plastic cylinder that holds a nicotine cartridge. This gets nicotine into your system quickly—as with a cigarette—but the dose is small and controlled, and doesn't include the 3,999 other chemicals in tobacco smoke.

### Nasal spray (by prescription; Nicotrol NS)

While this method gives you the fastest and highest hit of nicotine, it can be the most irritating to the nose, eyes, and throat.

Note: In clinical studies, all replacement methods worked equally well. In real life, people seem more likely to stick with the patch (pardon the pun). If you need extra help, you can combine treatments; several studies have found that the patch plus bupropion (see below) works better than either alone.

## Nonnicotine Options (by Prescription):

### Sustained-release bupropion (Zyban, Wellbutrin SR)

When combined with counseling, this drug can double your odds of quitting. Women often use cigarettes to self-medicate depression. Nicotine raises serotonin levels, and so does the antidepressant Wellbutrin—marketed for antismoking therapy under the name Zyban. (This change of name signifies that the drug is prescribed to treat smoking, not depression, which can affect insurance coverage and reimbursement.)

Other prescription medications, such as Catapres (clonidine), most often used for high blood pressure, and Pamelor (nortriptyline), a tricyclic antidepressant, help with smoking cessation, but are not FDA-approved for that use.

first days and weeks. Check out the Surgeon General's site (www.surgeon general.gov/tobacco) and the CDC's (www.cdc.gov/tobacco), as well as the American Lung Association (www.lungusa.org/tobacco) and the Massachusetts Department of Public Health (www.trytostop.org). Quit-net.com has tips plus online support from other quitters (free membership, fees for personalized support), while Smokeclinic.com attempts to re-create a quit-smoking clinic experience online.

Here are some tips to help you free yourself from cigarettes:

- Plan a quit day.
- Make a list of why you want to quit and all of the ways it will improve your life.
- Make notes about where and when you smoke: Who do you smoke with? What triggers your smoking? How can you change your routine to reduce those triggers? If you've tried to quit before, analyze the circumstances that led to relapse (people, places, cravings, feelings, etc.).
- Keep at hand other things you can hold in your hands (or put in your mouth), such as pens, carrot sticks, fat-free popcorn, or herbal tea.
- Plan what you might do to distract yourself when a craving hits (pop nicotine gum, call a friend, sniff an aromatherapy sachet, get very busy with something else).
- Schedule time to pamper yourself and work off stress (long walks, hot baths).
- Remember, success in preventing relapse is linked to confidence, commitment, and motivation. Think about smooth skin and healthy lungs. Visualize yourself not smoking at important events next year, and having fun with the people you love in the many healthy years to come.

Every woman has her own compelling reasons to quit. Some of my patients have quit because they want to get pregnant, and the safety of a developing fetus becomes paramount. Tracy, a patient in her early thirties, proudly marched into my office the other day and announced to my nurse that she had finally quit smoking. We all congratulated her, knowing she'd tried to quit several times. She did it with Zyban and a nicotine inhaler, after I threatened to take away the birth control pills she was using to alleviate her cramps. (Remember, smokers have an increased risk of developing blood clots when they take the Pill.)

The clincher, however, was the intervention of her best friend. She walked Tracy to the garage, turned on the car engine, and suggested that she put her mouth around the tailpipe and breathe in deeply. Horrified, Tracy asked, "What? Are you trying to kill me?"

"No, but your cigarettes are. You're inhaling their carbon monoxide and hydrogen cyanide!"

If Tracy's quitting image works for you, use it.

## BREAST CANCER

### *"I Have a Lump . . . It's Probably Nothing"*

. . . Said Sylvia when she took me aside at a board meeting to ask for an appointment. I offered an immediate exam in the privacy of the ladies' room. So there we were in the stall, her blouse and bra looped over the door, as I palpated an ominously hard, marble-sized mass in her left breast. I knew this was more than a "nothing." Sylvia's last mammogram, nine months before, showed no signs of cancer. I offered words of temporary comfort: It could be a fast-growing cyst, a local infection, or a bruise that caused blood to collect. "To play it safe," I said, "let's schedule an ultrasound."

The radiologist informed me that the mass was solid and looked suspicious. A biopsy revealed a cancer that had already spread to six lymph nodes.

Sylvia and her husband were distraught. How could this happen? She'd done everything right: yearly mammograms, breast self-exams, and doctor checkups. Shouldn't these have detected the cancer at an earlier stage? I understood their anger, realizing that the usual cautionary phrase "No exam is perfect" would not assuage their frustration. The disease had beaten our technology.

Sylvia bravely embarked on the most aggressive course of therapy available: mastectomy, massive chemotherapy, radiation, and breast reconstruction. She refused to cloister herself at home and mourn her condition. She was an active grandparent. I saw her at board meetings and charity events, and marveled at her energy and optimism. Sylvia kept her life on track—and more than three years later, she is cancer free.

Our detection system is not perfect. But it's the best we have right now and—along with new therapies—has led to a significant decrease in breast cancer deaths. During the past two decades, while the number of women diagnosed with breast cancer did not go down, the number of deaths from breast cancer decreased by roughly 29 percent.

### The mammogram controversy

Should a woman have routine mammograms to screen for breast cancer— and at what age should she start? This has long been a source of controversy. Most of us thought it was settled, and followed the recommendations of the American Cancer Society (ACS): Starting at age 40, a woman should have yearly mammograms.

One morning in October 2001, a front-page article in the *New York Times* shattered women's trust in this rule of breast health. The report cited an analysis published in *The Lancet* concluding that there was no good evidence that women screened with mammograms were less likely to die of breast cancer—and, as a matter of fact, were more likely to die of other diseases. The Danish authors had reviewed the seven major studies used to support mammography, and dismissed as invalid five of the largest ones, saying that they were flawed and failed to meet their personal standards of proof. In other words, they faulted 80 percent of the trial evidence, and their analysis of the remaining 20 percent found no benefit to mammograms.

A closer analysis of these objections discounted their practical significance (e.g., in one study of 133,000 women aged 40 to 47, the mammogram group was an average of five months older than the control group). The study that most supported their claim of no mammogram benefit was later found, by a group of international experts, to have major flaws of its own, involving poor-quality mammogram films.

A thorough review by the U.S. Preventive Services Task Force subsequently concluded that mammograms significantly reduce breast cancer mortality (based on pooled trial results, women over 50 who had mammograms every twelve to thirty-three months were 23 percent less likely to die of breast cancer than women who did not). And if this were not enough to settle the issue, a huge long-term study involving one-third of the women in Sweden found that when women were followed long enough (more than ten years), with mammograms every 1.5 to 2 years beginning at age 40, breast cancer deaths were reduced by as much as 44 percent. The average time it takes for cancer to grow to a size that can be detected (sojourn time) is shorter the younger you are. That means that women in their forties should *not* wait two years between screening mammograms.

All of this categorically supports the ACS recommendation that you *begin mammograms when you're 40, and continue to get them yearly*. All we're talking about here is a five- to ten-minute procedure, including a few uncomfortable seconds of pressure (it's necessary to spread and flatten the breast tissue to get a useful image).

There has been one change: The ACS no longer recommends that you get a baseline mammogram between ages 35 and 40. Despite this, if you have relatives who developed breast cancer at a relatively young age, or you are at high risk, talk to your doctor about starting mammograms in your late twenties or early thirties and repeating them at shorter intervals.

*What about "false positives"?* The younger you are, the more likely your breasts will be dense, and your mammogram image hard to accurately interpret. This has been used to argue against mammograms for women in their forties, because it can result in a higher rate of "Come back and let's see what's going on": This usually means additional X rays, an ultrasound, or even a *stereotactic,* or ultrasound-directed biopsy. For the latter procedure, a radiologist uses the image (from the mammogram or ultrasound) to place a special needle or other biopsy instrument into the abnormal area of the breast, removing a tiny core of tissue for microscopic analysis and diagnosis.

Are younger women having too many "unnecessary" biopsies? The fact that a biopsy is negative doesn't mean it is useless—if there is no other way of finding out whether that abnormality on your mammogram is cancerous. If the biopsy finds an early-stage cancer, then your chance of recovery is extremely high. My stance on this debate is obvious: Don't look back in regret because of inadequate screening.

## Other breast tests

*Breast self-exam.* Just as you should be aware of what's happening to your body, you should be aware of changes in your breasts. Some very well publicized studies have found that a breast self-exam (BSE) may not contribute to early detection and reduced mortality from breast cancer. Nonetheless, every clinician has patients who "caught" their breast cancer through self-exam. I maintain my recommendation to check your breasts for new lumps, skin dimpling, or bloody secretions from the nipple. (If you aren't sure how to do BSE, check the ACS website, www.cancer.org.)

If you find a lump, don't panic. Most are not cancerous, especially in women under 40. Benign *fibroadenomas* account for 10 percent of lumps, cysts for 25 percent, and fibrocystic changes (where the breast simply feels dense in one area) for another 40 percent. If you find a painful lump at the beginning of your menstrual cycle, you can wait for your next period, then check to see if the lump has disappeared. If, however, this is a brand-new lump or does not change over the course of your cycle, it warrants further assessment.

Any new pain or change in breast contour, such as indentation or dimpling, can signify tumor growth and needs to be brought to the attention of your physician for appropriate tests. (I had a patient whose daughter noticed an indentation on the lower part of her breast when she raised her arm to try on a new blouse. Neither she nor I felt a lump or change in density, but her ultrasound was abnormal and a biopsy revealed breast cancer.)

If you are over 40 and/or your periods have stopped, a new lump should always be investigated by a doctor within weeks of your feeling it.

Another point of contention is: When should we *stop* having mammograms? Since women aged 75 to 79 have the highest incidence of breast cancer, it makes sense to keep on screening; mammograms done every two years in women between 70 and 79 would prevent an estimated 1.4 breast cancer deaths per ten thousand women.

The average life expectancy of a 70-year-old woman in the United States is 15.4 years. If you reach 80, you can expect to live another 9.1 years. So, if you're relatively healthy in your seventies and eighties, you want to make every effort to slow your clock down. My personal recommendation for any woman over 70: Get a mammogram at least every other year.

*Clinical breast exam (CBE).* Between the ages of 20 and 39, you should have a breast exam done by a health care professional every three years—and yearly from 40 on. I would hope that clinicians' fingers have done the walking long enough to detect a lump. However, don't expect Wonder Woman's X-ray fingers. Lumps that feel soft and round can still be malignant; those that feel hard could be a harmless accumulation of fibrous, dense tissue.

Ideally, you should have your CBE just prior to your mammogram, so any concerns can be brought to the attention of the radiologist for further evaluation. Conversely, if you've had a normal mammogram (like Sylvia) but you and/or your doctor feel a lump, you need additional imaging. Even if the imaging is normal, you should be closely followed; if the lump remains, a biopsy may be warranted.

*Digital mammograms.* These bring your breasts into the computer age. A traditional mammogram produces a black-and-white image on a sheet of film; a digital mammogram is displayed on a computer screen. Digital is not necessarily more accurate, but it can be read faster and may require less recall for additional views. The main advantage is that, unlike film, it can't get lost. The image can also be sent to another computer to be read by other radiologists, or to a central computer programmed to detect abnormalities. While the benefit of the latter is still under study, if your mammogram was done at a facility that doesn't specialize in breast exams, having a second review might increase diagnostic accuracy.

*Ultrasound (sonogram).* Ultrasound can augment mammograms but should not be your sole screening procedure. It won't "see" the minute spiderlike calcifications that are a mammographic hallmark of most early cancers. Many radiologists (especially on the East Coast) believe that all women with dense or lumpy breasts should have a comprehensive ultrasound exam together with their mammogram. This is because women with dense breasts are at higher risk for cancer, and their mammograms are harder to read. Your insurance may not cover breast ultrasound (unless a specific reason is given), and this added test can double the cost of your annual breast exam.

The current norm is to perform an ultrasound in an area where a lump is felt or an abnormality is seen in the mammogram. This separates the true cysts, which are filled with fluid, from worrisome solid masses. Cysts are usually benign and can be left alone, but if they are painful or large—or if your doctor wants to make sure they are "just" cysts—they can be removed or aspirated with a needle.

I'm biased regarding breast scanning with ultrasound. My breasts were extremely dense and difficult to visualize. An ultrasound found an area that appeared abnormal; a biopsy showed many cells that were atypical but not yet cancerous. I chose additional surgery and, finally, a bilateral subcutaneous (skin and nipple sparing) mastectomy, with reconstruction. It could be argued that I would never have developed invasive cancer, and that this test caught cells in an "uncertain" stage. However, I am grateful I discovered their presence and had the option to prevent a future cancer.

*MRIs (magnetic resonance imaging) and PET scans (positron emission tomography).* These costly investigational tools are currently used in women at high risk for genetic breast cancer (see page 266), or those in whom a cancer was found and who need additional studies to make sure other small cancers are not missed. MRI and PET scans are not used for general screening purposes.

*Ductal lavage.* This requires passing a small catheter into the ducts of the breasts, rinsing them with fluid (lavage), and checking that fluid for abnormal-looking cells or other substances that suggest precancer or early cancer. This could lead to a prescription for Tamoxifen or another breast cancer prevention drug (see page 270). Results might also indicate the need for aggressive follow-up such as MRI or PET scans. The dilemma for the surgeon is: Which ducts should be lavaged? If there are abnormal cells in the fluid, from whence in the ducts did they come? Should a biopsy be performed, and if so, where? At this time, ductal lavage is not considered a universal screening technique but has potential for high-risk women and may in the future become easier and more accessible.

## Who Is at Risk for Breast Cancer?

### Known risks

*A past history of breast cancer.* If you've had it before, you are at higher risk for recurrence.

*Your family history.* Your chance of developing breast cancer is greater if close female relatives—your mother, sister, and/or daughter—have a history of breast cancer, especially if diagnosed before age 50. Breast cancer among your father's female relatives also increases your risk.

Just as lack of a family history does not mean you are *not* at risk (nine out of ten women who develop breast cancer have no family history), having a family history does not mean you are destined to get cancer. If you have a first-degree relative (mother, sister, daughter) with breast cancer, your increased risk of eventually developing it yourself (compared with a woman with no family history) is just 5.5 percent. Even if you have *two* first-degree relatives with cancer, your risk increases by only 13.3 percent.

*Hereditary factors (BRCA 1 and 2 genetic mutations).* There is a hereditary form of breast (and ovarian) cancer, but it is rare. Five to 7 percent of

### What Are the Odds?

The older you are, the greater your odds of developing breast cancer. The chart below (from the National Cancer Institute) shows the typical American woman's odds, decade by decade:

| | |
|---|---|
| From age 20 to 30 | 1 in 2,000 women |
| From age 30 to 40 | 1 in 250 |
| From age 40 to 50 | 1 in 67 |
| From age 50 to 60 | 1 in 35 |
| From age 60 to 70 | 1 in 28 |
| Ever getting breast cancer (by age 85 or older) | 1 in 8 |

breast and ovarian cancers may be traced to mutations in BRCA1 or BRCA2.

In noninherited cancer, two copies of a gene that controls abnormal cell growth have to be "hit" or mutated in order to instigate a cancer. This double hit usually occurs in just one group of cells, in one type of tissue. With hereditary cancer, you inherit a single abnormal copy of the gene from one of your parents, and it will be present in every cell of your body. Years later, all it takes for hereditary cancer to develop is for the remaining healthy copy of that gene to be damaged—either through an inherited tendency to "go bad" or general wear and tear. Unfortunately, if one gene copy is mutated, the other tends to be less stable.

The most studied hereditary breast cancers are due to inherited mutations in BRCA (BReast CAncer) 1 or BRCA2. An estimated one in eight hundred American women have mutations in one of these two genes; over a thousand types of mutations have been found. Some are harmless mutations, but others lead to production of abnormal BRCA protein that fails to suppress the replication and growth of potentially malignant tumor cells. If your mother or father carried this mutated gene, you have a 50 percent chance of inheriting it. It's possible that one of your parents has the gene, but it was not "expressed" (it never triggered the condition). And if your father carried the gene, you'd have to look to his close female relatives for evidence of its presence.

If you carry a mutated BRCA gene, your lifetime risk of getting breast cancer is 50 to 80 percent, and your risk of developing ovarian cancer by age 70 is 15 to 25 percent. Because each body cell contains this gene, it can instigate tumor-suppressor mishaps elsewhere, especially in the colon, pancreas, stomach, or prostate. If you or members of your family have this mutation, the risk for cancer in these organs is also increased.

*Your reproductive and menstrual history.* If you started menstruating early (at 11 or younger), had a late menopause (after 55), and never had children or had your first child at 30 or older, you have an increased risk of breast cancer.

*Race/ethnicity.* Caucasian women are slightly more likely to develop breast cancer than African-American women, but the latter have a higher mortality rate once diagnosed—in part because diagnosis is often delayed, but also because their tumors tend to behave more aggressively. Asian, Hispanic, and Native American women appear to have a lower risk.

*Breast cell abnormalities (found on biopsy).* If a biopsy shows atypical hyperplasia (an increased number of abnormal, but not cancerous, cells)

## Should You Have Genetic Testing?

According to the American Society of Clinical Oncologists, you should consider testing if you:

- Have two or more first- or second-degree relatives (on the same side of the family) who developed breast cancer before age 50, or ovarian cancer at any age.
- Are diagnosed with early-onset breast cancer, or ovarian cancer at any age.
- Are of Ashkenazi (eastern European) Jewish heritage, and have a personal or family history of early-onset breast cancer or any ovarian cancer.
- Have a family history of male breast cancer.
- Have a relative (first, second, or third degree) who has tested positive for a BRCA1 or BRCA2 mutation.
- Have evidence that your father may carry a mutated gene (relatives on his side with early-onset breast cancer or ovarian cancer, or a significant family history of other cancers).

There is one lab in the United States (Myriad, at www.myriadtests.com, or 800-469-7423) that performs these tests. If your family history warrants your being tested, check with your insurance carrier; they may pay for it, but it could mean your genetic analysis will become part of your permanent record. (According to Myriad's Web site, they release test results only to the doctor who requested them, even when an insurer pays, unless the patient consents in writing to release the results to another party.) A 1997 law prevents use of genetic information to deny group health insurance, but protection for individual policies is still a question that may need to be resolved in the courts.

or lobular carcinoma in situ (LCIS, abnormal cells in lobules of the breast), your cancer risk is higher. Also, two or more breast biopsies for other benign conditions could hint at an underlying problem that increases your cancer odds.

*Breast density.* Breast cancers usually develop in glands rather than fatty tissue. There seems to be a correlation between breast tissue density and risk of cancer: Dense breasts and higher cancer risk may be inherited together. As we get older, our breasts typically lose density as fat becomes the dominant tissue; we go from firm and perky to soft and droopy. The good news is that this makes tumors easier to spot on mammograms, as white areas within a gray background. If breast tissue doesn't change, it means an increased risk for cancer, and reduced odds that a mammogram will pick up a white abnormal area amid white normal tissue.

*Radiation therapy (X-ray therapy).* If you had radiation therapy in your chest area (e.g., for Hodgkin's disease), your odds of developing cancer increase. The younger you are when you have X-ray therapy (especially under 30), the greater the risk.

*Alcohol.* Finally, a risk you can do something about. Based on a pooled analysis of data from four countries (including the Nurses' Health Study), women who have two to five drinks a day face a greater than 40 percent increased risk of developing invasive breast cancer (compared with nondrinkers).

Alcohol raises blood estrogen levels, perhaps because it limits estrogen breakdown and increases its production. It's possible that bursts of estrogen that occur after you down a drink are more harmful to the breasts than constant exposure to lower levels of estrogen—whether natural or pharmacologic. Also, new research suggests that HRT plus alcohol has a greater effect on breasts than either factor alone. If you are on HRT, it might be a good idea to limit your alcohol consumption. In general, and for many reasons, women should not be imbibing more than one drink a day.

*Weight gain.* Adding pounds, especially after menopause, seems to increase your breast cancer risk. Fat cells produce more estrogen; after menopause, estrogen's effects aren't checked by progesterone production. A gain of 40-plus pounds in later life may double breast cancer risk in women who do not use HRT. A spare tire around the middle may be worse for the breasts than heavy hips and thighs.

## Less-certain risks

*Diet.* It's not clear that diet has an effect on this disease. Breast cancer is less common in countries such as Japan where soy intake is high and the typical diet is low in fat. When we try to extrapolate these findings to American women, neither high soy (foods or supplements) nor low-fat diets after puberty seem to make a difference in the risk of developing breast cancer.

*Lack of exercise.* Strenuous exercise when you're young may provide some protection, perhaps because it suppresses ovulation. We're not sure that physical activity as an adult lowers your risk; until we know for sure, I suggest that you stay on that treadmill and pump that iron, because exercise gives so many health benefits. It also decreases midabdominal fat, which *is* a risk factor.

**These do *not* increase risk**

*Birth control pills.* A very conclusive study of 9,200 American women aged 35 to 64, published in 2002 in the *New England Journal of Medicine,* showed that birth control pills did not increase risk of breast cancer—no matter the race, age, or weight of the woman, or the duration or type of Pill used.

*Breast implants.* Implants may make it harder to feel a lump (especially if the implant becomes encapsulated or hard), and make it slightly more difficult to interpret your mammogram. But there is no evidence that implants increase breast cancer risk.

*Antiperspirants and underwire bras.* Despite what you might have read or heard, there is no evidence that either of these increases your risk.

## What Can You Do to Prevent Breast Cancer?

If a patient asked me, "What—in one sentence—can I do to prevent breast cancer?" I'd have to answer, "Since you can't choose your relatives, or when you got your period, or when it's going to stop, keep your weight down, limit alcohol consumption, and make use of our twenty-first-century techniques for early detection." If she was at extremely high risk, I'd add, "Consider the following. . . ."

*Prevention with prescription.* Tamoxifen (Nolvadex) belongs to a category of drugs called SERMs, or selective estrogen receptor modulators, which promote or inhibit estrogen action in cells. In the breasts, tamoxifen acts as an anti-estrogen, blocking estrogen receptors.

For women who have estrogen-receptor-positive breast cancer (diagnosed through biopsy), taking tamoxifen for five years after initial breast cancer therapy reduces recurrence in the same breast by 46 percent, and development of a new cancer in the other breast by 50 percent. Most important, tamoxifen has been shown to reduce death from breast cancer by 26 percent.

What about prevention before the cancer occurs? If you are high risk (i.e., your chance of developing breast cancer in the next five years is greater than 1.6 percent), you may be a candidate for tamoxifen therapy.

Studies have shown it can decrease risk by 44 percent in high-risk women under the age of 49, and 50 percent in women who are older.

If previous breast biopsies confirmed your risk and showed lobular in situ cancer, or atypical hyperplasia (meaning that the cells were heading toward becoming cancerous), tamoxifen may reduce your risk by more than 80 percent. There are, alas, side effects. Rarely, tamoxifen promotes development of endometrial cancer, abnormal clots, and cataracts. Frequently, it makes menopausal symptoms worse. Some of my patients say it causes weight gain, although this is not cited as a complication in the medical literature. So, we're certainly not advising that every woman take it, "just in case."

*Aromatase inhibitors* (Arimidex, Aromasin, Femara) work by blocking one of the last steps in estrogen production at the tissue level: in fat cells and even breast tissue. Many researchers think that conversion activity, not the actual level of circulating estrogen, constitutes the most crucial breast cancer–estrogen connection.

The early response to these aromatase inhibitors for prevention therapy after nonmetastatic breast cancer has been at least as good as, and sometimes better than, tamoxifen. However, because we don't have long-term follow-up of women who have been treated with this class of drugs, the current recommendation is to first go with tamoxifen. A recent study of over 5,000 women who were treated for breast cancer and subsequently given tamoxifen for five years showed that those given Femara for an additional two and a half years were half as likely to develop a new or recurrent breast cancer as the women who were given a placebo. The results were considered to be so significant that the study was discontinued and *all* the women were given Femara. However, doctors don't know how long Femara should be used, or if women who finished their tamoxifen years ago should now start taking this drug. The aromatase inhibitors don't increase risk for endometrial cancer, blood clots, or cataracts, and are the alternative method if tamoxifen is not well tolerated or there are concerns about its side effects. But they, too, can cause unwanted effects: menopausal symptoms, nausea and vomiting, aches and pains, and shortness of breath.

*Prevention through surgery.* Removal of both breasts (bilateral mastectomy) remains an option for women at extremely high cancer risk. In most of these surgeries, the skin is left, and the breast tissue below is removed (subcutaneous). Reconstruction can be done either with implants inserted under the muscles or with tissue moved from other areas of the body. This is a radical procedure that may be chosen by women who are positive for a BRCA gene mutation, have widespread precancerous changes, or had invasive cancer in one breast and a high risk for recurrence in the other. Bilateral mastectomy reduces the risk of death from breast cancer 90 percent to 100 percent, depending on whether the nipples are also removed, as well as the individual woman's risk.

There is one more preventive surgery that has been shown to decrease the risk of breast cancer: *removal of both ovaries (bilateral oophorectomy)*. This procedure eliminates a substantial source of estrogen production and may decrease breast cancer risk by 20 to 50 percent in premenopausal women. It has been shown to decrease breast cancer by 50 percent in women who are carriers of the BRCA1 mutation.

## Ovarian Cancer

Your lifetime risk of getting this cancer is "only" 1 in 70. If you have reached the age of 40 and haven't been afflicted, the chance decreases to 1 in 100. Yet ovarian cancer is insidious, and there are no effective screening methods. It is also the most fatal of all gynecologic cancers. This year, 23,300 women will be diagnosed with ovarian cancer, and only half will be alive five years later.

*Your risk for ovarian cancer increases if:*

- You've never had a full-term pregnancy.
- You used fertility drugs—unless this was followed by a full-term preg-

### Ovarian Cancer Statistics

- Most ovarian cancers are found after menopause (median age of diagnosis is 61). Familial ovarian cancers due to BRCA mutations usually occur before the age of 50.
- Women who had breast or colon cancer, or have a family history of these cancers, are at higher risk.
- Women with a BRCA1 mutation have a lifetime risk of between 16 and 63 percent of developing ovarian cancer. Women with BRCA2 mutation have a lifetime risk of 16 to 40 percent.
- However, only 5 to 10 percent of ovarian cancer patients have a significant family history of cancer.

nancy. Unresolved infertility by itself can increase risk by two or threefold.
- Your diet is high in animal and milk fat.
- You consistently used talcum powder "down there." Until twenty years ago, some powders contained asbestos (a known carcinogen), and particles could migrate up through the vagina.

## Reducing your risk

*Birth control pills.* Right now the Pill is our best ovarian cancer prevention strategy. By preventing ovulation, the Pill helps prevent mutation of cells activated during ovarian cycles. It decreases risk from 40 percent (with less than two years of use) to 80 percent (with 10-plus years of birth control pill use). Many epidemiologists feel that all women should take the Pill at some point during their reproductive lifetime.

*Tubal ligation or hysterectomy.* These procedures "cut off" ovarian contact with contaminants that could cause irritation and cellular changes. These surgeries can decrease cancer risk by one-third to one-half.

*Pregnancy and breast-feeding.* Having two children decreases your risk by 40 percent. You benefit even more if you breast-feed, since that, too, suppresses ovulation.

*Removal of the ovaries (bilateral oophorectomy).* This makes sense if you have a BRCA gene mutation, and should be performed as soon as you've finished having babies. The surgery is fairly simple, and usually done through a laparoscope as an outpatient procedure. (The bigger issue for younger women is the loss of hormones produced by their still-functioning ovaries.)

Removal of both ovaries can decrease ovarian cancer risk by 75 to 90 percent. Unfortunately, it's not 100 percent, because cancer cells may already be present in the ovaries or pelvis by the time the surgery is performed. Moreover, the cells lining the abdominal cavity each contain the BRCA mutation and may later become cancerous, mimicking an ovarian malignancy. But this very rare event shouldn't dissuade a woman with a BRCA mutation from doing all she can to prevent ovarian cancer through surgery. Another plus: Bilateral oophorectomy in BRCA-positive patients has been shown to decrease the risk of breast cancer by 50 percent.

After age 40, if you are not BRCA positive and have no significant family history, you probably have a 1 percent chance of developing ovarian cancer over the rest of your life. Should you have your ovaries removed "just in case" if you are advised to undergo a hysterectomy?

Before menopause, you have to weigh the fear of abrupt and often severe menopausal symptoms (see chapter 2) versus the fear of future ovarian cancer risk (which, by the way, has been diminished by the removal of your uterus).

At or after menopause, the seesaw is weighed toward ovarian removal. Your ovaries have already ceased female hormone production, so your body will undergo less shock. You will need to consider whether you want hormone replacement therapy even if you don't have your ovaries removed. And the ovaries can usually be easily removed during a vaginal or abdominal hysterectomy. You will, however, lose an important source of male hormone with surgical removal of menopausal ovaries. Loss of libido may occur, making testosterone supplementation an issue.

### Detecting ovarian cancer

On the few occasions when I've found an ovarian tumor while performing an ultrasound, my heart has dropped. By the time a patient comes to see me complaining of symptoms (and I see this ultrasound picture) the disease is usually advanced. The physical complaints are so very nonspecific—abdominal discomfort or enlargement, feeling full when you haven't eaten much, fatigue, needing to void frequently, and shortness of breath—signs of almost anything and everything.

### Screening tests

Alas, they are currently inadequate. By the time a pelvic exam shows that the ovary is enlarged, the tumor has spread. Just 1 out of 10,000 early ovarian cancers will be found with a hands-on approach. Routine Pap smears may find malignant ovarian cells that were shed through the uterus, but this, too, is rare—and by then, the tumor has spread.

A blood test has been widely touted on Internet sites for the past fifteen years: "Get your *CA-125* tested. You could have ovarian cancer!" CA-125 is a protein that may be produced by tumors of the ovaries, stomach, and intestines—but levels are also increased during your period, if you have fibroids or endometriosis, and for no reason at all (it's elevated in 1 percent of healthy women). Also, its level increases in only 50 percent of early ovarian cancers. This means that the test will have many "false-positive" and "false-negative" results. CA-125 is more likely to be elevated in late-stage cancers, and will go down in response to treatment. Thus, the current medical consensus is that CA-125 is best used as a marker of therapeutic success.

*Ultrasound.* Helps us make a diagnosis, but should it be used, like mammography, to screen all women? Probably not. It can pick up cysts and growths, but can't distinguish benign ones from malignant ones—and once something is found, it needs further exploration. Roughly sixty-seven women would have to undergo surgery in order for just one to receive a correct diagnosis of ovarian cancer. A combination approach might be best: Test for CA-125 and, for those women with elevated levels, perform ultrasound. The American Cancer Society recommends this type of combined screening only for women with a strong family history of ovarian cancers.

We've got to do better, and the hope is we will in the near future. Scientists are profiling and categorizing molecular protein patterns in women who had ovarian cancer. In small preliminary tests, the abnormal pattern predicted ovarian cancer 94 percent of the time (versus 34 percent for CA-125). Although further research is needed to confirm these results, and there is no current recommendation for use of this test for screening purposes by any gynecologic or cancer society, the test (called Ova Check) has become available through some commercial labs. Blood is sent for analysis by a special computer that detects the *protein array* pattern seen in known ovarian cancers. It costs about $130 and until it becomes the standard of care, will not be covered by medical-insurance carriers.

## Uterine Cancers: The Cervix and Endometrium

### "The Scarlet Pap"

Dana was married for twenty years, and had two children. Her pleasantly unremarkable family portrait was suddenly defaced by her Pap smear, which showed a high-grade *squamous cell intraepithelial neoplasm* (precancerous cells). We know that most precancers and cancers of the cervix (93 to 100 percent) are due to the *human papilloma virus*. HPV is sexually transmitted at the touch of a penis or scrotum (through skin-to-skin or skin-to-vagina contact).

The unfortunate microbial truth is that when you sleep with a person, you are sleeping with the viruses and bacteria of everyone that person has slept with, the people they in turn slept with, and so on. Unless you're both first-time lovers, the chance of getting one of these microbes is astoundingly high. There are over thirty types of genital HPV, divided into "high risk" and "low risk" types—based on how likely they are to cause cancerous mutations in the cells lining the cervix.

Dana asked me how she could possibly have a sexually transmitted virus. Although the virus usually disappears (especially in younger women) after two years, it seems to be more tenacious and harmful as we get older. I suggested that in her case it might have been dormant for many years. Dana then informed me that she had never had sex with another man, and that she was her husband's first sexual partner. Although I felt my suspicions rising, I muttered something about unknown ways and means of infection.

The next day, I received an angry call from Dana's husband, questioning the accuracy of the test, the therapy that Dana would need, and whether this precancer would recur and have an effect on her future health.

After asking to speak to Dana (to gain her permission to pass on this information), I gave him the facts. He called me back the next day, and confessed that her HPV infection was "all his fault"; he had been seeing prostitutes. He intended to go into therapy for sexual addiction.

I treated Dana with a LEEP (loop electrosurgical excision procedure), using a small loop device carrying a special electric current to remove the abnormal tissue from her cervix. It did not rid her of the virus, but it did get rid of the precancerous cells on her cervix. So far, her subsequent Pap smears have been normal. They are still married, and she reports that they're making progress in therapy. When they have sex, her husband uses condoms.

Early diagnosis pays off. The death rate in the United States from this cancer has been reduced to just 4,100 women in 2003—the majority of whom either skipped their Pap smears for five years or never had one at all.

## How Pap smears work

The Pap is a complex test. Cells from the cervix are gathered with a brush and spatula, and are either smeared onto a slide (the traditional method) or placed in fluid, which is later filtered so that the residue of cells can be dispersed on the slide (a fluid-based Pap). The cells are stained and then viewed through a microscope.

The test sounds fairly simple, but it requires careful collection of the cells from the inner canal and outer surface of the cervix, good lab processing, and accurate professional interpretation. It's the beginning of the screening process, not the final diagnosis.

If abnormal cells are found, the Pap should be followed by *colposcopy* (using a special scope that magnifies the cervix) and a biopsy of the areas that appear abnormal. Most of our concern is with abnormalities of the squamous or epithelial cells on the surface of the cervix. These are classified using several terms:

- *ASCUS* (atypical squamous cells of undetermined significance). This means mild changes were seen. Of the 50 or 60 million Pap smears done on American women every year, 3.5 million show some sort of abnormality; most have been labeled ASCUS. Depending on the lab, only one in ten inconclusive Paps represents an actual precancer.
- *LSIL* (low-grade squamous intraepithelial lesion). This means mildly abnormal cells (also called "mild dysplasia," or cervical intraepithelial neoplasia, CIN 1) were found. These are usually linked to a low-risk HPV (human papilloma virus) infection.
- *HSIL* (high-grade squamous intraepithelial lesions). This means moderate to severe dysplasia (CIN 2 or CIN 3) and carcinoma in situ (cancer cells confined to the surface of the cervix)—generally due to a high-risk HPV infection.
- *Squamous cell carcinoma*. Cancer cells are present, and may have invaded the cervix.

What happens if your Pap test shows a slight abnormality? In 2002, new guidelines were published to help distinguish between worrisome and ignorable changes. In the past, you'd be told to either undergo colposcopy or come back and repeat the test every four to six months. Only after two negative Paps would you be "cleared" for ordinary follow-up. That's a lot of extra visits, not to mention cost and stress. Now, if your Pap shows ASCUS, a second test should be done to check for the presence of high-risk HPV; if present, this requires follow-up. And you certainly need follow-up if your Pap shows a high-grade lesion.

Note that the Pap test does not screen for ovarian or uterine cancer. Some endometrial cancers may be picked up by a Pap, but we don't count on this test for a diagnosis of this type of cancer.

In the past, we initiated Pap smears at age 18 or at the onset of sexual intercourse, but we now know it probably takes three years from initial HPV infection to develop high-grade lesions of cervical cancer. Moreover, while HPV is so contagious that it's now found in over 70 percent of young, sexually active adults, most of these infections are temporary; in adolescents and young women, 70 to 90 percent will disappear after two years. Even if the viruses cause low-grade lesions in these young women, 90 percent of those will spontaneously regress.

## How Often Do You Need a Pap Smear?

It's taken five decades to get most women to accept the dictum "Get a yearly Pap smear." While you need your yearly pelvic exam, you may not need an annual Pap smear. New American Cancer Society guidelines have relaxed the Pap screening schedule for *low-risk women* as follows:

*Young women:* Begin three years after the onset of intercourse, and no later than age 21.

*Between the ages of 21 and 30:* Repeat conventional Pap smear yearly, or liquid Pap every two years (if normal).

*Over age 30:* Repeat every two or three years if the previous three Pap smears were *all* normal.

*After age 70:* Stop if you've had three normal Pap tests in the last ten years.

*After hysterectomy:* No need for Pap smears if the hysterectomy was done for benign disease and the cervix was removed.

In short, performing Pap smears too soon (or too frequently) in young women may pick up early lesions that *would go away on their own*—leading to unnecessary stress and costly tests, biopsies, and treatments. Also, these could result in a "preexisting condition" label when the young woman applies for health insurance, and make her feel "branded."

If you've had three consecutive normal Pap smears and you are "low risk," you can safely wait two, probably three, years between Pap smears since you are not likely to experience cervical cellular changes from HPV. The crucial term here is "low risk." That leaves out a lot of women: those who've had previous high-grade lesions, have new or multiple sexual partners, have nonmonogamous partners, are HIV positive, have a history of DES exposure during their mother's pregnancy, are on chemotherapy or steroid therapy, or are smokers. All these conditions (with the exception of DES exposure) increase the risk of HPV infection, or the vulnerability of cervical cells to HPV-instigated mutations.

After 70, if you've always had perfect cervical health, an abnormal Pap is so unlikely (absent a new sexual partner) that you can stop.

Note that stopping Pap smears does not mean skipping gynecologic exams. Women need routine checkups to assess menstrual and hormonal problems, get advice about contraception and hormones, receive breast and pelvic exams, and be appropriately screened for other sexually transmitted infections. Remember, after the age of 70 women are most likely to develop breast, ovarian, or colon cancer, and to have problems with pelvic support and bladder control (which can be helped). Stopping Pap smears does not mean stopping gynecologic exams.

## How to minimize your risk of cervical cancer

- Use condoms with all new partners. (Since the HPV virus causes warts in less than 1 percent of infections, seeing "nothing" does not equate with a "healthy" penis!)
- Don't smoke. Smoking enhances replication and longevity of the HPV virus, and increases the chance it will cause mutations in the cervical cells.
- If your partner has multiple HPV-caused lesions (warts, which you or he can see with the naked eye, or which are diagnosed by a physician after applying a vinegar solution), he should be treated. But realize that once you share your vaginal and his penile flora, you probably will share them for a very long time.

## Treatment of cervical precancer and cancer

The key to our success against cervical cancer is early therapy, before invasive cancer occurs. Low-grade lesions can be destroyed by freezing (*cryosurgery*). High-grade lesions that have not invaded the underlying cells are often treated with LEEP in the doctor's office. If there is a possibility that cancer and/or invasion of cancer cells deep in the cervix has occurred, a procedure called *conization* may be needed (a cone-shaped portion of the cervix is removed). If the cancer is found to have spread, a hysterectomy plus additional treatment (radiation, chemotherapy drugs, lymph node resection) should be performed. For early stage invasive cancer, these treatments help 92 percent of women live at least five years (and often far longer) after diagnosis—and our therapies continue to improve.

## *The Other Uterine Cancer: Endometrial Cancer*

Endometrial cancer, which develops in the lining of the uterus, is the most common cancer of our reproductive organs—but the least fatal. Of all the gynecological cancers, this has the best prognosis: If diagnosed at an early stage, 96 percent of women who undergo appropriate therapy will be alive (and without recurrence) five years later. Moreover, this cancer usually gives the warning sign of abnormal vaginal bleeding. If we investigate with the right tests, we can diagnose it at a precancerous or early stage. The overall five-year survival for all stages of endometrial cancer is 73 percent.

**Risk factors**
Known risk factors include:

- *Overproduction of estrogen; underproduction of progesterone.* As noted in the chapters on hormones, endometrial cancer risk increases when the healthy estrogen/progesterone balance goes awry, and estrogen predominates. This occurs with the abnormal or infrequent ovulations associated with polycystic ovarian syndrome (PCOS—see page 9), as well as long-term estrogen exposure associated with early menarche and/or late menopause.
- *Obesity* also causes excess estrogen, as fat cells convert other hormones to estrogen compounds. Estrogen conversion may explain the increased risk seen in diabetic women, and those who have a diet high in animal fat.
- *ERT.* Unopposed estrogen replacement therapy (without progestin) increases the risk of endometrial cancer by five to eight times.
- *Previous cancers and/or treatments.* A history of breast or colon cancer seems to increase risk, perhaps due to genetic changes associated with certain BRCA mutations. Treatment with tamoxifen (see page 270) can also increase risk.
- *Age.* Ninety-five percent of endometrial cancers are found in women over 40; the average age at diagnosis is 60.

*Rita's Story*

Rita felt uncomfortably hormonal in her late forties, and consulted a physician who specialized in "creating the right and natural hormone milieu to combat aging" (there are quite a few of these in L.A.). He prescribed estrogen drops and a progesterone cream to augment her hormone levels, even though she was still having periods. She took the drops for three years, but at some point quit using the cream. She didn't worry about the "progesterone issue" because she bled every two months and even spotted irregularly, indicating (in her words) that her uterus was "doing its healthy self-cleaning."

When the bleeding continued for four weeks, she came to see me. An ultrasound revealed that her endometrium was thickened and uneven. An endometrial sampling found a well-differentiated cancer (the cells still looked like endometrial glands, indicating a fairly nonaggressive cancer). I performed a total hysterectomy, removing both tubes and ovaries as well as appropriate lymph nodes in a combined laparascopic vaginal procedure. The cancer had not spread, and she was essentially cured.

Rita's hot flashes were now severe. Although I told her that surgery for early endometrial cancer did not rule out subsequent estrogen therapy, she was understandably scared and chose to cope without medication.

## Protecting yourself from endometrial cancer

- Whatever your age, don't ignore irregular periods. If they are due to lack of ovulation, treat them with progestins or progesterone every one to two months or take birth control pills.
- Weight control: If you become obese, consult your doctor about routine pelvic ultrasound monitoring, especially if your periods are heavy or irregular.
- Taking birth control pills for two or more years, especially in your late thirties or forties, will reduce risk by 40 percent or more.
- If you take estrogen replacement, add some form of progestin.

## Diagnosing and treating endometrial cancer

The most important factor for early diagnosis is the recognition that abnormal bleeding at *any* age needs to be assessed. If a vaginal ultrasound shows uneven, white, thickened areas within the uterus, further testing should be done. Saline (saltwater fluid) can be injected through a catheter into the uterine lining to determine if these white areas are polyps, fibroids, or an abnormal endometrium. If the latter is found, a tissue biopsy should be done. A local anesthetic is injected into the cervix (a paracervical block); then a thin cannula (hollow tube) is inserted through the cervix into the endometrial cavity to scrape off and withdraw cells.

If cancer is found, the usual treatment is a total hysterectomy (uterus and cervix). The ovaries and some lymph nodes should also be removed, since this is where the cancer cells initially spread. Testing these tissues allows the surgeon to "stage" the cancer and decide if additional therapy is needed. If the cancer is contained within the uterine lining, the initial surgery should suffice. If it has invaded a major portion of the uterine muscle, or spread to the cervix or other pelvic organs, then radiation, chemotherapy, and/or high doses of progestin may be necessary.

## Colon Cancer

From age 50, there is frequently a gender separation of care by "generalist" physicians: Men are directed to begin colon cancer screening, while all below-the-waist care for women is delegated to a gynecologist. It's as if our digestive tract ends with our stomachs, and the only lower abdominal organs that can malfunction are our uterus and ovaries. And we women tend to have an "I don't feel anything is wrong, therefore I don't need to be tested" attitude when it comes to our lower gastrointestinal tracts. Or, like Nicole (at the start of this chapter), the "yuck" factor makes us put it off.

In fact, for women over 50 that first colorectal screening is probably more important than a Pap smear—and close in importance to a mammogram. Colorectal cancer is the third-leading cause of cancer deaths in women (after lung and breast cancer). One in eighteen women will develop this cancer in her lifetime—and 25 percent of those who get it, will die from it. In fact, we are far more prone to this cancer than we are to any malignancy of our pelvic reproductive tract.

Most colorectal cancers develop over eight to ten years, from benign growths called "polyps." This is one of the very few cancers that provide ample opportunity to detect and remove a growth before it becomes cancerous.

There are several options for screening an average-risk woman. (You are such a woman if you have no family history of colon cancer and no personal history of inflammatory bowel disease or polyps.) These should be started at the very least by the age of 50:

- Annual fecal occult blood testing plus flexible *sigmoidoscopy* (every five years)
- Double-contrast *barium enema:* X rays done after you drink a thick liquid, which coats your insides to give a clearer image (every five to ten years)
- *Colonoscopy* (at least every ten years).

I'll discuss these in more detail later, but first let's look at . . .

**Colon cancer risk factors**
Even though eight out of ten women who develop colon cancer have no defined risk, your risk can increase if you:

- Have a first- or second-degree relative with colon cancer, especially if he or she was younger than 60 at the onset of illness.
- Have had large, multiple, or precancerous polyps found in previous exams.
- Have a history of *ulcerative colitis* (also called chronic inflammatory bowel disease, or Crohn's disease).
- Smoke cigarettes. The cancer-causing agents in smoke are swallowed and get into your digestive system. Smoking contributes to 12 percent of fatal colorectal cancers, and smokers are 30 to 40 percent more likely to die from colorectal cancer.
- Have undiagnosed rectal bleeding or a change in bowel habits.
- Eat a diet rich in red meat and animal fat, which promotes overproduction of irritating bile acids.
- Have abdominal obesity (a "spare tire").

## Ways to reduce your risk

- *Cut down on red meat and animal fat;* eat more fruits and vegetables.
- *Take folic acid supplements;* the suggested dose is 400 mcg a day. Research shows this may decrease colon cancer risk after fifteen years of use, especially if you have a genetic predisposition.
- *Get more exercise and lose weight.*
- *Stop smoking.*
- *Calcium.* Calcium binds irritating bile acids. A high-calcium diet or calcium supplements (1,200 mg of elemental calcium per day) has been shown to reduce colorectal adenomas by 15 percent after one year.
- *Aspirin.* This pain reliever inhibits enzymes (COX-1 and COX-2) involved in the production of inflammatory substances that trigger early mutation and growth of colon cancer cells. In the Nurses' Health Study, women who used aspirin two or more times a week had a 44 percent lower risk of ever developing colon cancer after using it for more than twenty years. However, there is no current recommendation of how much aspirin to take or how often. Too much aspirin may actually injure the intestinal tract, causing ulcers and bleeding. My suggestion is, as long as you are not aspirin sensitive and don't have side effects that preclude your taking this over-the-counter but potent medication, consider starting low-dose aspirin at least three times a week when you are in your midfifties (for heart, brain, and colon protection). Before that, feel free to take an occasional aspirin for headache or pain.
- *Other NSAIDs* (nonsteroidal anti-inflammatory drugs) may also offer

mild colon cancer protection, but studies are too few to justify official recommendations.

- *COX-2 inhibitors.* These newer drugs (Celebrex, Vioxx, Bextra) may prove to be more potent anti-inflammatory modes of protection against colon cancer, with fewer side effects than aspirin, but the proof is not yet definitive. We also have to consider the cost-benefit analysis: COX-2 inhibitors require a doctor's prescription and are much more expensive than aspirin.
- *Estrogen therapy.* ERT may help decrease the production of irritating bile acids and tumor growth factors.

It was once thought that fiber and vitamins might help ward off colon cancer. Adding fiber to your diet is good for regularity and general nutrition, but there are conflicting reports on whether it protects against polyp development or recurrence. No protective effect has been found from supplementation with vitamins A, C, D, or E.

### Colon cancer screening

In the past, you were given a bill of clean colon health if fecal occult blood testing and sigmoidoscopy were negative—no blood in the stool, and no polyps seen through the flexible lighted scope inserted into your sigmoid colon (lower third of the colon). But 40 percent of colon cancers develop above the reach of the sigmoidoscope, and 75 percent of people who have polyps and/or cancers in this unseen area appear to be totally polyp free when just their lower colon is scoped. So, many physicians, myself included, feel that to screen appropriately, we need to view the entire colon.

A barium enema X ray, which requires no anesthetic, gives us an image of this portion of the digestive tract. But it's uncomfortable, can miss important lesions, and requires follow-up with a colonoscopy and a biopsy if something suspicious is found. (So now you've had to go through two preps and two procedures.)

The state-of-the-art "look, find, and remove" approach is colonoscopy. This procedure is performed at special clinics or outpatient facilities under mild sedation. Preparation includes ingesting clear liquids for twenty-four hours before the procedure (a lot of apple juice and Jell-O), and drinking a bowel-cleansing medication that causes diarrhea. This is the part that's unpleasant, but we've all had bouts of diarrhea and know what to expect, and it's over in a few hours.

Because sedation is given, the procedure itself should be painless.

(When I had it done I remember asking the doctor when we would start and being told that the procedure was over and I was fine.)

The numbers speak for themselves. Fecal occult blood testing of stool by itself (assuming a follow-up with a colonoscopy of everyone who tests positive) can prevent 15 to 33 percent of colon cancer deaths. Sigmoidoscopy, again followed by colonoscopy if polyps are found, can prevent 50 percent of these deaths. But the true "life saver" is colonoscopy, which, if performed on low-risk adults, can prevent *over 90 percent* of colon cancer deaths.

If you haven't grown polyps by your fifties, and there is no family history, you may be at extremely low risk of ever growing them; a colonoscopy every five or even ten years should suffice. If, however, you have been identified as a "polyp grower," depending on the biopsy results, you will need this test at least every three years. Removal of polyps prevents them from becoming cancerous.

Despite these stats, only one-third of us undergo appropriate colorectal screening. We may get on the gyne table for Pap smears, but any exam involving the lower end of our G.I. tract elicits disgust and denial. This dainty reticence can lead to a much greater bodily invasion: removal of part of the colon, *colostomy* (a surgical opening in the abdomen created for the stool to pass), and even death.

## Osteoporosis

Among the teens in my class at the School of American Ballet, Kelly was a standout. We all envied her extensions; she seemed to have no joints and could raise either leg high above her head. Her arabesques were perfect, and she floated as she pirouetted across the room. Kelly was all muscle and, we thought, exquisite bones.

Yes, her abdomen stuck out, but maybe that was due to her arched back. Her skin had a minor orange tinge, but perhaps that was a family trait; besides, makeup took care of it. She never seemed to be bothered by menstrual cramps or the need to change tampons like the rest of us. (I now understand that she was anorectic.)

I lost touch with Kelly when I went to college and then medical school. I heard she had become a well-known dancer. But in her forties, Kelly's bones gave out. Today, in her fifties, she is crippled by osteoporosis. This beautiful dancer now requires a walker to traverse a room.

Osteoporosis ages our bones and shrinks our bodies, the world we

## Is There a Virtual Colonoscopy Compromise?

Some women procrastinate because they don't want to be "put under," or don't have someone to drive them home after the procedure. Others worry about trauma to or perforation of the colon during the insertion of the scope (it's amazing how many "This happened to..." horror stories abound). Perforation is a rare complication that, if it occurs, is more likely to happen during biopsy or removal of a large polyp. I assure my patients that if they're in the hands of a physician skilled in colonoscopy, this concern should not prevent them from going through the procedure.

In recent years, "virtual" colonoscopy has been touted as a "no sedation, no invasion" alternative to the probe: creating a picture of the colon through multiple X rays of the colon with computerized tomography. However, know that you need to have the same bowel-cleaning preparation for a virtual colonoscopy as you would for the actual one. (In the future, it may be possible to swallow a substance that "tags" food so the scanner can distinguish between a polyp and something you ate. But right now, stool and polyps are indistinguishable.)

Also, during the scan, the colon is inflated with gas to separate the walls so that growths can be detected. This can be quite uncomfortable. The image may miss small and medium-sized polyps (less than one centimeter). This "miss" may be corrected if very high tech scanners using three dimensions (rather than the conventional two) are employed. Finally, a virtual scan gives images but does not diagnose or treat cancer. If a polyp is seen, you will have to schedule a true colonoscopy for verification and biopsy—which means another bowel prep and another medical bill. (As of this writing, Medicare and most insurers do not cover virtual colonoscopy.)

Since your first colon investigation establishes whether or not you form polyps, I recommend that you have a real colonoscopy. If you are polyp free, you might consider a virtual screening (with an experienced radiologist—not at a shopping-mall body-imaging center) for follow-up in the years to come.

move through, and our lifespan. None of us likes to imagine our future selves as hunched-over "little" old ladies (sweet or otherwise). Yet, we have to realize that our most age-vulnerable bones are the vertebrae in our spinal column. As they lose bone mass, they collapse, creating the curvature called "dowager's hump." As the vertebrae buckle, they press on the nerves emanating from the spinal cord, causing severe pain, muscle weakness, and even paralysis. The rib cage loses its support, constricting the heart, lungs, stomach, liver, and intestines so they can't function properly.

Upper-body support is just part of the story. Even minimal trauma can result in fractures of the hip, rib, wrist, ankle, and pelvis. Twenty percent of women who fracture a hip—and face medical complications from the trauma, surgery to replace the broken joint or insert pins to support it, and a prolonged recovery—will be dead within a year. Another 25 percent will need long-term or lifetime nursing care, and half will no longer be able to walk without a cane or walker.

Initially, this is a silent disease. We don't feel that our bones are becoming porous, until they break or collapse. Our internal support crumbles while we concentrate on our external appearance. How often do you wonder, "How are my bones doing today?" as you step on the scale, apply skin cream, or blow-dry your hair?

Your past may not include intensive athletic training or dieting (with irregular or absent menstrual periods), but that doesn't exempt you from the very real threat of bone loss as you get older.

### The making, and not breaking, of your bones

Your bones amass 90 percent of their mineral content by age 18. This engineering feat is achieved through a very active breakdown-and-building process, which occurs in three-month cycles. Bone-eating cells called *osteoclasts* drill small cavities that are then filled and expanded by bone-building cells called *osteoblasts*.

With proper nutrition, calcium, and estrogen production, the filling outpaces the drilling, and your bones increase their density until your early thirties—your age of peak bone density and the baseline from which your bones will be judged in the future. From here, filling may not compensate for drilling, due to declining osteoblast function, and you gradually lose bone mass. In your forties, this occurs at a rate of 0.5 percent per year. And with the estrogen loss of menopause, bone loss accelerates 2 to 3 percent a year for the first five or ten years postmenopause.

If you were bone-smart from childhood through your twenties, and your parents bestowed upon you good bone genes, you will reach a personal best at 30 sufficient to withstand the later loss. But if you start low, and lose more, you may be among the 40 percent of women whose fragile bones are likely to fracture.

**Assessing your osteoporosis risk**
Bone up on the following:

If you are Caucasian or Asian and over fifty . . .

- There is a 20 percent chance that you already have osteoporosis.
- There's a 50 percent chance that you are *osteopenic* (have low bone density—on the path to osteoporosis).
- Your lifetime risk of developing an osteoporotic fracture is 40 percent.

The figures are lower for black and Hispanic women.
You are at particular risk if:

- You already have a diagnosed vertebral fracture.
- You weigh less than 125 pounds.
- You didn't get your period for six months or more when you were younger—especially if you were thin, participated in competitive sports, or had a chronic disease.
- You had early (before 45) menopause.
- Your mother broke her hip.
- You smoke or abuse alcohol.
- You have a medical condition such as hyperparathyroidism (overactive parathyroid), Cushing's syndrome (overproduction of adrenal hormone), or intestinal malabsorption.
- You have taken (or are taking) oral steroid medication for more than three months.
- You chronically use(d) steroid inhalers.
- You are taking too much thyroid medication.
- You have rheumatoid arthritis or diabetes.
- You have a history of clinical depression. (This may affect growth hormone and bone formation.)

**How and when to get your bone density tested**
The bone "gold standard" is the dual-energy X-ray absorbtiometry (DXA) done on the hip and/or spine. You lie on a table with your clothes on (a nice change), and an image of your bones appears on a computer screen. The computer calculates bone density based on the way the energy waves are absorbed by different areas of the bones. It's quick—less than ten minutes—and safe. The amount of radiation is much less than that from a mammogram. It costs between $130 and $250. (Medicare pays a portion.)

The results are given as a standard deviation (SD) from the average of "ideal" women of your race who have reached their peak bone density, in their early thirties. This is called the T score. A comparison is also made with women in your age group; this is called the Z score. A decrease of one standard deviation corresponds to a 10 to 15 percent bone loss beyond the average for the group with which you're being compared.

"Osteoporosis" has been defined by the World Health Organization as a bone density T score at or below –2.5 SD. *Osteopenia* is the term assigned to T scores between –1 and –2.5 SD. These are very arbitrary labels, so when your score goes from –2.4 to –2.6, it doesn't mean that the affected bone will break today, or even in the future. These numbers simply indicate a continuous increase in risk. The hip measurement may be the most relevant guide to whether you'll break any bone. Your lifetime risk of fracture approximately doubles for each decrease of one standard deviation. At the age of 50, if you have a zero T score (i.e., it hasn't changed since you were 30), your lifetime fracture risk is calculated to be 10 percent. This increases to 33 percent if your T score is –2.5, and 49 percent if it's –3.5.

Since your insurance carrier may balk at paying for a DXA scan of your hips and spine unless you already have a diagnosis of osteoporosis or are over age 65, your doctor may initially screen you with a smaller machine that scans your arm or heel. This costs less than $45. If you score well, it probably means the rest of your bones would pass more extensive testing. But if your score is low, you should proceed to the nearest DXA machine for a full hip and spine evaluation. (At this point, your insurance carrier should acknowledge the medical need and cover the scan.)

A body scan, or quantitative computer tomography, also evaluates bone density. It takes three-dimensional pictures, but exposes you to at least ten times more radiation than a DXA test, gives results that are not as clear for predicting fractures, and costs more.

There is one more method to peer inside your bones: ultrasound, which measures the speed of sound waves passing through bone so that calculations can be made of whether the bone is dense or porous. The heel is usually checked by a portable "just step right up and see" device. If you test low, you should follow up with a DXA of your hip and probably your spine.

**When should you start bone testing?**
The internal crumbling of our support system progresses silently until, like Humpty Dumpty, we fall or just apply the wrong pressure. When to test bones depends on your risk factors—and who you ask. The National

Osteoporosis Foundation states that BMD (bone mineral density) testing should be done on:

1. All postmenopausal women 65 or older, regardless of additional risk factors (even if they have been on osteoporosis therapy, but never had an official BMD test)
2. Postmenopausal women younger than 65 with one or more additional risk factors for osteoporosis (see page 288)
3. Postmenopausal women who have had a fracture of any type as an adult after age 45

I use these recommendations for my patients, and I'll often add urine and blood tests for women who have osteoporosis at an earlier-than-expected age, in order to see if their bone loss occurred in the past or is ongoing. First, I have the patient collect her urine for twenty-four hours; if its calcium content is low, that indicates poor calcium absorption through the G.I. tract. I then test the urine and blood for markers of bone resorption (substances released when bone is broken down). If these tests show active bone loss in a relatively young patient, I test her parathyroid hormone levels (see below).

## How to Treat Your Bones So They Treat You Well

All of the available therapies work by stopping the hole-drilling (resorbing) cells from excavating tiny cavities, and allowing the bone-filling cells

### Hyperparathyroidism: The Disease That Eats Up Bone

The parathyroids are glands that sit on both sides of the thyroid, near the base of the neck. They regulate the amount of calcium in your bloodstream. If the calcium level falls, parathyroid hormone is secreted, and instructs the bone-eating cells to go into action so that this mineral is released from the bones to go where it is needed.

Calcium is essential for all muscle contractions, including those of your heart, as well as the function of your vascular and nervous systems. If the parathyroid becomes overactive, bone is literally eaten up, causing blood calcium levels to become dangerously high. This disorder is usually treated by surgically removing the parathyroid glands.

(primed with calcium) to fill in these porous areas. Hence, these medications are called "antiresorptive drugs." Note that the ones that are listed under prevention will help support the therapies listed as treatment.

## Prevention

*Calcium.* The most essential age-defying mineral is calcium. Our daily requirement increases from 1,000 mg between ages 25 and 50, to 1,200 mg over 50, and 1,500 mg if we're not using ERT/HRT or older than 65. Why? Over the years, our intestines absorb less calcium, especially as our estrogen levels plummet. Typically, our sun exposure also decreases and our "older" kidneys produce less vitamin D, contributing to poor calcium absorption. Our parathyroid glands have to work harder to ensure that blood levels of calcium remain adequate and "strip" our bones in order to do so. Since most of us get less than 600 mg a day in our diet, we need to turn to, and take, calcium supplements.

To figure out the amount of elemental calcium you're getting per tablet, always look at the back of the bottle; the numbers on the front are often confusing and even misleading. More is not better; doses of calcium greater than 2,500 mg a day can cause kidney damage. And don't try to take all your calcium at once; you can't absorb more than 600 mg at a time.

If you are calcium deficient, taking supplements may reduce your risk of bone fracture by 10 to 15 percent. But if you have low bone density and you are experiencing the rapid bone loss of early menopause, or you already have osteoporosis, supplements are not enough. However, calcium should be added to whatever you take or do to enhance bone strength, since it's the cement needed for all bone work, be it construction or support.

*Vitamin D.* In order for calcium to be absorbed by your intestine and incorporated into your bones, you need vitamin D. This "sunshine" vitamin is made in your skin after exposure to certain wavelengths of sunlight. You need only fifteen minutes a day for ample D production, but as soon as you don your clothes or apply sunscreen, you block this effect. Milk and some cereals are fortified with vitamin D, but yogurt and cheeses are not. Small amounts of D are also produced by your kidneys, but this decreases with age. You need 400 IU (international units) most of your life, but if you are over 65—or exposed to limited sunlight at any age—take 800 IU. Since vitamin D is long-acting, you don't need to get it at the very same time you take your calcium. Your multivitamin has 400

## Types of Calcium Supplements: Good, Better, Best?

*Calcium carbonate* (Calci-Chew, Caltrate, Os-Cal, Oyster Shell Calcium, Rolaids Calcium Rich, Tums, Viactiv, and many more). This is the most concentrated form of calcium you can take, which means that you may be able to make do (depending on your daily requirements) with one to three tablets or chews a day. Here are the carbonate facts:

- Well absorbed, if you have normal amounts of stomach acid (which decreases with age, or with acid-lowering medications).
- Should be taken with food, and in divided doses (500 to 600 mg at a time; more than that is not absorbed).
- Should not be taken at the same time as iron supplements (which decrease calcium absorption).
- May cause constipation or bloating, less so if you take it with lots of water.

*Calcium citrate* (labeled as calcium citrate or Citracal brand). This is the most easily absorbed calcium, but it is less concentrated and requires more tablets than calcium carbonate to achieve your required daily dose. These are the citrate facts:

- Well absorbed, even with low levels of stomach acid.
- Should be taken *between* meals.
- Will not cause, and may even prevent, kidney stones.
- Should not be taken at the same time as iron supplements.
- Causes less gas or constipation than calcium carbonate.

**Other calcium supplements:**
- Calcium phosphate (Posture). This is similar to calcium carbonate, but more expensive.
- Calcium lactate (Calphosan, Phos-Cal) and gluconate (Kalcinate). These have low elemental calcium content, and require consumption of many tablets.
- Calcium hydroxyapatite (Bone-Up capsules). This is made from cow bones (bone meal), combined with other minerals, protein, and glucosamine. It should be taken in divided doses with meals. Six capsules supply 1,000 mg of calcium.

IU, and calcium tablets often contain extra D, so you can easily reach your daily goal. But don't consume over 2,000 IU per day.

*Estrogen.* Estrogen is good for your bones, whether you produce it or take it. With postmenopausal use, it initially increases spine density by 4 to 6 percent, and hip density by 2 to 3 percent. It maintains these increases after three years of treatment. But once you stop estrogen, menopausal bone loss restarts and your gains may disappear. Even low-dose estrogen seems to be effective, which is a boon in our current state of worry about "taking too much." ERT/HRT probably does its best bone work if you start during the first five to ten years after menopause.

Most studies have shown at least a 25 percent reduction in the risk of hip fracture for women who *ever* used ERT/HRT, and a 34 percent reduction for nonspine fractures for women who *currently* use it. The WHI study (see chapter 2) showed that after five years of HRT, the risk of hip and spine fractures was reduced by one-third, and the rate of other osteoporosis-related fractures went down by 23 percent. (Keep in mind that the average age of study participants was only 63, and follow-up may not have been long enough to assess the true benefit.)

Currently, the Food and Drug Administration (FDA) and the National Institutes of Health (NIH) have approved ERT/HRT for prevention, rather than treatment, of osteoporosis.

*What about magnesium?* This mineral is often included in calcium supplements; their labels suggest it's necessary for protection of bone health and absorption of calcium. Our average magnesium intake (280 mg) is probably enough to sustain appropriate calcium absorption. In studies, use of calcium alone proved just as beneficial as calcium plus magnesium (over 800 mg a day). If you have a gastrointestinal disease, or are over age 70 and have established osteoporosis, you should take an extra 500 mg of magnesium a day. (Your calcium or multimineral supplement may already include this.)

*What about progesterone cream?* To date, manufacturers' claims that natural progesterone cream prevents osteoporosis have not been substantiated. Clinical trials in which these creams were added to estrogen did not show that they increased the bone-protecting effects of estrogen. The exception may be a high-dose, high-potency oral progestin called Megace, which is used to treat recurrent or metastatic cancer of the breast and endometrium.

## Treating Osteoporosis

### Bisphosphonates

These medications act like our natural phosphate compound but resist being broken down by enzymes. Once absorbed into the bone, they are there to stay, and stop osteoclast action. There are currently three bisphosphonates commonly used for treatment of osteoporosis.

*Alendronate (Fosamax).* This has been approved by the FDA for postmenopausal osteoporosis prevention and treatment. In early menopause (two to four years after periods stop), a half dose (5 mg a day, or 35 mg a week) has been found to increase spine and hip BMD by 1 to 4 percent after two years. This drug, like the other bisphosphonates, seems to work best if your BMD (bone mineral density) is at least two standard deviations below that of an average 30-year-old, or you have established osteoporosis. The full dose can increase bone density by 6 to 10 percent after three years, and decrease hip and spinal fracture by up to 50 percent. If you don't have osteoporosis, there seems to be no significant effect on new fracture rates.

To treat osteoporosis, Fosamax can be taken as a daily 10-mg pill, or weekly as one 70-mg pill. Because it is poorly absorbed, it should be taken on an empty stomach with 8 ounces of water. Wait at least thirty minutes after taking Fosamax before eating or drinking anything. Do not lie down after taking the pill (you don't want the tablet to remain in one place on the way down and cause an erosion). You should not take Fosamax if you have reflux or ulcer problems.

*Risedronate (Actonel).* Approved for prevention and treatment of postmenopausal osteoporosis, it increases bone density between 3 and 6 percent in three years, and decreases spine fracture by 30 to 45 percent. In postmenopausal women in their seventies with osteoporosis (again, this seems to work better if you have the disease), just one year of therapy reduced their risk of vertebral fracture by as much as 65 percent, and hip fracture by 40 percent, but failed to do so in older women who did not have osteoporosis. This medication can be taken daily at a dose of 5 mg, or as a once-weekly pill of 35 mg. Like Fosamax, it should be taken with water only, and you should stay in an upright position for thirty minutes postingestion. It can cause heartburn and stomach upset, but some studies suggest these are less severe than with Fosamax.

*Didronel (Etidronate).* This is approved in Canada for osteoporosis prevention and treatment in postmenopausal women (but that use is not

FDA-approved). As the first bisphosphonate on the U.S. market (for another bone disease), it was prescribed by many doctors and was found to increase bone mineral density by 4 percent in the spine, 2.3 percent in the hip. It appeared to reduce risk of vertebral fracture by 37 percent, but did not reduce hip fracture. Too much of this drug can cause abnormal bone production, so it should only be taken for fourteen days every three months, at a dose of 400 mg per day. It does not seem to have gastrointestinal side effects.

*SERMs* (selective estrogen receptor modulators). These drugs act like estrogens in some parts of the body (e.g., bones and certain organs) and oppose estrogen in others. SERMs include raloxifene and tamoxifen, but only *raloxifene (Evista)* is approved for osteoporosis prevention and treatment in the United States. In postmenopausal women, it increases BMD in the spine and hip by 2 to 3 percent over three years and reduces the risk of vertebral fracture in such women with known osteoporosis by 45 to 50 percent. So far, it has not been shown to reduce fracture risk at other sites.

Like estrogen, Evista also lowers total cholesterol and low-density lipoprotein (but it does not raise the "good" HDL levels). Unlike certain oral estrogens, it does not raise triglycerides. This may translate into a meaningful cardioprotective effect in those postmenopausal women who are at high risk for cardiovascular disease (see page 232). There are also very encouraging data that raloxifene decreases breast cancer risk by 65 percent over four years when used by women with osteoporosis.

Raloxifene is prescribed as a daily 60-mg tablet. It does not cause gastrointestinal upset but, like estrogen, can increase the risk of deep-vein clots. The most common side effect is hot flashes. For women who already suffer from this symptom, this may be cause for pause when weighing which medication to take for their bones.

### Some other osteoporosis medications

*Calcitonin (Miacalcin nasal spray).* Our thyroids produce calcitonin, but not enough for postmenopausal bone protection. A synthetic form of salmon calcitonin (fifteen times more potent than our body's "home-made" product) was first developed as a shot but is now available as a nasal spray under the brand name Miacalcin. It stops bone resorption, but to a lesser degree than the other treatments listed above. It is indicated only for women who are at least five years postmenopause. Studies have found that this medication increased spinal BMD by 3 percent, but no significant effect has been seen in the hip. Calcitonin may reduce the risk of new vertebral fracture in postmenopausal women with osteoporosis, but there are questions about the dose required to do this. So, most experts don't view calcitonin as a first-line therapy and prescribe it only for women who can't take other osteoporosis medications.

*Parathyroid hormone: Teriparatide (Forteo).* This is the most effective bone builder currently available for women with severe osteoporosis. It represents the dichotomy of medicine: Too much of a hormone may cause harm (e.g., hyperparathyroidism activates bone-eating cells), but small amounts can be beneficial. In this case, small spurts of recombinant human parathyroid promote bone remodeling by increasing the number and action of the osteoblasts, which then "lay down" bone at an accelerated rate. Forteo is given as a daily injection under the skin with a disposable pen device that can be used for up to twenty-eight days. Studies have shown that after nineteen months, this therapy can reduce the incidence of new vertebral fractures by almost 70 percent (in women who have already had that type of fracture), and of nonvertebral fractures by over 50 percent, compared with placebo. It costs about $600 a month for daily injections, which are given for no longer than two years—sounds expensive, but in the long run, it's cheaper than surgery, prolonged hospitalization, and nursing home care.

*Testosterone (male hormone).* Adding male hormone to estrogen may be more effective than estrogen alone in building bone density, especially in the femur (the long bone in the thigh).

*Tibolone (Livial).* This synthetic hormone has estrogen, male hormone, and progestinlike properties. Currently unavailable in the United States, it's very popular in Europe for treating menopausal symptoms and bone loss due to lack of estrogen and menopause.

*Statins.* In the lab, statins inhibit bone-eating cells, but we're not sure whether this translates into a real-world, whole-bone benefit.

## Combination therapies

On occasion my patients and I are disappointed to find that one therapy has not improved the measurement of their bone density. Results may seem low or absent because of a slight variation in a machine's calibration, and comparing results from different machines may erroneously give the impression of bone loss. Moreover, it can take over two years to see a positive change resulting from treatment. However, even no change is positive; remember, without the medication, bone loss would have progressed and bone mineral density would have decreased, not stayed the same.

There is evidence that combining estrogen or Evista with any of the bisphosphonates causes favorable though modest increases in BMD, compared with use of any of the agents alone. We don't yet know if this translates into better fracture protection.

## Osteoarthritis: When Joints Wear Out

It's hard to feel young when you can't stand up straight without pain. The most common form of arthritis, osteoarthritis (OA) is a leading cause of life-constraining disability. This disease involves the progressive destruction of cartilage, the hard but slippery tissue around your joints that absorbs shock and lets bones glide smoothly. If you develop OA, your surface layer of cartilage starts to wear out and lose elasticity. Your joint linings (*synovia*) get irritated, dry up, and the bones rub against one another—causing swelling and pain, and limiting motion. To add to the joint destruction, tiny pieces of bone or cartilage can break off and float around in that joint space.

Many of us have these changes without the concomitant discomfort. If we were to X-ray the joints of everyone over 65, half would have this damage, but only a third of the group would feel it. The joints that get the most wear and tear are the ones likely to undergo these changes: our hands, knees, hips, and spine. After age 45, we women are more likely to suffer than men, as our joints' clock seems to be affected by our hormonal clock.

My husband often quotes a phrase that was passed down in his long-lived family: "Every time you wake up in the morning and don't hurt more than when you went to sleep, be thankful." His ancestors must have had osteoarthritis, and rightly noted that the pain was more severe in the morning, before their joints began their daily functioning.

I'd estimate that 17 percent of my patients over 45 have significant joint pain—enough that I have direct speed-dial between my office and my favorite rheumatologists and orthopedic surgeons. So far I've been lucky; nothing hurts. But every time I see a patient with severe osteoarthritis, I question whether I want to take the chance of injury or joint stress from skiing or running. And yes, I bless the fact that I awake in the morning without pain.

### Risk factors and symptoms

Osteoarthritis can result from a combination of cartilage fatigue, joint injury, stress from carrying extra weight, and a profession or sport that stresses joints. There seems to be a genetic component to some hand and knee arthritis. The symptoms: joint pain (steady or occasional), stiffness in your joints after sitting or sleeping, joint swelling, or hearing or feeling "crunching" as bones rub together.

### Diagnosing osteoarthritis

After a physical exam, your doctor will order an X ray to assess bone damage, bone spurs, and cartilage loss. However, there may not be a direct correlation between these findings and your pain or disability, and early disease may go undetected. Blood tests or tests of fluid drawn from the joint may be necessary to rule out other disorders, such as infections or autoimmune disease.

### Managing osteoarthritis

There are no treatments available that can reverse cartilage damage, but it is possible to relieve symptoms and minimize further damage.

### Nondrug treatments

*Rest and stress management.* There's an expression I learned from my parents: "Don't be a shtarker." Taken from the Yiddish, it means don't overdo. Work those joints, but don't push them to the point of increased pain. If the physical demands of your job are a problem, an occupational therapist may be able to help you find ways to work around your symptoms.

*Splints and braces.* Judicious use of splints or braces (while sleeping or during certain activities) can be helpful, but overuse can actually promote weakness and stiffness. Consider getting special shoe inserts that redistribute your weight to better protect joints.

*Weight loss.* An extra 10 pounds puts twenty or thirty pounds of force on the knee with each step. Taking off weight can be critical to improving your symptoms.

*Acupuncture.* There is some evidence that acupuncture can improve knee pain and function, when used as a supplement to other therapies.

*Hot or cold packs.* Applying heat (a hot pack, hot towel, or hot shower) can help reduce pain, or you may get relief from an ice pack or cold pack (you can even use a bag of frozen vegetables wrapped in a dishtowel).

### Managing arthritis with medications

The trick here is to balance pain relief with its potential side effects. Never combine medications without consulting your doctor; they can cancel each other's benefits or cause dangerous interactions. Discuss

## Is It Safe to Exercise?

Just sitting there is the worst thing you can do for your osteoarthritis. In a study of patients over 45, simple home-based exercise significantly reduced pain and increased function. (And the more closely they stuck with the program, the greater their reduction in pain.)

Start with walking: The more you walk, the more you can do so without pain. Swimming, using exercise machines, and even biking can be beneficial— but don't begin an exercise program without developing a plan with your physical therapist or physician. It's important to learn to warm up safely and to know when not to put strain on a joint. Your exercises should include:

- Strength-building exercises. For example, building up your quadriceps (thigh muscles) will help arthritic knees.
- Exercises to stretch and work joints and improve range of motion.
- Aerobic exercise to help control weight.

ways to minimize side effects (e.g., if you should take the medication with food, or add another drug to protect your stomach). Here are your options:

*Acetaminophen (Tylenol).* This is considered first-line therapy, and can work well to relieve mild to moderate pain when there is minimal inflammation. Regular use can be dangerous, however, if you have liver problems, consume too much alcohol, or use blood-thinning medications.

*Nonsteroidal anti-inflammatory drugs (NSAIDs).* These reduce pain and inflammation by inhibiting an enzyme called cyclooxygenase, which comes in two forms, COX-1 and COX-2. (COX-1 may protect the stomach lining, whereas COX-2 is an active participant in the process of inflammation.) NSAIDs, such as aspirin, naproxen (Aleve), or ibuprofen (Advil, Motrin IB), are available over the counter. Prescription NSAIDs include diclofenac (Voltaren, Cataflam, Arthrotec), meloxicam (Mobic), and naproxen (Anaprox, Naprelan).

Some of these drugs also seem to offer protection against colon cancer, and aspirin may be good for your heart. However, because they suppress COX-1, they can cause stomach problems (including bleeding and ulcers) and are best taken with food or in enteric-coated pills. Your doctor may also add a stomach-protective drug such as misoprostol

(Cytotec), a histamine blocker (Tagamet or Zantac), or a proton-pump inhibitor (Prilosec, Prevacid).

*COX-2 inhibitors* (Bextra, Celebrex, Vioxx). These are a subtype of NSAIDs that work by suppressing only the COX-2 enzyme. This preferential blocking may make them easier on your gastrointestinal system. The downside is that these drugs may not be good for your heart, and of course newer prescription drugs are more expensive than older (or over the counter) medications.

*Creams.* Topical creams, sprays, or rubs containing capsaicin or methylsalicylate can temporarily relieve pain. Menthol, oil of wintergreen, camphor, or eucalyptus oil can also make your joints feel "comforted."

*Injections.* For intractable pain, hyaluronic acid (Synvisc, Hyalgan) can be injected into knee joints. Corticosteroid injections into joints can reduce severe inflammation but should not be used more than two or three times a year.

*Estrogen.* There is evidence that ERT can slow the progression of joint disease. Low estrogen levels may promote arthritis. Although it's not officially listed as a menopausal complaint, I've noticed that many of my patients feel joint achiness at the onset of menopause, and that this is relieved once they start estrogen therapy. Joint discomfort may recur after ERT is discontinued.

*Supplements.* There is some evidence that vitamins D, C, E, or beta-carotene may help slow disease progression. A large NIH trial is under way to test whether supplements of glucosamine and chondroitin sulfate might minimize joint damage (see page 195). (These are components of normal cartilage, naturally present in food.) Don't take this route without medical supervision.

*Surgical treatments.* If your mobility is seriously limited and you are in severe pain, you may choose to undergo surgery in which the knee or hip joint is replaced with a metal, plastic, or ceramic prosthesis. These can last for ten to fifteen years (or longer as the prostheses improve). A soft synthetic implant that can substitute for worn-out knee cartilage was recently approved for use in Europe, and is being used in trials by a few specialists in the United States.

**Treatments that don't work**
Promises, promises . . . have been made in treating arthritis, some in good faith, others in hopes of faithfully making money. In the past, the orthopedic surgeons did a procedure that "cleansed and flushed" (*debridement*

*and lavage*) the pieces of bone and scar tissue out of the knee joint. We all thought it helped. However, when this was compared with sham surgery (a small incision made, and nothing else done), lo and behold there was no difference in the outcome!

Beware of treatments promoted with words such as "natural," "cure," or "no side effects," or claims that the medical establishment is blocking the availability of a breakthrough, or ads offering testimonials instead of research evidence. This goes for medications, objects, and chiropractic manipulations. For more information, check reputable Internet sites such as the NIH's National Center for Complementary and Alternative Medicine (http://nccam.nih.gov), or Quackwatch (www.quackwatch.org).

**Better joints down the road . . .**
In the future, arthritis sufferers may get relief through gene therapy or stem cell transplantation. One day we hope to be able to grow new cartilage cells from your old ones, and inject them back into your joints if and when they become worn out.

## Coping with Thyroid Disorders

Hypothyroidism (underactive thyroid) becomes more common as we get older—and can literally slow us down while speeding our age clocks forward. The butterfly-shaped thyroid gland, found at the base of your Adam's apple, secretes a hormone that influences the growth and development of all your tissues, and regulates metabolism for the entire body. Once the thyroid gland ceases to make enough of its hormone, metabolism slows down.

This condition occurs in 5 to 10 percent of all women, and our female hormones are partly responsible. As they fluctuate during puberty, periods, pregnancy, and perimenopause, they may trigger an autoimmune reaction, so that antibodies mistakenly attack and destroy thyroid tissue. As women, we are five to eight times more likely than men to develop hypothyroidism, especially between our pregnancies and the onset of menopause. Indeed, the severe drop in estrogen and progesterone after a delivery causes 5 percent of women to become hypothyroid.

**Risk factors**
You are at increased risk for developing hypothyroidism if you have a family history of thyroid disease, or have an enlarged or uneven thyroid,

rheumatoid arthritis, diabetes, high cholesterol, or another autoimmune disease such as lupus—or if you just had a baby.

## Symptoms of hypothyroidism

These can vary from none (the disorder is discovered with a blood test) to a feeling that you've entered the twilight zone and don't recognize your body! Symptoms often include:

- Lethargy
- Weight gain
- Cold intolerance
- Constipation
- Dry skin
- Mental impairment
- Depression
- Irregular periods
- Menopausal symptoms

## Diagnosing hypothyroidism

The diagnosis is made with a blood test for TSH (thyroid stimulating hormone), which is secreted by the pituitary gland in the brain to stimulate the thyroid to produce thyroid hormones (thyroxin). If the thyroid doesn't do its job, the pituitary puts out more TSH.

The thyroid hormones are called T3 and T4. Most of these are bound to proteins in the blood; only unbound or free thyroid works on the cells. So, checking the free thyroxin index (FTI) or free T4 is sometimes used to assess the actual "working" levels of thyroid hormone and to monitor replacement therapy, especially during pregnancy.

It's imperative that we diagnose an underactive thyroid in pregnancy. This condition can increase risk for miscarriage, fetal death, premature labor, and pregnancy complications, and can also decrease a child's I.Q. later in life.

*Who should be tested?* If you are contemplating getting pregnant, or are in the beginning of your pregnancy, you should definitely be tested. Otherwise, begin routine testing between the ages of 35 and 40. TSH levels should then be checked every five years, since hypothyroidism develops slowly. If you develop symptoms, the blood test should be done sooner. Nearly every woman who comes into my office complaining of weight gain hopes to prove it's not her doing, but a "glandular thing."

Only rarely do an elevated TSH and a low thyroid hormone level explain those unwanted pounds.

### Thyroid-boosting treatments

Once the thyroid doesn't produce enough of its hormone, replacement is usually needed for the rest of your life. (The exceptions to this include pregnancy and incorrect initial diagnosis.) There has been much debate about the virtues of synthetic T4 hormone (levothyroxine) versus "natural" thyroid extract. The gold standard, and the therapy that has been successfully used for decades, is levothyroxine; the best-known brand is Synthroid. A few years ago there was a major Synthroid scare when it was "discovered" that eight million Americans use the drug daily—and it had not been FDA-approved. Not exactly the manufacturer's fault; Synthroid was developed before 1962, when current approval requirements were not an issue. In 1997, the FDA required that all brands of levothyroxine submit new drug applications (which have since been approved). There can be minor differences among brands, so if you switch from one brand to another, your TSH level should be checked.

*Treatment in pregnancy.* TSH levels should be checked every six weeks. The dose may need to be adjusted as the pregnancy progresses, and again after delivery (when perhaps it can be lowered or even stopped).

*Treatment for nonpregnant women.* Starting therapy if your TSH is over 5.5, even if you don't have symptoms, may make you feel "peppier." Thyroid therapy should definitely be prescribed if your TSH is greater than 7. The initial dose of levothyroxine ranges between 0.075 mg and 0.112 mg, depending on your body weight. Have your TSH levels rechecked after six to eight weeks to see if your dose is appropriate. It may take even longer to feel back to normal, so be a patient patient. Once the right dose is found, it usually remains stable for years and TSH levels need only be checked every six to twelve months.

*What about natural thyroid?* This contains large amounts of T3, which is broken down more quickly than T4, so a pill a day may not keep thyroid levels stable. It is prepared from animal thyroids obtained in slaughterhouses and may, indeed, vary in purity.

*Can thyroid medication interact with other drugs?* Yes. And this can change or cancel its level and action as well as that of the other drug. It should not be taken with antacids, calcium carbonate (Tums, Caltrate, calcium-containing Rolaids), or iron because it won't be properly absorbed. So, take these supplements at least four hours before or after your thyroid medication. Thyroid also changes the effectiveness of antiepileptic, anticoagulant, and anti-diabetic meds, digitalis (given for heart conditions), and tetracycline. If you take an SSRI antidepressant (Paxil, Prozac), the dose of thyroid may need to be increased.

### Too Much of a Good Thing?

Less common than hypothyroidism—but affecting about two million women—is hyperthyroidism. An overactive thyroid can cause fatigue and insomnia; nervousness and tremors; rapid heartbeat, palpitations, and shortness of breath; diarrhea; sweating, intolerance of heat, and hot flashes; frequent or heavy periods; infertility; and weight changes (usually loss, but sometimes gain through increased appetite). Slightly bulging eyeballs can be a sign of Graves' disease, a type of hyperthyroidism.

This disorder usually emerges between the ages of 20 and 40, and is diagnosed with a blood test for TSH, which will be abnormally low. Treatment options include medications to calm the thyroid down, or destroying the overactive cells with radioactive iodine. The latter causes the thyroid to cease all work—and an ongoing need to take thyroid hormone supplements.

If the symptoms include swelling or nodules (the "goiter" we used to see before iodine was routinely added to salt), part of the thyroid may need to be surgically removed.

## THE HEALTH-SPAN LIST: YOUR ROUTINE MEDICAL TESTS AND WHEN TO HAVE THEM

Let me say up front that this list is not as overwhelming as it seems.

- You need to visit your internist/family practitioner/primary care doctor, and probably your gynecologist once a year; many of these tests fit into your annual checkups.
- Most of the blood tests can be done at the same time.
- Eye exams can initially be performed by an optometrist; you might need to see an ophthalmologist if there are problems.

- The dermatologist is both your anticancer and cosmetic friend.
- Most radiology facilities can do mammograms and tests for bone mineral density in one appointment.
- You need to visit the gastroenterologist/proctologist once every five to ten years after age 50 (unless you have problems).

In sum, you'll probably end up taking your car for servicing more often than your body; let's keep our priorities straight. A small investment in early detection can save you years of healthy life.

## The "Slow Your Clock" List

### Monthly
Breast self-exam (at home)

### Annually
Pelvic exam
Clinical breast exam (by health care practitioner)
Skin self-exam (at home)
Age 21 to 30 (or if at high risk): Pap smear
After age 40: Mammogram; rectal exam
After age 50: Fecal occult blood test (if you "only" had sigmoid-oscopy)
After age 60: Urinalysis

### Every two years
Blood pressure (annually after age 50)
Skin exam by dermatologist

### Every three years
After age 30: Pap smear (if at low risk, after three negative tests)
Fasting blood glucose test (two-hour postmeal, or fasting insulin if at risk for insulin resistance or type 2 diabetes)
Eye exam (annually after age 65)

### Every 5 years
Fasting blood lipid levels (total cholesterol, HDL, LDL, triglycerides) and C-reactive protein
From 35: Thyroid test (TSH)

From age 40: Electrocardiogram (add echo stress test if at cardiac risk)

From age 50: Colorectal cancer screen: sigmoidoscopy (plus yearly stool check for occult blood) or *preferably* colonoscopy (every five to ten years, depending on risk)

**Onetime tests (repeat if necessary)**

At age 65: Bone mineral density (do earlier if at risk; do every two years if undergoing therapy)

**As-needed tests**

STD testing (sexually transmitted diseases): after new partner, before pregnancy, before a new sexual relationship

**Immunizations**

Every 10 years: Tetanus booster

Once at 65: Pneumococcal

Annually after 65: Influenza (or sooner at your doctor's discretion)

**Warning signs that should send you scurrying to the doctor**

From outside to inside:

- A mole that changes color, grows, or bleeds
- A breast lump, change in breast contour, or unusual breast pain; brown or bloody discharge from the nipple
- Vulvar or vaginal irritation or itching that does not go away, despite over-the-counter remedies
- Chest pain or any pain above the waist, especially if occurring during exertion or stress, accompanied by nausea and vomiting and shortness of breath
- Coughing that continues more than two weeks—earlier if it includes discolored or bloody sputum
- Shortness of breath with minimal exertion or stress, or when at rest
- Any change in heartbeat pattern or rhythm
- Unexplained weight loss or weight gain; loss of appetite
- Unusual, prolonged, or heavy vaginal bleeding
- Delayed menstrual period before your midforties, especially if accompanied by pelvic pain

- New, unusual, or unremitting pain in any part of your body, from head to toe
- Change in bowel habits (unexplained constipation, diarrhea); rectal bleeding
- Frequent need to urinate together with unusual thirst
- Unexplained abdominal bloating
- Any infection (signs include fever, chills, coughing, sore throat, burning with urination, diarrhea) that does not resolve quickly
- Frequency of, urgency of, or pain with urination
- Uncontrollable loss of urine with coughing, sneezing, change in position, exercise
- Inability to prevent urination after urge to void
- Unexplained fatigue or malaise (just not feeling well); dizziness; fainting
- Severe, unusual headaches that don't respond to over-the-counter pain medications
- Difficulty thinking or remembering, even if transitory
- Numbness, even if transitory, in any part of the body
- Mood changes that last more than a couple of weeks

**The future of early detection**
Our ultimate disease detection will emerge through genomic science. Finding the "genes of risk" may put each of us on molecular notice so that we can modify our behavior, take appropriate medications, and get the right surgery—or even gene replacement. Some of these tests already exist and are used in risk assessment for breast, ovarian, and colon cancer; cholesterol abnormalities; certain anemias; nerve disorders; and even Alzheimer's. But for most of us, the goals of slowing our clocks down and living longer and better depends on our personal astuteness in recognizing our inherited and behavioral risks, early symptoms of disease, and the importance of tests for early detection. The life you improve and lengthen can be your own.

# 7

## Looking Young from the Outside In

I've devoted most of this book to our inner bodies and how to get the most out of medically proven and approved therapies that slow the clock of organ dysfunction, disease, and disability. These chapters belong on the "critical list." But clock-related questions like "Where did my smooth, clear, nonsagging skin go, and how do I get it back?" are also of major (if less potentially mortal) concern. So let's get superficial!

### THE SKIN'S CLOCK: TICK, WRINKLE . . . TOCK, SAG . . . TICK, SPOT . . . TOCK, BAG

Our skin is an amazing organ (yes, it is an organ) stretching over approximately eighteen square feet: a water-resistant, heat-maintaining, protective shield that grows, regenerates, folds, expands, supports, nourishes, and defines our bodies. It is our first line of defense against bacteria, viruses, radiation, oxidation, and the other environmental hazards we must survive. Like the rings of a redwood tree, it's a measure of our age. Or is it?

The sun, not time, is our skin's greatest adversary. Its rays cause over 80 percent of the changes that cry out "old age" before we are biologically there. This is called *photoaging,* an apt term for those of us who look yearningly at the photos of our faces (and necks and chests) from years past.

In order to understand the rays of age, let's go through a quick physics primer: *Ultraviolet B rays* (UVB), are short-spectrum rays (in the range of 290 mm to 320 mm) that cause superficial, immediately noticeable damage to our skin. UVB "irritates" the melanocytes in the bottom layer of our outer skin or epidermis, and causes them to produce melanin pigment. Many of us avidly pursued melanocyte proliferation in our youth as we tried to achieve that "healthy" tan. A recent study in the *Archives of Dermatology* found that college students still prefer taxing their melanocytes to produce a tan, rather than leaving them pale and at ease.

There's even greater tissue devastation when red, not brown, becomes the predominant skin color due to sunburn. These insults depress the skin's immune system and vastly increase the likelihood of potentially deadly malignant melanomas, which now occur in one out of ninety Americans.

## Skin Cancer: It's Not Pretty

Almost half of all new cancers in the United States are skin cancers, affecting one million of us each year. There are three common types of skin cancer: basal cell, squamous cell, and malignant melanomas. The first two are often found on sun-exposed areas: head, neck, backs of hands. To detect these early, be alert for new or growing spots or bumps, or sores that don't heal. Basal cell carcinomas, the most frequent type, are slow-growing and seldom spread. Squamous cell carcinomas are a bit more aggressive but are less deadly than melanomas.

Since 1980, the incidence of melanoma among light-skinned Americans has nearly tripled. So named because it starts in the melanocytes, melanoma is the seventh most common cancer in women, and causes over three-quarters of skin cancer deaths.

Fortunately, melanoma can usually be cured through surgery if caught before it spreads. Once it invades the lymph nodes, the five-year survival rate goes down to 30 or 40 percent.

## You Are At Risk for Melanoma If You:

- Spent a lot of time in the sun, especially as a child or teenager.
- Experienced multiple blistering sunburns (three or more of these in childhood quadruple your risk).
- Have fair skin, blue eyes, red or blond hair, and develop freckles easily. But dark-skinned people are *not* immune.
- Have two or more family members who've developed melanoma.
- Have a lot of moles.

But wait—we have to get on another wavelength. *Ultraviolet A (UVA) rays* are longer (320 to 400 mm) and penetrate deeper than UVB rays. They are a product of not just the midday sun but all natural light, which reaches your skin through window glass, clouds, smog, and some sunscreens. (In fact, 40 to 80 percent of the sun's UV rays pass through clouds, 80 percent are reflected by the snow, and 17 percent by the sand.) These are also the rays that are offered, for a price, at tanning salons, whose ads should really read: "Look browner now, and prunier later."

### Why UV Radiation Causes Skin Aging

To "ride" these waves, you need to get more familiar with your outer covering. Skin has three basic layers (from bottom to top):

- The *subcutis,* or bottom layer, is a shock absorber and heat conserver.
- The *dermis,* or middle skin layer, is where hair follicles, blood vessels, sweat glands, and nerves are kept in place by skin-supporting fibers made of a protein called collagen. The bottom of the dermis and the subcutis form a supporting base of collagen and fat cells.
- The *epidermis,* or top layer, contains *melanocytes* (pigment-producing cells) and *keratinocytes* (which produce a protein called keratin). The bottom of the epidermis (the basal cells) is where little keratinocytes come from. As they rise to the top, they give their lives to protect you; the part of the epidermis that you see, the stratum corneum, is made entirely of dead cells. These are sloughed off and replaced by the next rising crop of keratinocytes.

## Show and Tell: Detecting Skin Cancer

Know your moles and other pigmented marks—even the ones on your scalp; on the back of your neck, genitals, or buttocks; and between your fingers or toes. To spot the more dangerous spots, ask yourself:

- Is it asymmetrical (one half not like the other)?
- Does it have a ragged or irregular border?
- Are there color variations within the mole?
- Is its diameter larger than that of a pencil eraser?
- Is it changing in size, color, shape, or texture (becoming bumpy, scaly, or crusty; or bleeding)?

If you see any of these characteristics in a new or existing mole, call your doctor.

UV radiation has been found to stimulate production of hydrogen peroxide, which triggers a breakdown of collagen, thus damaging the structural integrity of your skin. Cumulative collagen damage is the most likely contributor to photoaged skin. To add insult to injury, UV also impairs the synthesis of new collagen. Tiny amounts of scar tissue build up over time and eventually become visible as wrinkles.

A 1997 article in the *New England Journal of Medicine* showed that surprisingly small amounts of exposure to sunlight (a few minutes here and there, over several years) can lead to premature skin aging. This is far less than the exposure required to produce any visible reddening of your skin.

We don't all photoage at the same rate. This depends primarily on the degree of sun exposure, skin pigment, and skin type. Those of us who have outdoor lifestyles, live in sunny climates, and are lightly pigmented show the greatest degree of photoaging. Cigarette smoking doesn't help (see page 316). The causes of chronologic aging are less clear. Over time, there appears to be an increase in damage from the metabolism of oxygen in the cells' energy units (*mitochondria*); this damages DNA, proteins, and fat in the membranes of cells. Thus, the skin thins, fine wrinkles occur, the fat under the skin disappears, blood vessels become more fragile, and we bruise more easily.

## Sun Versus Time: How Skin Really Ages

What would your skin look like if you never went out in the sun? You would still see signs of chronologic aging (known as *intrinsic aging*): fine wrinkling, thinner and more fragile skin, and some loss of subcutaneous fat tissue. Little purple-red spots are also caused by time.

Photoaging, also called *extrinsic* (outside cause) *aging*, looks quite different. The skin becomes sallow or mottled, coarse, and leathery, with deeply furrowed wrinkles. UV rays also trigger a sag-promoting process called *solar elastosis*: The skin thickens due to accumulation of abnormal elastic fibers—which are haphazardly organized and granular—at the expense of normal, resilient collagen. If you want to see what photoaging has done to your skin, compare the color, texture, and wrinkles of your face or neck with your less rayed tush and inner arms.

Other marks of sun damage include:

- Age or liver spots (*lentigines*)
- Dilated blood vessels on your face, creating broken-looking "spider veins" (*telangiectasias*) or red bumps (*cherry angiomas*)
- Thick, rough, reddish growths (*actinic keratoses*), and raised brown or black spots (*seborrheic keratoses*)

If it's too late to avoid sunlight for life, there are still things you can do to clean up some of the damage and prevent more of it (see page 313).

## The Role of Skin Type

The FDA and the American Academy of Dermatology have relegated you to one of six skin types. If you fall into one of the first three categories (i.e., you're light-skinned), you are most prone to photoaging and should use a sunscreen every day, no matter what: rain, shine, or clouds. Even if you are not in one of these "most likely to crisp and wrinkle" categories, if you or anyone in your family has a history of cancerous lesions, skin cancer, or sun damage (most of us have this), the same strict precautions apply.

### Find your closest type

- Type 1: You burn easily, never tan, have red hair and freckles. Especially common among those of Irish, Scottish, or Welsh descent.

- Type 2: You burn easily but can get a minimal tan. You have fair skin and hair and blue eyes.
- Type 3: You sometimes burn but can get a light brown tan. You're dark-haired and Caucasian or Asian.
- Type 4: You minimally burn and usually tan to a moderate brown. This type is more prevalent among Caucasians of Mediterranean descent, or light-skinned people of African, Asian, Hispanic, Indian, or Middle Eastern ancestry.
- Type 5: You rarely burn (lucky you!) and tan well. You are of Middle Eastern, Asian, Hispanic, Indian, or African descent.
- Type 6: Your skin never burns and you're sun-insensitive. You are probably of African descent, with deep skin pigmentation.

## What to Do About Photoaging

### Preventing further damage

There is no such thing as a safe tan. Even the slightest change in pigment is indicative of skin cell injury. The UVA rays from tanning booths ultimately inflict the same (if not more) damage to the skin as that caused by natural sunlight. If you want the bronzed-goddess look, it's much safer to fake it. Use rayless self-tanning creams or sprays containing *dihydroxyacetone* (DHA), a substance that interacts with proteins in your outer (dead) skin layer, and stains it brown—for a few days, anyway. These creams do not penetrate the pores and don't inflict any damage.

*Limit exposure to rays—or wear protective clothing.* This first admonition is so commonsense as to be comical in this guide for the intelligent woman, but most of us don't follow it. I call it the "ten to three" coverup rule. Why? Burning UV rays are out in greatest force at midday. Avoid spending time in the sun during these hours—or if you must, wear protective clothing: long sleeves, long pants, a hat, a scarf, or a collar around your neck.

I was recently in Australia, which has the world's highest rate of skin cancer due to its latitude, depletion of the ozone layer, and the genetic makeup of its mostly light-skinned population. They sell marvelous sun-protective hats and lightweight clothing that can be worn in and out of the water.

Clothing's sun protection varies by style, fabric (tightly woven or thick ones block sun better), and whether and how much UV-protective chemical treatment is used on the fabric. A number of manufacturers now offer sun-protective clothing (Solumbra, REI, Sunveil, and UV Aquawear, to name a few); you can easily find outlets via an Internet search. Sun-protective fabrics are rated according to ultraviolet protection factor (UPF). Unlike sunscreen SPF ratings, the UPF considers both UVA and UVB radiation. A "very good" rating with a UPF protective factor of 25 to 35 is equivalent to SPF 25 or 30; "excellent" is UPF 40 to 50+, equivalent to SPF 30+. A UPF 50 is supposed to mean that only one-fiftieth of UV rays can penetrate it and reach your skin. (While these are U.S. government standards, compliance by manufacturers is voluntary.) By comparison, an ordinary polo shirt might rate a measly 6.

Protective clothing is the best protection, but don't forget sunscreen. Unless you're wearing a total face mask, or a hat that comes down to your chin, your face will nearly always be exposed. Nor is the rest of your body safe; clothing moves, is shortened for style, and may not screen out all rays—or you may remove it to go in the water or just because you're hot.

*Always wear sunscreen.* Consider investing in three types for different sun-exposure scenarios:

1. Daily wear, even when you're not planning to be outdoors in the sun. Apply sunscreen to your face, neck, and hands. It should contain zinc oxide, titanium dioxide, Parsol 1789, or another broad-spectrum sunscreen, and have a minimum SPF rating of 15. There are many excellent over-the-counter products, which include Cetaphil Facial Moisturizer SPF 15, Clinique City Block SPF 15, and Olay Complete UV Protective Lotion. Slightly stronger formulations are sold through dermatologists' offices.

2. High-sun outdoor activities and sports mandate an SPF of 30 or more. Even though its description is not totally accurate (you have to reapply it after sixty to ninety minutes), choose a product labeled "water-proof" or "sweatproof" that contains 4 to 7 percent zinc oxide, Parsol 1789, or titanium dioxide. Brands include SkinCeuticals Sport SPF 45 and waterproof Coppertone Sport SPF 45.

3. If you're not swimming or under intense equatorial sun, but are spending extra time outside, this is when you're at greatest risk for casual sunburns. Go for the less expensive family-size bottles. Once more, an SPF of 30 to 45 is best. Examples include Coppertone Shade Sunblock

## Deciphering Sunscreens

*SPF* stands for "sun protection factor." It multiplies the amount of time you can be exposed to sun wearing the sunscreen and not get a burn, as compared with the time in which your unprotected skin would be burned. Example: You're fair-skinned and ten minutes is enough to turn you red. An SPF of 5 increases that time to 50 minutes. An SPF of 20 multiplies your burn time by 20: in other words, 200 minutes. However, the SPF protection does not increase proportionately with the number on the bottle: SPF 15 absorbs 93 percent of burning rays, and SPF 30 goes up to 97 percent but is not twice as effective as SPF 15.

Unfortunately, the SPF deals only with UVB rays and actual burn time. (Older, traditional sunscreens were formulated solely to block UVB.) SPF doesn't give us skin-aging time, which occurs at the astounding rate of just minutes a day. And there is no FDA-approved system for rating UVA protection on the label. Instead, look for a statement that your lotion blocks both UVA (those photoaging rays) and UVB (those burning, browning, and skin-cancer-causing rays).

For best protection, choose a sunscreen that reflects (rather than absorbs) UV radiation and contains zinc oxide or titanium dioxide. In the past, such creams were greasy and left a whitish film on the skin, but today's improved versions are more pleasant and less opaque (no more white stuff on the lifeguards' noses). Next best, look for a label that says "broad spectrum," which probably means it includes Parsol 1789 (also called *avobenzone*).

In general, sunscreen begins to work thirty minutes after it goes on, so apply it before you venture outdoors, not after. Since even waterproof screens usually lose their effectiveness within ninety minutes if you perspire or swim ("water resistant" ones last only forty minutes), remember to keep smearing it on. Few of us apply sufficient amounts evenly to all exposed surfaces; the typical slap-on-and-go approach leaves chinks in our antiray armor. Dermatologists recommend that you use a full ounce (enough to fill a shot glass) to cover your body and face.

Sometimes people are sensitive to a particular chemical in sunscreen (such as PABA) and develop skin irritation. If this happens, look for a different active ingredient, or ask a dermatologist to recommend an alternative lotion.

Finally, listen to the weather forecast, which now often includes a UV index, especially in sunny West Coast areas. An index of 8 or above signifies a high level of UV. Remember, there's always a daytime star beaming brightly, even behind clouds. There is no such thing as a rayless day.

Lotion SPF 45, Banana Boat Kids sunblocks, or a reputable high-SPF drugstore brand.

## Other In-Your-Face Insults

Smoking vies with UV radiation as a prime cause of accelerated skin aging. The thousands of chemicals in cigarette smoke wither the minute blood vessels that supply the skin with oxygen and nutrients. These toxins alter the function of fibroblasts, cells that regenerate the collagen in your skin. The free radicals in cigarette smoke (oxygen molecules in search of a lost electron) thicken and break the skin's stretchy elastin fibers. This leads to a loss of tone, and wrinkles. Smoking literally embalms your dermis: The formaldehyde and ammonia in smoke fix and "preserve" it. Inhaling those toxins also deactivates the ovaries' estrogen, further contributing to the loss of your skin's collagen and fluid content.

When you purse your lips around a cigarette to inhale and exhale, you train your skin in wrinkle formation. Then, to shield your eyes, you squint and frown. Multiple fine creases appear around the lips, then fine lines around the eyes, followed by frown lines. These gradually deepen. Loss of water and elasticity causes sagging under the eyes, drooping lids, and fallen jowls. Add a tint of yellow, and you've created a ten- to fifteen-year advancement of your face's clock. If you make surgical repairs while you're still smoking, they take longer to heal because the skin is oxygen starved and the fibroblasts are unable to lay down collagen effectively. Finally, cigarette smoking is associated with psoriasis, squamous cell carcinoma, and an increase in death rates from malignant melanomas.

These are more than superficial reasons to stop! And note that secondhand smoke inexorably, albeit more slowly, gives a similar hue and droop.

*Weight changes.* There is a French expression that translates to "Suffer your fanny for your face." As you get older and lose elasticity, weight loss can leave you with stretched-out skin. Make every attempt not to gain weight in the first place—but if you do, take it off slowly and allow your skin time to get used to its less fat-filled form. If you're considering plastic surgery after weight loss, give yourself at least nine months before doing it. Whatever you do, don't yo-yo; it's a fast route to stretch marks and folds.

*Lack of sleep.* Ever notice how much better your skin looks after a good eight or nine hours of sleep? Sleep is the ultimate mender, allowing your immune system time to repair the damage caused by daily activities.

For skin, it's a time to regenerate collagen and ward off free radical attack. Fluid that is normally pooled in your lower body when you stand or sit can recirculate (no longer fighting gravity) and enter the vessels supplying your neck and face, and "fill up" the cells of your skin. This rehydration and improved blood flow temporarily diminishes the crevices that appear as fine wrinkles, and give you a glow that can last for hours (similar to that created by exercise). If you don't let your body get the rest it needs, there are many telling signs: depression, fatigue, increased vulnerability to infection, achiness—but those on your face may be hardest to conceal.

*Alcohol.* For some women, even moderate amounts of alcohol create a crimson facial hue. Alcohol dilates blood vessels and increases blood flow to the skin; this is especially noticeable in fair-skinned women who tend to blush. Alcohol consumption can trigger hot flashes in perimenopause and menopause. An alcohol flush may also be due to an allergy to the sulfites in wine, or sensitivity to its tannic acid content, which is higher in red wine than in white. Finally, many women aged 30 to 50 develop a skin condition called *rosacea,* and alcohol consumption may make this worse.

## Your Skin Is a Mirror of Your Health

Skin reveals much more than just your age. As it does with every other organ, systemic disease takes its toll on the skin. Make use of this most visible and accessible organ, and monitor its condition from head to toes. If your color turns blotchy or sallow, or you note unusual bruising, scarring, lumps, bumps, or rashes, call these to the attention of a dermatologist and/or your primary care physician. Skin changes can reveal diabetes, autoimmune disorders, and other treatable illnesses.

## Prescription "Cream on" to Dream on About Youth?

I, like all doctors, have the power of prescription. One of the phrases I dread hearing from a patient is, "While you're at it, could you write me a prescription for . . . ?" because I am then assuming responsibility for any potential side effects. And of course I don't want to admit that I may not be familiar with the drug or the prescribed regimen (there's nothing as embarrassing as asking a patient what it is or how to spell it).

Rosalyn pulled out a list of prescribed skin creams, and asked me to write renewals for each of them; she had not yet met her insurance deductible limit and wanted to save the extra cost of a visit to her dermatol-

## Rosacea: The Redness That's Not Your Fault

Rosacea is a type of fine, bumpy adult acne that appears on the "blush" areas of the cheeks and on the nose. Alcohol and excessive heat, including that generated through exercise, can aggravate it.

**To get rid of the red:**
- Limit yourself to one alcoholic drink a day. Try white wine instead of red, or wine that has minimal or no sulfites.
- Check with your dermatologist; if you have rosacea, it can be treated with an antibiotic topical cream, lotion, or gel.
- Don't try to scrub away rosacea with hot water or abrasive, drying cleansers.
- Consider a gentle laser treatment (see page 325) if the redness doesn't fade, and you're incessantly and/or unsuccessfully camouflaging with heavy makeup.

Remember, whatever you do to bring out your true, paler color will ultimately be ruined if you don't stay out of the sun.

ogist. At 42, she was a California-bred, lifelong sunbather, as attested by her skin: fine lines etched her face and dark spots mottled her neck, arms, and legs. Blood vessels were becoming noticeable on her cheeks and around her nose.

"I'm going to Hawaii, and when I come back I want to start these," she proclaimed. A discussion involving the whole first part of this chapter ensued. I agreed to prescribe retinoic acid only on the condition that she wear a hat, sit in the shade, and use oodles of sunscreen.

We both knew she'd probably disregard my advice. "I'll be good, but what's the point of going if I can't be in the sun?" She'll have to go back to the dermatologist, deductible or not. They have a bright future together.

Here are the most commonly used remedies for skin damage that are *available by prescription* or through dermatologists or skin care specialists. While definitely helpful, they may not be the answer to all of our clock-slowing skin desires. (I'll cover nonprescription alternatives later in this chapter.)

### Retinoic acid or tretinoin (Renova, Retin-A, Avita)

This synthetic derivative of vitamin A is considered a *keratolytic* drug: It loosens and removes the outer keratin-filled layer of skin (exfoliation). The only topical prescription medication approved by the FDA to treat mild or moderate photoaged skin, retinoic acid was initially used for mild acne. (It increases the rate of cell division and turnover, so that pimples run their course and disappear more rapidly.) When a secondary gain was found and proclaimed, it grew from an adolescent skin therapy to a "use at any age or as you age" cream or gel—applied to reduce fine wrinkling, pigment changes, and skin roughness due to sun exposure. Tretinoin thickens the epidermis and evens out melanin (pigment) distribution. It increases collagen synthesis and inhibits the enzymes responsible for collagen degradation. It has even been shown to stimulate formation of new blood vessels that nourish the skin. A multicenter randomized study found that after twenty-four weeks of use, Renova significantly improved fine wrinkling, roughness, and mottling in 79 percent of individuals. Other studies have shown that if tretinoin works, spots begin to fade after six to eight weeks, and fine lines decrease in three to six months.

Tretinoin is not a sun-damage cure. Once treatment is discontinued, the effect is lost. So if you start, and it helps, keep going. It may also help shield you from the sun's wrinkle wrath; there is good evidence that pretreating skin with tretinoin prevents a UV-caused increase in enzymes that contributes to collagen breakdown.

*Maximizing benefits, minimizing side effects.* Potential side effects include skin irritation (especially among fair-skinned women), dryness, and peeling. Remember, tretinoin is not a sunscreen; indeed it may increase sun sensitivity and cause redness.

Apply tretinoin only at night; light inactivates it. First-time users should use a low concentration (starting at 0.025 percent) and apply sparingly (no more than a pea-sized amount for your entire face). Creams may be milder than gels. Cleanse your skin before use, then wait twenty to thirty minutes before applying the tretinoin. Be careful not to get it into your eyes, mouth, or nose. Use it every other night at first, until you are sure that your skin is not irritated, then nightly.

You can use tretinoin in conjunction with other exfoliant products, as long as you apply them at different times of the day. If you don't see a visible effect after six months, it probably won't happen. Consult with your doctor about other options.

*Tazorac (tazoratene).* This is another retinoid (vitamin A derivative) that has been approved by the FDA to treat psoriasis and acne. Like Retin-A, it also helps (but is not approved for) photoaging; studies have found it effective in reducing fine wrinkles and mottled pigmentation. It reduces inflammatory damage in the skin and can help skin cells develop and multiply. I've used the 0.1 percent gel or cream under my eyes (I alternate it with Retin-A) and have noticed an improvement (okay, on some days it's just a halt) in fine-line appearance. Like Retin-A, Tazorac causes dryness and irritation. Tazorac should never be used during pregnancy.

## Alpha-hydroxy acids (AHAs)

These are not new. Derived from fruit and milk sugars, they've been used by famous beauties (we have the historic references, not the pictures) as far back as Queen Cleopatra of Egypt. Older formulations seem to have come literally from the bottom of the barrel: the sediment left from fermented grapes. Today, they are referred to as fruit acids, but many of the products are produced in a lab. Their action is not well understood. Some researchers believe that AHAs exfoliate and combat photoaging by increasing skin thickness, elasticity, and collagen content, and help retain moisture in dry skin. Others feel that their major effect is simply to weaken the linkage of cells in the outer layer of dry skin so that they shed, leaving this outer layer more flexible. When the acids are used in high concentration, as in skin peels (see page 323), they cause irritation and sloughing of the outer layer of skin. Exfoliation will not make you lose your wrinkles, but after several months your skin may feel smoother and pigment irregularities may be less noticeable. AHAs are mixed into a moisturizer; there are experts who think that the latter deserves the credit for skin improvements. Certainly, if you stop using the AHA, the effect will dissipate.

AHAs come from many food sources:

- glycolic acid (from sugarcane)
- tartaric acid (from grapes)
- lactic acid (from tomato juice and sour milk)
- malic acid (from apples and pears)

Glycolic and lactic AHAs have been the favorites of skin chemists, but there are some new acids on the block:

*Alpha-lipoic acid.* This is said to have antioxidant properties, and may protect collagen from degradation. ALA is touted as better and longer lasting than other AHAs because it is soluble in both water and lipids (fats).

*Beta-hydroxy acids.* Salicylic acid (originally derived from willow bark) has been placed in this category, but pure chemists would disagree. It may be gentler than AHAs, but also less effective.

## Maximizing benefits, minimizing side effects

The degree of exfoliation (and sense of stinging) depends on the concentration and acidity. To achieve a visible result, the concentration should be 8 percent or higher (some nonprescription creams may meet this criterion). The pH of the cream should range between 3 and 5; anything lower makes the product irritating. A higher pH may sting less but won't exfoliate as well. It's hard to ascertain the pH from the label on the jar; this is one reason to ask your dermatologist to prescribe or recommend your first AHA product.

Clean your face thoroughly and wait twenty to thirty minutes before applying the product to be sure your skin is completely dry. It's a good idea to test a new product on a small patch of skin first to check for stinging, burning, pain, redness, or even bleeding. If you overdo these products, irritation can actually increase your risk of photodamage. Once you begin using AHA, don't even think about going outdoors without putting on sunscreen. If after four to six weeks you don't notice results, and there's no irritation, either increase application to twice a day or try a stronger product.

## Estrogen skin cream

Studies show that estrogen preserves collagen content and thickness (see page 52). Estrogen cream has been used extensively to help prevent thinning or—to use the gruesome word—atrophy of the skin of the labia and the vaginal mucosa. Many of my patients complain that their facial skin aging has accelerated as they "lose" their estrogen's "skin-plumping powers" during perimenopause and menopause. Years ago, I started to suggest that they try using the estrogen cream I was prescribing for "down there," up there on their face and neck. I did the same. Over time, I changed the formulation from the commercially available Premarin and Estrace creams to one that I had compounded with a cream that would moisturize facial skin.

I'm not going to tout this as my invention or even contribution to skin support. But my patients have remarked on its effect. I've used it consistently and for what it's worth, my wrinkles are minimal despite my age and my childhood, adolescent, and young adulthood propensity for sun worship. Because of its 0.3 to 0.5 percent estriol content, this cream is not going to appear on cosmetic counters. You'll need a prescription from your physician filled by a reputable compounding pharmacy.

## MORE AGGRESSIVE "WRINKLE BEGONE" MEDICAL THERAPIES

### Chemical Peels

These are akin to a controlled burn, or if they are light, a smoldering. The caustic chemicals cause the skin to peel off so that new skin emerges with more evenly lined-up collagen, giving a softer, smoother, more uniform appearance.

Initially, peels can cause some less-than-comely skin changes. For three to fourteen days (depending on the type), expect redness, swelling, even blistering, followed by brown crusting and peeling as the old skin is shed and the new appears.

This treatment is not new; it's been around for fifty years, which may not be a bad thing; presumably dermatologists and skin specialists now have lots of experience with it.

Here's what a peel can do:

- Diminish fine lines around the eyes and lips
- Even out pigmentation

Best results are seen in light-skinned and light-haired women (dark skin is more likely to develop discoloration or scarring).

What it can't do:

- Treat deep wrinkles or sagging skin

Precautions (for moderate to deep peels):

- The acute skin stress may cause a recurrence of herpes type 1 (the virus that causes cold sores). To prevent this, most specialists prescribe an antiherpetic medication such as Valtrex, to be taken two days before and five days after the peel.

Treatments that may improve results:

• Retinoids or AHAs used before treatment can help the chemical peel substance penetrate deeper, and hasten healing.

## Superficial (light) chemical peels

These peels have been touted with the come-on "Take your lunch break and skin break, and return to the office looking younger, fresher, and glowing." The glow is actually a temporary redness and swelling that can last for a few days. The advantage of a light peel is there is no downtime, and it's virtually painless. However, most women need three to ten peels in order to get results that are visible for more than a few days. The most commonly used peeling agents are:

*Glycolic acid.* These solutions range in concentration from 20 to 70 percent; the lower the dose, the lighter the peel. The acid is applied with a brush, gauze, or Q-tip, timed, then neutralized with a special solution and followed with a moisturizer and sunscreen.

*Salicylic acid.* Solutions range in concentration from 15 to 30 percent. These have a preset time of activation and don't require a neutralizer. Because salicylic acid is fat soluble, it penetrates acne plugs better than other chemical peels. A commonly used light-to-medium peel is called Jessner's solution (a mixture of salicylic acid, lactic acid, and resorcinol).

*Trichloracetic acid (TCA).* This is a fairly strong chemical (I was taught to use it on vulvar skin to treat warts), but a 15 to 20 percent solution is considered "light." It works well but leaves more redness than many other peels. It normally requires five to seven days to heal, so it probably should not be included in the classification of "lunchtime peels." I still recall a peel event that occurred several years ago, when a colleague had this done. She thought she could return to work the next day—but had to cancel all her patients for the next week!

## Medium peels

These often combine salicylic acid and TCA 35 percent, or glycolic acid and TCA 35 percent. Other combinations or percentages are also available. You will feel a burning sensation and may need to take an over-the-counter painkiller. Your skin first appears white, then becomes red and swollen, and there may be some scabbing. Many physicians suggest starting with a superficial peel, to see how your skin reacts.

## Deep peels

These are usually done with phenol, which is a very caustic substance. A sedative, or anesthetic, is necessary. And because it can cause an irregular heartbeat if absorbed, cardiac monitoring should be available. The burn is quite deep, and in addition to blisters there may be some bleeding. Healing can take up to six months.

A deep peel can cause dramatic lessening of wrinkles around the eyes and mouth but will not clear deep scars or acne pockmarks. Some very undesirable side effects can occur, such as fading of pigment (so that your face is lighter than the rest of your body) or uneven darkening (especially if you are dark complected). Today, this procedure is rarely performed.

*Cost:* A superficial peel costs $100 to $200. A deep peel costs about $3,000, with medium peels somewhere in between.

### *Dermabrasion and Microdermabrasion*

Think of this as electric polishing or "sanding" of the skin. A rapidly spinning wheel textured like fine sandpaper is used to remove the superficial layer of skin.

*What it can do.* Treat facial scars (including those from acne), remove vertical wrinkles around the mouth that cause lipstick to "bleed," or remove tattoos.

*What it can't do.* Remove wrinkles entirely or produce baby-smooth skin.

*Precautions.* Dermabrasion is painful and requires sedation or a local anesthetic, as well as an experienced and skilled practitioner, and it can be quite bloody. Frankly, it is viewed as outmoded since the introduction of laser treatments (see below).

In the mini-form, *microdermabrasion,* only the outermost layer is "sanded down." This results in only mild redness—but also milder skin changes that may not last very long. But it can be refreshing and will leave your face really clean.

## Laser Resurfacing

A laser beam consists of a single wavelength of light. Depending on its color (wavelength), intensity, and the duration of pulses, a computer-controlled laser can precisely cut, destroy, or vaporize skin tissue, and seal small blood vessels (preventing bleeding). With the advent of dermatologically directed lasers, we've surfaced from chemical peels into the high-tech world of the twenty-first century.

Like peels, laser therapy promotes the emergence of new skin whose surface should be smoother, more even in color, and devoid of acne pockmarks or raised scars. Unlike a peel, there is more control over the depth and degree of burn. Depending on the wavelength used, the laser can target selected types of tissues (such as dark age spots) without harming the surrounding skin.

*What it can do.* Expect a 40 to 60 percent reduction in wrinkles. Laser resurfacing can be done on delicate areas, such as around the eyes, with more control than peels. Depending on who you talk to (the most enthusiastic being the laser surgeons), laser resurfacing can turn your skin clock back by a decade or more. And the results can last up to ten years. To achieve this outcome, a repeat treatment is often needed after one year.

*What it can't do.* Lift sagging skin or smooth out the crepiness of the neck.

*Precautions.* Again, darker-skinned women are more likely to have side effects such as uneven or pronounced pigmentation.

There are several types of lasers. The two most commonly used today are the CO2 laser and the erbium (Er):YAG laser.

### The CO2 (carbon dioxide) laser

The CO2 laser emits short pulses of high-energy laser light, which vaporizes skin layer by layer. Some form of anesthesia is advisable, either conscious sedation (similar to that used for colonoscopies) or general anesthesia. If you prefer to stay alert, a local anesthetic can be injected into the facial nerves. Expect your skin to look burned, with significant swelling, bruising, and oozing. It takes seven to ten days for the new skin to appear and heal enough so that you feel comfortable about appearing in public.

Rarely, there can be more serious and even permanent risks. If the laser surgeon is not experienced, uses the wrong type of laser or an incorrect setting, or goes too deep—or if infection occurs—there can be permanent scarring. Sometimes, even when the procedure goes well, the skin becomes unnaturally light.

## Melinda's Story

Melinda, 51, came to see me as a new patient for menopausal symptoms. Her hair was combed forward so that bangs covered her forehead, and her cheeks were partially obscured by pageboy curls. She wore a hat with a wide brim, and large dark glasses. The visible skin looked red, thin, and taut. I thought she was a burn victim. She was, but this burn was caused by a laser-resurfacing procedure done two years earlier.

Melinda was a nurse and had seen some women achieve exceptional results from laser therapy. She hoped it would clear her acne scars and the fine wrinkles she'd acquired from years of California sun. She chose a dermatologist who claimed to have performed multiple laser procedures. Unfortunately, this turned out not to be the case. Melissa suffered second- and third-degree burns, requiring extensive care at a burn treatment center. After hearing her story, I have to admit that I was less than enthusiastic about encouraging or referring any other patients for this procedure.

Several years have passed; Melinda is doing much better after multiple treatments. And I have been reassured by dermatologists and plastic surgeons whom I respect that an experienced practitioner using the right machine with the right settings makes a burn like Melinda's highly unlikely. Still, it serves as a warning: Make sure your laser surgeon is qualified and experienced (see page 327).

### Erbium (Er):YAG laser

This kinder, gentler laser treats mild to moderate wrinkles. The Er:YAG laser produces energy of a wavelength that is absorbed by water (the major component of skin cells) so that the heat is scattered and doesn't penetrate deeply, allowing greater precision in the removal of thin skin layers than with the $CO_2$ laser. It may be especially well suited for fine skin around the eyes or on the neck. The healing process is faster, and there is less redness and trauma than with a $CO_2$ procedure. Obviously, the odds of scarring are smaller.

### The rainbow of other lasers

Depending on their wavelength/color, these are used for specific lesions.

*The argon laser* emits a yellow light absorbed by the red pigment in blood and the brown pigment of melanin. It's used to treat spider veins, benign sun freckles, cloasma (pigmentation caused by pregnancy or birth control pills), rosacea, birthmarks, and even "red nose syndrome." One downside: It can depigment an area of skin so that it becomes too pale. It should not be used on dark skin.

*The Nd:YAG laser* uses infrared or green light, absorbed by brown marks such as liver spots. It's also used to remove tattoos.

*The Q-switched Ruby laser* uses bursts of red light to remove tattoos, brown spots, and freckles.

*Nonablative lasers.* "Nonablative" implies that the skin is not destroyed—and indeed, with these lasers the top layers remain undamaged. The beam heats and stimulates cells below the surface layer, causing them to produce more collagen. This treatment is helpful for fine lines and mild to moderate sun damage but is not the laser of choice for deeper wrinkles. Healing is rapid, and there's virtually no downtime. Because the treatment is new, we don't have good data on how long its effects last or how often a redo is necessary.

### How to get laser-fine therapy

The FDA approves manufacturers' lasers for specific procedures but does not oversee training of physicians who do the procedures. It's appropriate to interview a prospective laser specialist and to inquire where the doctor has trained, which types of laser the doctor works with (since one kind is not right for everyone), and how often the doctor uses each type of equipment. Ask whether she or he owns or rents the equipment (if she owns it, she is more likely to know how to use it). Request to see before-and-after pictures, and try to get permission to speak to previous patients. You can also ask about membership in or accreditation by an appropriate medical society: the American Society for Dermatologic Surgery, www.asds-net.org/index.html; the American Academy of Dermatology, www.aad.org; the American Academy of Facial Plastic and Reconstructive Surgery, www.facial-plastic-surgery.org; or the American Society of Plastic Surgeons, www.plasticsurgery.org.

*Cost:* Roughly $1,500 to $3,000, depending on how much of the face is lasered (this does not include anesthesia or operating room fees). The cost may be higher if your treatment extends to the neck, hands, or other parts of your body.

**Laser hair removal**
It's possible to permanently remove body hair with lasers, and bid goodbye to your shaver or depilatory cream. Laser heat energy destroys the hair follicles, and the hair will not grow back. Several kinds of lasers are used; these include the long-pulsed alexandrite, the diode, and the Nd:YAG. A laser can also be used on facial hair—but as with other laser treatments, there is a risk of increased pigmentation for dark-skinned women.

## Making Vessels Less Apparent

Lasers have become a boon to women concerned about unsightly or painful veins. In the past, the usual treatment for spider veins (those small red or blue vessels that form intricate patterns on your legs) was *sclerotherapy,* using tiny needles to inject them with a solution that causes them to collapse, scar, and eventually disappear. While this is effective, depending on the solution used, there could be side effects such as skin ulceration, brown stains—and, rarely, allergic reactions or blood clots.

Lasers have been used to treat superficial facial veins for nearly twenty years, and can now be used on larger leg veins with success rates similar to sclerotherapy. Over several sessions, longer-pulse lasers can close leg veins with minimal discomfort. If you have darker-pigmented skin, opt for the Nd:YAG laser, which is less likely to create blotches.

*Varicose veins* (bulging blue veins, caused by backward blood flow in damaged vessels) are not only unattractive but often hurt. The traditional treatment requires surgery; the vein is tied off and then removed or "stripped." New techniques make it possible to treat the distended vein "locally" without removal, using either a laser fiber, which is threaded into the vein, or radiofrequency technology. Both methods essentially heat and seal the vein. A local anesthetic is needed.

Recently, one of my patients who had already undergone vein stripping found that, to her dismay, she'd developed new varicose veins—and decided to try the laser procedure. She was still healing when I saw her, but it was evident that the veins had become extremely black-and-blue and were destroyed. She looked forward to the results but recounted that the procedure was painful, as was the first week of recovery.

## Intense Pulsed Light (IPL) Technology: A New Light Way to Turn Back Your Skin Clock?

A laser uses coherent light, which consists of a single wavelength (think parallel) so that the beam is focused and intense. IPL uses a noncoherent, nonlaser, broader beam not limited to a single wavelength and filtered through a special flashing lamp. The intensity, wavelength, pulse speed, and duration can be varied, depending on the type and depth of the skin problem that is treated. Currently, there is little published research, but biopsies taken after the procedure have shown thicker, better collagen. Small studies of Caucasian and Asian patients undergoing IPL have shown good results for the treatment of pigmentation, broken blood vessels, and poor skin texture.

The makers and practitioners of IPL talk about "skin rejuvenation" and say that patients feel they have reduced their facial age. The procedure causes minimal discomfort (a slight stinging sensation) and limited downtime (a few hours of redness). But it takes five to six treatments, three weeks apart, to get results. Charges range from $100 to $300 per treatment.

## WRINKLE FILLERS

An alternative to creaming, rubbing, burning, heating, or pulling wrinkles away is to fill them in. We don't like the term "plump" when applied to our bodies, but we adore it when it comes to our skin. Here's what is available to fill in the gaps produced by the sun, environmental insults, and our years of living.

### Collagen

*Bovine collagen injections* for "dermal augmentation" were first developed in the 1970s, and approved by the FDA in 1981. The three types currently used are made from the hides of closely guarded herds of U.S. domestic cattle. Their isolation protects them from contamination by foreign cows that could harbor "mad cow disease." The harvested collagen is purified, sterilized, and processed in varying viscosities, strengths, and formulations.

*Zyderm I* contains 3.5 percent bovine dermal collagen with a very small amount of lidocaine, which helps numb the injection site. Zyderm I is used to treat superficial wrinkles around the eyes and mouth, and in the forehead. It can also fill in acne scars and augment lips. Note that the FDA has approved this and other bovine collagen products for filling "contour deformities," but not for augmentation that enlarges normal facial features. In other words, collagen has not been approved for injection directly into the pigmented areas of the lips but can be used to correct wrinkles bordering the lips. Zyderm I is the least viscous and requires that extra amounts be injected (overcorrection), causing temporary swelling; this goes down as the fluid content is partially absorbed.

*Zyderm II* is almost twice as concentrated, containing 6.5 percent bovine collagen. It's used for coarse deeper wrinkles, acne scars, and lip augmentation. A smaller amount is injected and there is less initial swelling than with Zyderm I.

*Zyplast* is only 3.5 percent bovine collagen but is linked to another substance to form a dense latticework, which makes it viscous. It is more resistant to degradation than Zyderm, and can be injected into deeper layers of the skin to fill coarse wrinkles, including those from nose to lip (the nasolabial fold). It, too, is used to get fuller (really full) lips. What's injected stays, so overcorrection isn't necessary. Many skin specialists layer Zyplast with Zyderm I or II.

*Bovine collagen precautions:* You need to be tested to make sure you're not among the 3 to 5 percent of individuals who are allergic (enjoying a steak in no way ensures your ability to tolerate these injections). A collagen allergy can be serious, and can result in a rash, hives, joint and muscle pain, headache, and (rarely) even shock and breathing difficulties. The test involves injecting a tiny amount of collagen under the skin in your forearm and examining the area to make sure there is no redness, swelling, or itching that lasts for more than six hours. You should be given two skin tests two weeks apart—the last at least four weeks before you embark on treatment.

Even if you have two negative tests, you're not completely home free. Rarely, delayed hypersensitivity can occur, with swelling, thickening, redness, and tenderness where the collagen was injected. This reaction may require treatment—steroid injections or oral steroid medications—but it does go away after several months. Because collagen stays in the body and continues to be absorbed for months, it shouldn't be given to pregnant women or those who are about to get pregnant. After collagen treatment, you may have some mild bruising or swelling for a few days. You can immediately camouflage this with makeup.

*Cost:* Prefilled syringes come in various sizes. One cc is enough to fill one or both nose-to-mouth wrinkles, and costs about $350. Obviously, less is needed for superficial lines. Then, of course, you're paying for the time and skill of your doctor. Depending on where you live, who treats you, and how much is done, figure $300 to $1,000 per treatment.

### Other sources of animal collagen

*Fibril* is another injectable filler made from pigs' dermal collagen. It's produced as a gelatin-powder compound that is mixed with your blood and then injected.

### Using your own: autologous collagen and fat injections

Most of us have plenty of fat to spare, and we won't be allergic to it. So why not simply arrange a fat transfer? It's not quite that easy; we have to go through several intermediate steps.

In one procedure, the harvested fat obtained through liposuction is processed, mixed with sterile water, and frozen so that the fat cells rupture. This can then be stored for later use. The fatty content from the cells (triglycerides) is injected into the wrinkle, and in theory promotes an inflammatory response, which stimulates the deposition of new collagen.

In a second procedure (suck now, transfer now), the aspirated fat is rinsed, treated, and reinjected into the wrinkle for an instantaneous plump. This type of transfer is only used on deep wrinkles, and there are disadvantages. When fresh fat is injected, it often doesn't take; the cells are quickly destroyed and what remains, like bovine collagen, is inevitably

### The Collagen Clock: How Quickly Do I Lose the Wrinkles, and for How Long?

It may take two or three sessions, two weeks apart, to fill up those crevices and deeper wrinkles, so that you get the results you and your doctor want. You'll probably need to repeat a treatment every three to six months. The more you move the muscles around the area (especially around the lips), the faster the collagen is absorbed. Not talking, not eating, not frowning, and not smiling would help—but I frown at the notion.

absorbed. (Fat injections can last from just months to more than a year.) A large needle is required to push the fat into the wrinkle, and this can cause bruising and swelling. The dual "get it out and put it in" procedure is more costly than bovine collagen, averaging more than $1,000 per treatment.

*Autologen* is also self-made. This is prepared from a piece of your own excess skin after it's removed during a surgical procedure, such as a face lift or a tummy tuck. It's sent to the manufacturer, where three inches of harvested skin is processed to yield a sterile solution of 1 cc, containing 3.5 percent of your collagen. It won't cause a reaction and once injected back, it is less likely to be reabsorbed than fat or bovine collagen; it generally takes hold for a year or more. The cost will obviously have to include that of the plastic surgery procedure.

### Human collagen (but not your own)

*Alloderm,* made from processed human cadaver skin, is most frequently used in the treatment of severe burns, but has been adapted by some surgeons for use in augmentation of the nose and lips, or to fill in scars. A similar product, *Cymetra,* is micronized (processed into minuscule pieces) so it can be injected like collagen. It is viscous and requires a fairly large needle to inject.

*CosmoPlast* and *CosmoDerm* contain human collagen obtained from foreskins and grown in a laboratory. (I find the concept of where this comes from and where it's destined to go quite amazing, though it's often glossed over in the company's ads and websites.) This collagen has been widely used in Europe, and received FDA approval in March 2003. It's combined with an anesthetic to reduce injection discomfort, and can be used like bovine collagen. Unlike the cow product, it doesn't require pretesting for allergies. Because it's quickly absorbed, an excess amount (overcorrection of 50 to 100 percent) is needed for deep wrinkles. In studies presented to the FDA, this treatment lasts for three to six months. The less viscous CosmoDerm is used for fine lines; CosmoPlast is used to fill pronounced wrinkles and to augment lips. These cost about 25 percent more than bovine collagen ($500 per cc).

### A synthetic option: Gore-Tex

(I guess it *is* the ultimate moisture shield!)

*Expanded polytetrafluoro-ethylene* (e-PTFE) was FDA-approved for facial, plastic, and reconstructive surgery in 1993, and is marketed as Softform and UltraSoft in sheets, strips, and thin tubes. These can be implanted in depressed scars, nasolabial folds, and around the lips—but they can be felt and won't pass the kiss test. The implants are permanent, so it may be advisable to first try a temporary filler to be sure you like the newly plumped look. The average cost is $2,000 per treatment, not counting anesthesia (if needed) or surgical fees.

## Fillers That Await FDA Approval

"Fill 'er up" seems to be a worldwide skin goal. Several fillers used in other parts of the world have not as yet been approved by the FDA. Patients can obtain them in Europe and Canada, and many bring them back for "local" injection. I also understand that some dermatologists and skin specialists purchase them by mail (talk about stuffing your mailbox!) for use in their offices, claiming that they are safe . . . and sensing that they're unlikely to be prosecuted.

*Restylane.* This is made from hyaluronic acid, a natural component of connective tissue. Since we all have it, an allergic reaction to it would be rare. Currently used in seventy-two countries, including Canada and much of Europe, it should be approved in the United States by 2004.

Restylane is a viscous gel created by streptococcus bacteria through a fermentation process. It flows smoothly as it's injected (dermatologists love to use it), and because its absorption is slow, there is no need for overcorrection. Apparently, it remains in place for six months to a year, longer than collagen and human fat. It can be used for fine wrinkles, for smile lines and around the eyes, as well as for lip augmentation.

*Perlane.* This also is a hyaluronic acid product, but is thicker and may be even longer lasting. It's used for deep facial lines. Its makers are also seeking FDA approval.

Because these products have not been FDA-approved, there are no nationally established prices. In Canada one treatment costs about $600 U.S., but these prices are going up with demand. (In anticipation of approval, Restylane and Perlane are already being advertised on the Web at a projected cost of $750 to $1,000 per treatment.)

*Hylaform gel.* The manufacturer of bovine collagen (Inamed), anticipating upcoming competition, has made its own hyaluronic product—from roosters' combs (showing exemplary economy in putting all parts of a chicken to use). Even though Hylaform gel comes from an animal source, it's reported to be less likely to cause an allergic reaction, and to last longer than bovine collagen. Those who use it say there's less clumping and that it injects more smoothly than collagen. Overcorrection is not necessary. Hylaform gel is used to fill scars, wrinkles, and lips. FDA approval is pending.

*Artecoll.* This consists of polymethylmethacrylate (PMMA) microspheres suspended in bovine collagen. PMMA has been used for decades in a variety of medical devices, and so is considered safe. It's marketed in Canada, and an advisory panel has recommended that it be approved by the FDA, after which the manufacturers plan to sell it under the name Artefill. The collagen is eventually absorbed, leaving behind permanently implanted "beads." These then stimulate the surrounding tissue to form collagen. In one study, 65 percent of users reported improvements lasting more than two years, but there is some risk of permanent surface bumps from the beads.

*Rivederm and Intra.* More "beads," made of dextran suspended in hylan gel of nonanimal origin. These are used in the Netherlands.

*Silicone.* The man-made polymers once used for breast implants are now processed into a refined liquid. Silicone has been used for permanent correction of superficial wrinkles and scars. But it can cause foreign-body reactions or infections, can migrate to other parts of the body, and can be adulterated with dangerous compounds. The FDA has not approved the marketing of liquid silicone for any purpose—so doctors cannot legally advertise or inject the substance.

*Radiance (or Bioform).* This synthetic compound contains calcium hydroxyapatite, a component of our teeth and bones, formulated into an injectable paste. It's FDA-approved for treatment of vocal cord paralysis and urinary incontinence, but it has been used off label to fill out fleshy areas around the nose and mouth, as well as deep furrows in the brows. It may last as long as two to five years. One cc costs about $1,500. At that price, its chief drawback is both worrisome and costly; Radiance can migrate to other parts of the body, creating unwanted and expensive lumps.

## Wrinkle Blockers

*Botox, or botulin toxin type A (botulinum).* This is a neurotoxic protein produced by the same bacterium that causes botulism. Injected under the skin, it causes paralysis of small facial muscles by blocking nerve endings from releasing the neurotransmitter acetylcholine, the chemical that stimulates muscle cells: no acetylcholine, no muscle contraction. The toxin was first studied in the 1960s, for the treatment of *strabismus* (crossed eyes), then used to relieve *cervical dystonia* (neck spasms), and later for uncontrollable eye twitches.

Finally, it came to the fore on the forehead, where injections were found to decrease migraine headaches. Botox also was found to relax the muscles that cause frowns and drooping brows, and made those that were injected appear calmer and, yes, less wrinkled (anger management for wrinkles). Even before this toxin was approved for cosmetic use (specifically, temporary relief of vertical frown lines between the eyebrows) in 2002, Botox was injected 1.6 million times in 2001 for purely aesthetic purposes.

Dermatologists and skin specialists are injecting it off label elsewhere, wherever muscles move and lines and wrinkles are created: in the chin, at the corners of the mouth, on crow's-feet around the eyes; they are even using it to minimize "turkey gobble" neck. (Allergan, the maker of Botox, advertised that it could be used on "your toughest wrinkle," and was rebuked by the FDA for going beyond its approved use. Now it officially targets "your toughest frown lines.")

All this has raised concerns, without raising eyebrows, about the masklike, emotionless look appearing on the faces of women (and men) from L.A. to New York. Researchers at Indiana University found that after repeated Botox injections, some people were left with limited eyebrow movement, often making the brows look flatter and droopier.

When injected by a qualified dermatologist or plastic surgeon, Botox certainly has a place in helping us smooth away years of worry, stress, and feeling. But Botox "parties," with assembly-line injections by a doctor or nurse, minimize the importance of your individual needs—and make this look like a cosmetic gimmick instead of a medical procedure with real, known risks.

*So what are the risks?* A *British Medical Journal* editorial warned that Botox use was outstripping research on benefits and side effects. To date, the most common side effects in FDA-reviewed studies are headache, respiratory infection, flulike symptoms, droopy eyelids, and nausea. The "droop" should resolve (remember, this paralysis is temporary) after two to twelve weeks. Any mild bruising in the injection site usually goes away in three to ten days, and can be covered with makeup. Neck injections could temporarily affect the vocal cords. Like collagen, Botox should not be given to pregnant women or nursing mothers.

It may take five to seven days to notice results, two weeks for maximum effect, and a second set of injections to get complete wrinkle relaxation. Effects last for roughly three months, but may last longer after Botox has been used several times. The more you try to use the muscles in the injected area, the more likely it is to wear off.

The FDA says Botox should be injected no more than once every three months, at the lowest effective dose. The average treatment costs between $300 and $1,000, depending on how much is used, where it's used (despite FDA warnings), and who is injecting it.

## A Botox Story

I've seen many of my patients develop a "Botox" face. This was recently typified by Anne, a 67-year-old former actress and renowned beauty, who came into my office for her checkup. Yes, her hair was tightly pulled back (and not one gray root showed). But that did not explain her extraordinarily smooth forehead, so taut it glistened. Her usual wonderful smile seemed limited and superficial. I felt I was missing the real woman behind this ethereal smoothness. When I asked her how she was, she replied, "I'm happy as a clam." I couldn't help feeling the analogy was unfortunate. A little bit of this stuff probably goes a long way; too much erases the real you.

## Other Wrinkle Blockers

*Myoblock.* A second type of botulinum toxin (type B) is also used to produce a reversible muscle paralysis. It's cosmetically employed outside the United States, but is currently approved by the FDA only for treatment of *cervical dystonias* (a type of neck spasm), although off-label use is permitted. It requires larger doses than Botox, but takes effect more quickly. It may be an alternative for patients resistant to Botox's effects.

*Dysport.* Like Botox, this is made from type A toxin; its manufacturer claims that the injections are stronger and last longer, so that patients need repeats just twice a year. FDA approval is pending.

## Plastic Surgery

According to the American Society of Plastic Surgeons, 6.6 million Americans got some form of nip, tuck, or lift from a board-certified physician in 2002. The top procedures were nose reshaping, liposuction, breast augmentation, eyelift, and facelift; 85 percent were performed on women. The 35-to-50 age group had 45 percent of the procedures.

To keep this chapter at a readable length, I'll cover these procedures only briefly. For more in-depth current information, I suggest you go on-line. To learn more, and to find a board-certified plastic surgeon, check the websites of the American Society of Plastic Surgeons (www.plastic surgery.org) or the American Academy of Facial Plastic and Reconstructive Surgery (www.facial-plastic-surgery.org); the latter are primarily ear, nose, and throat specialists.

## Body contouring methods

*Breast augmentation.* I won't go into the psychosocial issues of why so many of us want fuller or reshaped breasts. I practice medicine in Los Angeles, where cleavage is a priority. The procedure is welcomed by many of my patients who have lost a lot of weight, or whose breasts sag after bearing and breast-feeding their children.

Augmentation is usually accomplished through use of saline (salt-water filled) implants that are surgically placed directly under breast tissue or beneath the chest wall muscle. (Silicone-filled implants can sometimes be used with special consents.)

The incisions to insert the implants are made under the nipple, the lower curve of the breast, or in the armpit. These usually fade over time, but in some women they can become raised and red, forming keloids. This scarring is more likely to occur in dark-skinned women and those of African descent, especially if they have existing keloid scars from surgical procedures or healed cuts elsewhere on their bodies.

The chief risks from implants should be divided into those that are immediate and those that occur later. In the first category, you need to consider infection and bleeding. When it comes to the second, well, there are quite a number of possible problems:

- Foreign body infection: If bacteria in your mouth (and there are more here than in any other part of your body) enter the bloodstream and get to the implant, they can cause a silent infection, and the reaction can lead to fibrous scar tissue forming around the implant, and *capsular contractions.* Many breast surgeons advise that you take prophylactic antibiotics whenever you have dental work performed to prevent this. Hardening of the breast due to scar tissue is thought to occur in up to half of women with implants, although it may occur less frequently if the outer shell of the implant is smooth rather than textured.

- Leak or rupture: This doesn't necessarily mean that the implant collapses. In a silicone implant, if the outer envelope remains intact, the gel can seep, or "bleed," into surrounding tissues. Studies have shown that an average of 89 percent of women can expect to have their silicone or saline implants intact after eight years, but that decreases to 51 percent after twelve years, and only 5 percent after twenty years. Many plastic surgeons talk about implant "shelf life" and the need for implants to be changed after years of use. Newer implants may have a longer shelf life; time (and exams) will tell.

- Loss of sensation in the nipple or breast: This is rare, occurring in less than 2 percent of women.

- Mammography problems: Mammograms may be more difficult to interpret, and ultrasound may be needed in order to get additional information, especially if there is thickening at the edge of the implant. Breast implants, however, don't cause cancer.

- The autoimmune question: The possible link between implants and autoimmune diseases has received extraordinary publicity—and despite the dearth of true scientific evidence, resulted in a $3.2 billion settlement in 1998 from one implant company, Dow Corning. Suits were brought for myriad reactions, including joint pain and swelling, skin rashes, headaches, swollen glands, muscle weakness, fatigue, general achiness, hair loss, memory problems, and irritable bowel syndrome. Even as the cases were being adjudicated, five major studies and at least that many minor ones found no association or only an insignificant link between silicone implants and these autoimmune responses. Some researchers have suggested that there may be a small group of women with genetic factors that make them susceptible to a syndrome resulting from exposure to silicone. Because of this legal morass, the FDA mandated that these types of implants could only be used with special consent for "redos" or for breast reconstruction after cancer surgery. This eleven-year silicone restriction was recently reviewed after further data were presented showing that there was no significant difference in the complication rates after saline and silicone implants and that many women preferred the "look and feel" of silicone. Although an expert panel voted to approve silicone implants, the FDA deferred a final decision. To get the latest information, visit the FDA website: www.fda.gov/cdrh/breastimplants/biavail.html.

*Breast lift (mastopexy).* This is a lift-up-and-shape after a fall-down-and-sag due to pregnancy, nursing, and the gradual conversion of glandular breast tissue to fat with age. Excess skin is removed, and the nipples repositioned. It's less likely to last in—and may not be appropriate for—large-breasted women. Depending on how much of a lift is performed and whether it is combined with breast reduction or implant insertion, the scar runs around the nipple and down to the bottom of the breast (a moderate lift) or can continue along the base of the breast like an upside-down T. These scars can sometimes make breast exams and/or mammograms more difficult to interpret.

*Tummy tuck (abdominoplasty).* Some women just can't lose the pendulous abdomen they are left with after they've had their babies. This surgery reconstructs their below-the-waist profile to fit the rest of their bodies and their clothes. Abdominoplasty is a major procedure, in which excess abdominal skin and fat are removed, muscles are tightened, and a new navel is created. The incision is large, forming a huge semicircle from hipbone to hipbone, curving down toward the pubic hair.

A new portable pain pump can now be used for the first few days after tummy tuck and breast surgery. The pump slowly infuses Marcaine, a long-acting anesthetic, into the surgery site.

## Liposuction

More than twenty years after its introduction, liposuction is now the most commonly performed aesthetic surgical procedure in America. This is *not* an alternative to weight loss, but rather a way to lose stubborn bulges as you lose weight in the rest of your body. Contrary to the popular belief that "if you take it out in one place, it will just come back in another," it won't. Liposuction permanently removes the fat cells under the skin in the treated area. If you lose additional weight, the remaining fat cells will shrink. If you gain weight, they enlarge but do not multiply or send emissaries to other parts of the body.

Liposuction won't work on the "apple" fat we tend to add on our waists and bellies as we age (which also increases risk for heart disease). That fat is accumulated under muscle, or in the abdominal cavity, not under the skin. It also can't help that bumpy orange-peel skin (commonly known as cellulite). There are several techniques to suction away unwanted bulges:

*Suction-assisted lipectomy (SAL).* This has been performed in just about every site of excess localized body fat: in the chin, neck, upper arms, abdomen, hip, thigh, and buttocks, and even in the knees, calves, and ankles. A *cannula,* or hollow tube, attached to a vacuum pump, is inserted under the skin through a small incision. SAL is also used to remove benign fatty tumors, those soft lumps that sometimes grow under the skin in various regions of the body.

This procedure has—when done on excessively large areas on the wrong type of patient (with underlying health problems) under prolonged general anesthesia—resulted in some very serious complications, including severe bleeding, infection, fluid loss (leading to shock), blood clots, fat embolisms (fat globules clogging major vessels), and organ perforation. Deaths have occurred.

Today, a *superwet* or *tumescent* technique is commonly used. A dilute solution containing a numbing agent and epinephrine, which contracts small blood vessels, is injected into the fat to help loosen it and allow for easier suction with less bleeding. Here, too, there have been complications, when too much fluid or local anesthetic is injected, or when too much fat is removed. Fluid can rush out of the vascular system to fill the now-empty space whence the fat was suctioned (known as *third spacing*), and can create severe electrolyte imbalance, a drop in blood pressure, and even heart failure. Depending on a patient's size, the "safe" limit for the amount of fat suctioned off is considered to be three liters; many surgeons feel this is best done under controlled general anesthesia.

There are no guarantees of "I love my newfound flatness." The overlying skin may look baggy or rippled or become discolored, and the final result may not be symmetrical.

*Ultrasound-assisted liposuction (UAL).* Ultrasound energy breaks down the fat and makes it easier to suction out; it may also help limit bleeding. It can, however, burn through the skin, causing wound complications. UAL is usually limited to areas of the hips, central body, and back.

The cost of a liposuction procedure depends on the type of anesthesia (local or general), facility (doctor's office, day-surgery center, or hospital), type of procedure and amount of fat removed, and the location and reputation of the surgeon. Costs can range from $1,500 to $15,000.

## Facial surgical procedures

"If it's good, you won't notice it."
—A BEVERLY HILLS PLASTIC SURGEON

We've all seen bad face-lifts, and may not notice the good ones. A *complete face-lift* (rhytidectomy) has a face-saving potential of ten to fifteen years, and can be done in women of all ages; plastic surgeons tell me they've done it successfully on women in their seventies and eighties. It's the ultimate fix, but it can also fix your face in a way that doesn't move or look natural.

A full lift is costly: $15,000 to $35,000 (with hospital and anesthesia fees), and requires at least two weeks of downtime. It can take months for the swelling to go down, and six months to a year for numbness to dissipate. Some women complain of fatigue for six weeks or more after surgery.

When patients ask me, "How much does this hurt?" I have to go by what former patients and plastic surgeons have told me. Pain increases if the surgery causes pulling or pressure on bone, as with chin implants and brow lifts. Otherwise, there is discomfort, but the pain is not usually severe unless there are complications. Prescription pain pills are needed for the first few days, after which Tylenol usually suffices.

Whenever I see a new patient, I take a medical history, which includes the question "Have you had any surgeries?" I then prompt the patient a bit, by adding, "Tonsils, appendix . . . ?" I hesitate to ask the obvious (or at times the not obvious): Why does she look so much younger than her stated age? My nurse has no such compunctions. As she chats with a patient, she'll say, "You look great! Have you had work done on your face?"

When it's good, it can be very, very good. And after witnessing phenomenal work, I will that evening, in the privacy of my bathroom, pull back at the corners of my face and neck to see, What if? (I haven't.)

Smaller procedures requiring less recovery time (and money) are becoming the "in" way to combat facial aging. After chemical peels and filler injections, an *eyelid lift* (blepharoplasty) is the most popular facial repair. Incisions are usually concealed in the natural lid creases. The excess skin on top is removed so the eyes look open and alert, but hopefully not startled. Often, this is combined with suction of under-eye fat folds, through a minute incision inside the lower lid.

A *"mini-lift"* transfers fat from the jowls or neck to plump up saggy cheeks or deep wrinkles. A *forehead or brow lift* will get rid of loose skin, and if there are pronounced vertical frown lines, part of the muscle that creates them can be removed. The incision is placed behind or at the hairline.

A brow lift as well as other tightening procedures can now be done *endoscopically*. Telescopic, thin surgical instruments are maneuvered under the skin through several small incisions to remove tissue and tighten muscles—but the result may not be as even as that obtained with a continuous incision. Most plastic surgeons hide these incisions in the hairline or behind the ears. And apparently, keloids very rarely occur on the face.

Facial procedures cause varying amounts of bruising and swelling. Make sure your expectations are realistic. Overenthusiastic nips and tucks may look better initially, but once the swelling goes down, they can leave you with that "wind tunnel" look. It is essential, as with any surgical procedure, to consult with a board-certified surgeon experienced in the type of surgery you want. Get referrals from doctors, hospitals, and friends you trust. Ask the surgeon about her or his training and years of practice. Make sure she is affiliated with a good local hospital, so in the event of any complications you can be referred there. Other questions should include:

- How new is the planned procedure?
- How does it compare in results and side effects with older, tried-and-true methods?
- Can I see before-and-after pictures, and speak to previous patients?
- What surgical facility do you use, and who will be present to administer anesthetic medications? (Certified nurse anesthetists are fine, unless you have underlying medical conditions such as heart disease, in which case an M.D. anesthesiologist may be more appropriate.)

Don't select a surgeon based on ads, gimmicks, or sales. Trust your instincts. Does the doctor seem caring? If what the surgeon promises seems too good to be true, invariably it isn't.

There are enormous societal pressures to stay young and beautiful. If your sense of self, joy in getting dressed or undressed, and pleasure in presenting yourself to the world, a loved one, or the mirror truly yearns for this enhancement, then go for it. But please be a cautious consumer, and remember that all these procedures are elective. You may end up looking better and younger, but your body's clock will tick on and will not slow down unless you care for it in the manner I've outlined in the body of this book.

## Do Your Hands Match Your Face?

Procedures that help photoaging on facial skin can also help your hands. These include microdermabrasion and chemical peels. If you have prominent or broken-looking veins, sclerotherapy, using saline injections, collapses the veins so they disappear. The same lasers used to treat fine facial wrinkles can be used on the hands. Those used for pigmentation problems, such as red or yellow lasers, can diminish or erase age and sun spots.

You can't stop washing your hands (while in the office, I wash mine twenty times a day), nor is it fashionable to don white gloves when going out. But you can put on a waterproof sunscreen and apply moisturizer morning and night.

### Miracle in a Jar?

I spent my first thirty-five years simply washing my face with soap (the same stuff I used on my hands). After the age of 16, I put on lipstick, and I graduated to eye makeup in my twenties. No, I didn't use sunscreen or moisturizer. I figured that humid air, the literal sweat of my brow, and my tendency to have oily skin would be enough to lubricate my skin. Since wrinkles were unacceptable, they would not dare appear on my face (after all, physiological realities do not apply to medical students and physicians!).

But as the skin under my eyes puffed a bit, I discovered laugh lines when I peered into the mirror to change my contact lenses, and encountered unexplained dark spots on my cheek; I saw the cosmetic light and began to apply foundation and powder. The magazine and television ads portraying 20-year-olds with perfect skin now caught my interest. I perused the cosmetic counters, and listened to youthful salespeople promoting liposomes that sink in, collagen that rebuilds, vitamins that slay those nasty free radicals, and the "same stuff that's in prescriptions" now available in a lovely, decorative jar. I, like most baby boomers, was on a quest to "cream on in order to dream on" that my skin's clock would cease to advance.

Welcome to the $6 billion world of skin creams and cosmeceuticals. The term "cosmeceutical" is a misleading misnomer. According to the Federal Food, Drug and Cosmetic Act, cosmetics are defined as "articles intending to be rubbed, poured, sprinkled or sprayed on, to introduce into or otherwise apply . . . for cleansing, beautifying, promoting attractiveness, or altering the appearance without affecting the body's structure or functions." Drugs are defined as "products intended for treating or preventing disease, and affecting the structure or any function of the body." Drugs are subject to premarket review and approval; cosmetics are not. This means that a true cosmeceutical would have to be regulated as both. Most often, it's not.

Some cosmetics are regulated as drugs and must meet standards for both categories. If your cream's label has an "active ingredient" at the top of the list, that particular substance had to be proven safe and effective for the stated use. Typically, that impressive-sounding substance—Parsol 1789 (avobenzone), zinc oxide, titanium dioxide, oxybenzone, octyl salicylate (octisalate), octinoxate, octocrylene, ensulizole—is a sunscreen. (There may be several, to cover both UVA and UVB rays.)

As a label, "cosmeceutical" is almost as popular with marketers as "natural"—but it is not a legal term. The claims that range from "anti-aging" to "an appearance of . . ." (less definite than "a decrease in . . .") are not supported by the large-scale, double-blind, placebo-controlled studies demanded for drug claims. Hype abounds, but it doesn't mean it's bound to be true.

Even though the "let's not upset the FDA" claims don't meet drug standards, there is some consumer protection. A self-regulating body called the Cosmetic Ingredient Review, sponsored by the Cosmetic, Toiletry, and Fragrance Association, has a panel of scientific and medical experts who evaluate the safety of cosmetic ingredients. Cosmetic firms can also participate in a voluntary reporting program, providing information to the FDA on manufacturing, product experience, and adverse reactions to a product. About 35 percent of companies do this, but once more, their reporting doesn't mean the FDA approves or endorses what's in the product or the product itself.

This said, many nonprescription products can bestow some noticeable benefit—perhaps because of their excellent moisturizing capabilities. Remember, if you add fluid to (or keep fluid in) the skin, it will be far less likely to show its creases, so fine lines appear less etched. But the lines reappear as soon as that moistening dries up.

Here's a quick primer on a variety of products touted to "prime time" your skin.

## Lower-than-prescription-strength, over-the-counter products

*Retinol.* Whether this less active form of retinoic acid works is questionable. It is certainly less irritating. Some small, short-term studies suggest a benefit similar to the prescription-strength product, but these studies were done under controlled laboratory conditions. You don't know how much, if any, retinol is in the jar on your shelf, or if the active ingredient is stable.

*AHAs (alpha-hydroxy acids).* An estimated 1,500-plus over-the-counter products contain AHAs (for a description of how these work, see page 320). The Cosmetic Ingredient Review Panel has deemed them safe if they have an AHA concentration of no more than 10 percent, a pH of 3.5 or greater—and either include a sunscreen or have labeling that directs consumers to use one. Make sure the product lists which type of AHA or chemical acids it contains, the concentration, and pH. Test it on a small patch of skin the first time you use it to make sure you don't get redness or irritation. Stop using the product immediately if you notice continued stinging, itching, burning, pain, or sun sensitivity. Some skin specialists are concerned that overuse of AHAs can thin the skin.

*Hydroquinone.* This is the only FDA-approved skin-whitening substance, used for bleaching age spots. The prescription-strength version is sold under the brand names of Eldoquin, Eldopaque (with sunscreen), and Solaquin, and contains a 4 percent solution; a milder version, Melanex, includes a 3 percent solution. Hydroquinone has been used for years to fade darkened areas on the skin by inhibiting melanocyte metabolism. But if you stop using it, the newly freed melanocytes rebound and increase pigment production as soon as your skin is exposed to sunlight. The spots return, and may be darker. Be sure to use a strong sunscreen.

Lesser strengths of hydroquinone have been added to many popular skin care products, touted to "brighten" the skin rather than bleach it (this avoids a druglike claim). It generally means there is far less hydroquinone in the product, and it may not be present at all.

*Kinetin* (0.1 percent N-furfuryladenine lotion, brand name Kinerase; available through dermatologists and on the Internet). Kinetin belongs to a group of plant hormones called cytokinins that regulate plant cell division and growth. There is no proof that kinetin does the same for human skin. The limited research to date (all manufacturer sponsored) report-

## Scrub Out the Old, In with the New: a Fallacy

Microabrasion, peels, or laser treatments are costly. Why can't we control small wrinkles (and budgets) with do-it-at-home exfoliation?

Your top layer of skin consists of dead cells, and scrubbing them away will not stimulate the production of new ones. At most, it might expose the newer cells so your skin looks smoother—and once those moribund cells are banished, the newly exposed skin is better able to absorb your moisturizer.

A "natural" scrub containing pulverized apricot seeds or walnut shells may not be the best choice. Seeds and shells have sharp edges that can cause microscopic cuts. Choose one that uses artificial, evenly rounded "microbeads." And note that reusable loofahs and sea sponges are conducive to bacteria growth.

Your skin is not the kitchen floor. Aggressive scrubbing can make broken blood vessels or acne worse. When you do scrub (gently), go crosswise to the wrinkles, not parallel. The latter will stretch and etch them.

It's best to exfoliate at night and, depending on the strength of the scrub and your rub, no more than once a week. Afterward, apply a moisturizer to your damp skin (and make sure that before the skin hits sunlight, it has been sunscreened).

edly showed that Kinerase improves fine wrinkles and blotchiness after twelve weeks of daily use, without causing irritation. Don't assume Kinerase is superior because it's sold through dermatologists; this was a corporate marketing decision, not a medical one.

*Copper peptide creams.* Copper can hasten wound healing by aiding collagen and elastin synthesis. Skin specialists theorize it may help with photodamaged skin repair. Some studies show that creams with copper minimally improve fine wrinkling and skin thickness. Copper is currently being marketed in over-the-counter creams. At least it's nonirritating.

*DMAE (dimethylaminoethanol) creams.* You may have seen DMAE marketed as a dietary supplement for improved mental and physical performance (it is a building block of the neurotransmitter acetylcholine). Preliminary studies of creams containing DMAE, sponsored by their makers, are said to show small improvements in sagging facial skin. We'll have to wait for more solid (or should I say supported?) results.

## Antioxidants (vitamins A, C, and E; coenzyme $Q_{10}$)

According to the FDA, there is no clinical proof that a vitamin applied directly to the skin can "nourish" the dermis, or have an effect similar to that achieved when the vitamin is absorbed with food or taken as a supplement. Some corporate-sponsored studies have shown benefits, but if manufacturers present convincing data to the FDA, their products must be classified as drugs—so they moderate their label claims. It's a Catch-22: If it works, it has to go through expensive and rigorous testing; if it doesn't work . . . then what's the point?

Because the FDA does not recognize health claims for vitamins added to cosmetics, they are concerned that a vitamin-fortified ingredient list will give a misleading impression of a nutritional or health benefit. It is okay, however, to list the vitamin's chemical name, for example, substituting tocopherol for vitamin E in the ingredient list, but using the phrase "vitamin E cream" on the product label. I was amazed to learn that chemists add vitamin E to cosmetic products to prevent deterioration of the product itself. In other words, it's an antioxidant for the chemicals in the cream, but not necessarily for the free radicals in your face.

Many dermatologists and manufacturers proclaim that they have figured out how to get antioxidant vitamins into the deeper layers of the skin, to improve skin texture and minimize wrinkles. We've already discussed vitamin A, so let's look at the other antioxidants: C, E, and coenzyme $Q_{10}$.

*Vitamin E.* Studies suggest that topical vitamin E, particularly alpha-tocopherol creams, can decrease skin irregularities, the length of facial lines, and the depth of wrinkles. In mice it also reduces UV-inducted skin cancer, but don't count on it to protect our human dermis from the sun.

*Vitamin C* (may be listed as "ascorbic acid"). Vitamin C by itself is unstable, but some newer products may have solved the stability and delivery problems by changing C into an ester and attaching it to a fatty acid. This helps get it into the tissues and decreases irritation. These C creams are thought to stimulate collagen growth. Adding vitamin E may help stabilize C and make it more effective.

Myriad products are available from dermatologists, cosmetologists, and high-end department stores. Here are some examples: Cellex-C Advanced C serum ($103 for 2 tablespoons), Avon's Anew Clearly C serum ($20 an ounce), and SkinCeuticals C serum ($74 an ounce). The limited evidence may not justify the high prices for such tiny bottles. Lower concentrations in less expensive brands are, however, probably even less likely to get in and do their C thing (if there is such a thing).

*Coenzyme $Q_{10}$* ($CoQ_{10}$ or ubiquinone). Since increased cellular oxidation is associated with aging—including collagen loss and wrinkling—and $CoQ_{10}$ has antioxidant properties (see chapter 5), a few researchers (and corporations) got the idea of adding $CoQ_{10}$ to face cream. A 1999 German study found that $CoQ_{10}$ cream did penetrate the skin, reduced oxidation and depth of wrinkles, and improved the skin's resistance to UVA radiation. How much of the active ingredient is in these OTC creams, and whether it is stable or effective, is as usual unregulated and unknown. You will have to be the final judge of which of these antioxidant creams improves your skin.

## Why Do We Need Moisturizer? What Does It Do?

Our bodies are like radiators, and constantly expel heat through the evaporation of water, which can total a pint a day. We lose even more moisture if we run a fever, reside in a hot or dry atmosphere—or (unfortunately) as we get older and our protective layer of skin thins and becomes less capable of retaining its inner fluid. Think of a moisturizer as additional skin armor that partially blocks exit of this fluid. A moisturizer can't thicken your skin or change its cellular structure—but it makes the skin look and feel softer so that wrinkles are less apparent. However, once fluid is allowed to evaporate from the skin, the basic wrinkle structure will be there in all its crevassed form.

### Types of moisturizers

The primary cream component (aside from water, often called *aqua*—I'm not sure why the Latin term is preferable) consists of some kind of oil or fatty substance that allows the cream to be evenly spread and coat your skin with a moisture-saving barrier. Types of oils include:

### Emollients that sink into the skin

*Vegetable oils* (you name the plant, they've made an oil). These range from nuts to avocado, olives, palm trees, rice bran, jojoba, carrot, and wheat germ. Some of these plants sound "wetter" than others, but that doesn't necessarily improve their moisturizing effect once they are processed.

*Animal oils.* Fish oils, lanolin (from the fatty coating on sheep's wool; these oils can cause allergic reactions, especially if wool clothing bothers you).

*Vitamin E.* The ubiquitous tocopherol is a good moisturizing oil (because of its properties as an oil, not as a vitamin).

### Occlusives that don't sink into the skin

*Mineral oils.* These include petroleum jelly (Vaseline is a brand everyone knows) and silicone oils from rocks and sand. These oils form an excellent occlusive shield, because their molecules are too large to be absorbed into the skin surface. Obviously, they can also clog pores, leading to pimples in susceptible individuals.

### "Oil free" preparations

*Collagen.* This is a protein that will form a good barrier against water loss, but it is not absorbed and will in no way add to or improve the collagen in the deeper layer of your skin.

*Humectants.* These draw moisture from your own tissues up to the skin surface or absorb it from the air (good for oily-skinned people). These preparations have large molecules and don't penetrate into the skin. In the humectant list, we have glycerin, mucopolysaccharides, hyaluronic acid, and propylene glycol.

Which should you choose? If you have dry skin, try a combination of emollient and occlusive. If your skin is oily, either skip the moisturizer and just use a mild cleanser, or use a humectant.

## What's in Your Moisturizer and Skin Cream?

There are more than five thousand different ingredients used by the cosmetic industry to ensure your youth and beauty. They are listed in descending order on the label, starting with the greatest amount in the product. So you can pretty much count on the fact that the evocative ingredients listed toward the end are barely present and will have very little influence on your dermatologic need, but may definitely influence your pocketbook.

One other secret: The manufacturer can ask the FDA to grant "trade secret" status to a particular ingredient, in which case it doesn't have to be specified on the label, but the list must end with the phrase "and other ingredients." The manufacturer must prove that the ingredient imparts some unique property to a product and that the ingredient is not well known in the industry.

## Other ingredients: animal, vegetable, or mineral?

*Liposomes.* These are pictured in the ads as little spheres that will pick up a dewrinkling substance, carry it into your skin, then break open and release it. While liposome spheres can indeed trap water- and oil-soluble ingredients, they are not necessarily a magical delivery system.

*Aloe vera.* The anti-irritant quality of this plant from the lily family is promoted in many skin lotions and creams. Unfortunately, it requires specialized processing, and a lot of plant is needed to produce a small amount. So, the good stuff is expensive and usually contains less than the 5 to 10 percent necessary to truly soothe your skin.

*Human placenta.* Baby-smooth skin is associated with babies, who in the womb are fed by the placenta. Ergo, placenta should be good for your skin. A huge industry was conceived in the 1940s, and placental tissue was washed and processed (and decontaminated with alcohol and preservatives) to provide ingredients touted to have amazing hormone- and tissue-growth properties that would remove wrinkles. If these claims were true, the placental hormones would be classed as a drug. The FDA decreed that human placenta cream was not only ineffective, but its manufacturers were making inappropriate claims. As a result, products that contain placental ingredients are supposedly stripped of their hormones; the placenta is offered purely as a source of protein—although how the protein gets into your skin is not clear.

*Collagen.* The collagen in creams is derived from young cows. Since collagen is part of our body's connective tissue, adding it to a cream, oil, or concentrate sounds good. However, the collagen is not water-soluble— and the FDA has not found evidence that it can penetrate your skin, let alone have an effect below the surface. (To review how collagen works as a wrinkle filler, see page 329.)

Another C word you'll see in skin products is *cerebrosides,* a kind of glycolipid (a fat substance chemically combined with a carbohydrate). Nutritionally this sounds like a nightmare, but in your skin, it's produced in the deeper layers. As it rises to the top layers, it is chemically changed to ceramides, which help form the network of membranes between cells that helps your skin stay supple and moist. The raw material used to make cosmetic cerebrosides comes from the brain cells of cows, oxen, and pigs,

# What the Chemist Knows:
## Common Ingredients in Creams and Lotions

Here is some information to help you decode what's in that product you're putting on your skin:

**Moisturizing ingredients:**
- Cetyl alcohol (fatty alcohol)—this keeps oil and water from separating, and makes the product foamy
- Dimethicone silicone—a skin conditioner and antifoam ingredient made from silicone
- Isopropyl lanolate, myristate, and palmitate
- Lanolin and lanolin alcohols and oil—these are extracted from sheep wool and can cause irritation if you tend to have allergies to animal products
- Oleic acid (olive oil to the nonchemists)
- Stearic acid and stearyl alcohol (unlike ethyl alcohol, which would encourage evaporation and dry the skin, these "fatty alcohols" help keep moisture in)

**Preservatives to prevent product deterioration:**
- Trisodium and tetrasodium edetate (EDTA)
- Tocopherol (vitamin E)

**Antimicrobials to prevent bacterial growth (you don't want your skin cream to be a culture medium for germs!):**
- The parabens (the family names are butyl, propyl, ethyl, and methyl)
- DMDM hydantoin
- Methylisothiazolinone
- Phenoxyethanol
- Quaternium-15

**Solvents to dilute or thin the product:**
- Butylene glycol and propylene glycol
- Cyclomethicone (volatile silicone)
- Ethanol (alcohol)
- Glycerin

(continued)

**Emulsifiers so that oil and liquid mix better:**
- Glyceryl monostearate
- Lauramide DEA (also a foam booster)
- Polysorbates

In addition, you may see color additives (usually made from coal or petroleum sources), substances to adjust acidity (such as citric acid), abrasive silica (for scrubs), and absorbent anticaking agents such as magnesium aluminum silicate and talc.

(Source: *FDA Consumer.*)

or from plant sources. When introduced in a moisturizer it's supposed to increase "luminosity" and "hydration," but industry studies have not been evaluated by the FDA with a yea, nay, or maybe.

For more information on cosmetic claims, problems, and ingredients, visit the Food and Drug Administration's cosmetics Web page at http://vm.cfsan.fda.gov/~dms/cos-toc.html.

## The Reichman Routine for Skin Care

I divide basic care into washing, moisturizing, sunscreening, and fortifying.

*Washing.* You don't need to spend a fortune to get your face clean. I suggest (and actually use) Cetaphil; this line includes cleansers for dry, sensitive, and normal-to-oily skin. Even though it is relatively inexpensive, some drugstore chains make their own generic version.

Clean your face in the morning and before going to sleep at night. If eye makeup doesn't come off with this gentle cleanser, one of the easiest and least expensive moisturizing cleansers for makeup removal is Albolene, which comes in big jars. I've noticed that this is a favorite of makeup professionals, and of actors who have to remove thick layers of makeup.

*Moisturizing and sunscreening.* Rinse with warm water and, while your skin is still moist, apply a moisturizer. In the morning, use one with SFP 15 or higher, ideally containing zinc oxide, titanium dioxide, or Parsol 1789—or a "broad spectrum" sunscreen combination. (Brands include Cetaphil, Aveeno, Neutrogena, Almay, and Nivea Visage.)

## "Hypoallergenic" Doesn't Mean It Won't Irritate

While it may be reassuring to see "nonirritating," "hypoallergenic," or "dermatologist-tested" on your skin cream label, there is no legal standard for what these terms mean, and no testing required to prove them. If you are prone to skin irritation or allergic reactions, approach all creams and makeup with caution until you have tested them on a small patch of skin, or ask an experienced dermatologist for recommendations on the least irritating products.

This skepticism should also extend to hair dyes, which generally are not tested for safety before marketing. Some of my patients have asked which product is best for restoring color to pubic hair. Although I have not made a scientific study of them, the male-beard-dyeing products formulated for short, coarse hair are easy to apply. Care should be taken not to let the dye touch the thin skin of the inner labia, the vaginal mucosa, or the skin around the opening of the anus.

When dyeing any hair, do a patch test first. Follow package directions, or put a dab of dye behind one ear and wait two days (try not to wash it off) to see if you develop any itching, burning, or redness. If you have a reaction, try different colors or brands until you find one that causes no irritation. Keep dye well away from your eyes. For those of us who are frequently coloring our roots, the bad news is that there is (mixed and inconclusive) evidence that years of dye use could slightly increase our risk of bladder cancer.

You can go for a more expensive and perhaps richer-feeling moisturizer. (I was once given a free bottle of La Mer cream, and little dabs seemed to anoint my skin with a glistening moistness. The advertisers claim the cream is made from an ancient European recipe that can ultimately reduce scars. I doubt it, but at $90 an ounce, I too can become captive to "expensive may be better.") You should be able to judge for yourself and use "mirror feedback" to assess the degree of hydration you're getting from a moisturizing cream. An expensive cream may absorb more quickly, smell better, and have ingredients from exotic sources but may not be any more effective than a less expensive product. If the cream does not contain sunscreen, add this before you leave the house. But don't apply creams with sunscreen to your upper or lower eyelids. The costly creams specially marketed for the eye area may have a lower concentration of active ingredients, and no added perfume to limit irritation. If you've had no problems using face cream near your eyes, there's no reason to add an extra product to your shelf or your face.

An overall body moisturizer after you step out of the shower in the morning (or like me, get out of the tub in the evening) should be applied when your skin is slightly damp. Because of the large amount you need to cover your body, go for an inexpensive product such as Cetaphil, Lubriderm, Curel, or Eucerin moisturizing creams. Use cream with sunscreen on your arms or other sun-vulnerable areas if you plan to go outdoors.

*Fortifying.* This is where you should talk to your skin specialist about prescription Retin-A, which can be used in conjunction with (but not at the exact same time as) a reputable AHA or antioxidant cream or solution. I also use an estrogen cream (described earlier).

## When Should You See a Dermatologist?

I recommend that my patients see a dermatologist at least every two years for a head-to-toe check to ensure there is no skin cancer. From a cosmetic standpoint, if you've suffered sun damage, or simply want to know what's out there to protect, enhance, or rehabilitate your skin, you should consult with a board-certified dermatologist more frequently. Remember, however, that the products sold in her or his office generate personal profit. A handful of big companies make most products sold in dermatologists' offices; they arrange to put their private labels on and sell them to patients. Even if your doctor's name is on the jar, it doesn't mean that she or he helped in any way to formulate or manufacture the product. It may, however, be excellent, and indeed may be less expensive than many you can buy at the cosmetic counter in high-end department stores. Don't hesitate to ask about the ingredients, and whether what they "may do" is worth the price. It's also perfectly acceptable to inquire about basic brands available at your local drugstore or supermarket.

You have probably noticed that I haven't addressed the role of cosmetologists, facialists, and those wonderful individuals in spas who perform facials to soothing New Age melodies. I would prefer that you discuss this with your dermatologist. In some cases, heat, poor cleansing with "squeeze as you go" extractions, and scraping during this process can break small blood vessels, and worsen rosacea and acne. There is often insufficient scientific evidence to support the myriad claims of what their products and treatments do for your skin. For many of us, the "time out" for our face and body, as well as the cleansing and moisturizing of a facial, do contribute to our sense of skin well-being. But beware: If you think it's difficult to resist the products in dermatologists' offices, the beautiful bottles and jars of fragrant creams, lotions, and masques marketed to you in your semidrowsy and relaxed state are even harder to resist.

Each of us looks at her face with different hopes and expectations. Realize that your skin has expectations of its own. Premature aging from sun damage is more than disappointing; it's the all-too-visible penalty for your failure to follow the skin's rules. Unfortunately, many of us didn't know these rules when we were younger, but now in our more mature wisdom we can avail ourselves of the tremendous advances in treating photo- and chronologic aging. Total reversal of the skin's clock may not be possible, but we may be able to set it back. Sun protection during the day will have the greatest impact on slowing down this external, visible time meter. And remember, beautiful people take care of their entire bodies, and are beautiful from the inside out.

# 8

## *Young and Healthy in Mind*

I stop midsentence for a search-and-rescue of the word I need to complete my thought."

"I'll walk into a room and forget why I'm there."

"I used to have an almost photographic memory—and now I can't remember what I read in yesterday's paper."

"I was at the top of my class in graduate school. Why can't I focus anymore?"

"I saw this happen to my mother."

With these or similar phrases, countless patients entreat me to prescribe the hormone, medicine, vitamin, or herb that will restore their memories, multitasking abilities, and mental coping skills.

Margie, at 45, was sure that perimenopause was causing her "to lose her mind." Her periods were regular and hormone tests were normal. She had ailing parents, a difficult teenage daughter, and an ex-husband who'd declared bankruptcy. She worked a ten-hour day, and when she plopped into bed she couldn't sleep. Her mind wasn't lost; it was overwhelmed.

Candace, 62, voiced concern because she was missing appointments, had difficulty recalling information, and was not functioning up to par in her job as a lobbyist (where it was critical to remember who knew who, gave what, and said what). She laughed nervously as she said, "It's probably just my age," but then admitted her fear that this signaled the onset of Alzheimer's.

## FEAR OF "MENTAL PAUSE"

Memory does change as we get older. As early as our forties, many of us notice that we process information a bit more slowly. Those "What *is* her name?" and "Where on earth are my keys?" moments become more frequent. It may take extra time and practice to learn a new skill or routine. And focusing on multiple concurrent tasks becomes more difficult at a time when we have more things to remember, do, and forget. We feel stressed, and stress takes its mind toll.

What's normal when it comes to memory? Neurologic and physiologic studies demonstrate that age can slow our ability to recall recent events or newly learned facts. It becomes more difficult to conquer new disciplines such as math, languages, or computers. There is even a distressing medical term to describe this: *age-associated memory impairment*. It occurs in 50 percent of us in our sixties, and 70 percent by the age of 70. This may be a predecessor to more severe forgetfulness, called *mild cognitive impairment* (MCI); roughly half of those with MCI go on to develop Alzheimer's within five years.

Before you conclude that any forgetfulness is a sign of MCI or worse—let me reassure you that mental decline is not inevitable. A recent Mayo Clinic study of people in their nineties found that half had no significant memory problems—and many were extremely sharp. Others who were noticeably forgetful about appointments or conversations were still able to live independently.

Nowhere is "use it or lose it" more important than in our abilities to think and remember. As you know, the schooling of our brains starts at a very young age, but you may not have been taught that this can also prevent the future degeneration of our brain cells. Your language skills, education, and intellectual level at the age of 20 may influence your risk of developing Alzheimer's disease in your eighties.

## IS IT NORMAL FORGETFULNESS,
## A "SENIOR MOMENT" . . .
## OR ALZHEIMER'S?

The increasing rate of Alzheimer's disease (AD) in our population is basically a marker of medical success, as we live long enough to get it: The greatest increase in this disorder is expected to occur in women over the age of 85. Currently, 4.6 million Americans have AD—and this number will likely triple to sixteen million by midcentury.

It starts with a whimper: Just 1 percent of Americans aged 60 to 64 have diagnosed Alzheimer's. From there on in, AD prevalence doubles every five years—until, for those of us who make it to 85 and beyond, that figure has exploded with a bang at 40 percent. What causes this mental loss? I was taught in medical school that as we age, brain cells die, the brain shrinks, and if we live long enough there's so much neuronal damage that AD inevitably ensues. However, neurophysiologists are currently unfolding a more complex scenario. We can actually add brain cells, and build and maintain synapses (communication links between our brain cells) as long as we live. In AD, loss of memory begins before brain cells die, as clumps of protein called *amyloid* hamper communication between the healthy brain cells. This has immense therapeutic significance. Researchers hope to figure out how to stop, remove, or disarm the amyloid debris (plaques) before brain cells die. This could halt or even prevent Alzheimer's.

Inflammation and oxidative damage probably contribute to the damage of AD: The body tries to get rid of amyloid plaque by sending in "garbage collecting" cells; this attack on plague causes neuron damage and death. And as all this takes place, there may be a reduction in the levels of important neurotransmitters such as acetylcholine. We also know that a cholesterol-carrying protein called *apolipoprotein E* (ApoE for short) helps protect the brain synapses from being damaged by amyloid. If you inherit a less robust form of ApoE, called e4, you are at increased risk of developing AD. But there is more to this disease than passive genetic risk.

## Risk Factors for Alzheimer's Disease

- *Genes.* The best predictor we have so far for AD risk is which of four common variations of ApoE you have inherited, but even this is not a sure thing. The ApoE-e4 form carries a 27 percent lifetime risk of developing AD—versus about 9 percent for individuals who don't have it. However, it doesn't seem to carry even this much risk for black and Hispanic individuals. And because most people who carry one or even two copies of ApoE-e4 will not get AD, and many people without e4 *will* get it, this is neither adequate nor prophetic as a screening test for AD.
- A *family history* of AD or dementia.
- *Stroke.* Undetected or "silent" strokes that show up on MRI scans are linked to a 2.3 times greater risk of AD or other types of dementia.
- *A previous head injury,* especially if you blacked out for an hour or more, or had posttraumatic amnesia. The brain's response to head trauma (and perhaps its attempt to help repair the damage) is to form amyloid plaques. This hallmark of AD has been found in children as young as 10.
- *Diet* (see page 360).
- *Smoking.* Smokers have twice the risk of getting AD (but when they quit, at whatever age, this risk is reduced).

## Medical Ways to Distinguish Between Mere Forgetfulness and the Onset of Alzheimer's

Seek a medical opinion if your forgetfulness seems to be getting rapidly worse (over just a few months), if people around you comment on it, and if memory problems interfere with your work or household management. You can start by consulting your family physician, but for a thorough assessment, you probably should see a neurologist or be referred to a memory clinic. The initial workup will include screening to rule out depression, and blood tests to check for thyroid problems, $B_{12}$ deficiency, abnormal lipids, high blood sugar, and chronic diseases.

We use scores and numbers in medicine, and multiple tests have been developed to assess our cognitive abilities (thinking and memory). One of the basic standardized tests that doctors use is the Mini-Mental State Examination (MMSE). This includes questions about orientation ("What is the day of the week?"), memorizing lists, counting backward, following directions, repeating a tongue twister, writing sentences, and copying drawings. The maximum score is 30 points. The MMSE is not an "Alzheimer's test": You might score low for a number of reasons, including test jitters, fatigue, or just having a bad day. Ask for a copy of your test results, and schedule a retake if you think it doesn't reflect your usual state of mind.

Brain scans such as magnetic resonance imaging (MRI) and computerized axial tomography (CT) can reveal signs of other conditions that might cause AD-like symptoms, such as previous mini-strokes, and can measure changes in brain size. So far, PET scanning (positron emission tomography) shows the most promise for detecting early-stage AD and tracking disease progress. Instead of brain structure, PET scanners take pictures of brain activity, showing the busy "hot spots" versus less active "cold spots."

Unfortunately, researchers disagree on the accuracy and meaning of scan findings. They continue to refine tests and search for other physical changes that could serve as AD markers. They have developed a dye which, when injected into the vein, is picked up by the plaque, so that it stands out in a PET scan. They are also measuring changes in the size of the hippocampus (a brain area important for storage and processing of memories) and are looking for spinal fluid proteins associated with AD. Although routine genetic testing for ApoE is not recommended, because most people who carry the e4 variation will not develop AD, you might consider the test if several relatives developed AD before the age of 65. This, plus an abnormal PET scan, is currently the most accurate way for you and your doctor to assess your risk, so that you can change your lifestyle and consider early use of medications (see page 362).

### Keep your wits about you as long as possible
Here are some of the ways we *think* will help you reduce your risk of Alzheimer's disease and other dementias:

*Eat a heart-healthy diet for brain protection.* The foods that protect your heart will nourish your brain. Several large European studies have linked hypertension and high cholesterol to increased AD risk. High cholesterol seems to trigger overproduction of amyloid in the brain. So fill your grocery cart with fresh fruit and leafy vegetables, whole grains, and polyunsaturated fats from vegetables, nuts, and fish.

Omega-3 fatty acids (including docosahexaenoic acid, or DHA) from fish oil boost levels of the neurotransmitter acetylcholine, needed for normal memory function. Not all fish are created omega-3 equal; farm-raised fish that don't move around much are less likely to help our brains and hearts than free-exercising ocean fish (which have less overall fat, but more omega-3). When you buy fish or order it in a restaurant, don't be embarrassed to ask where it came from.

There are also data showing that high blood levels of the amino acid homocysteine (see page 176) are associated with vascular disease and brain atrophy. You can reduce homocysteine levels by abstaining from red meat, substituting vegetable and nut oils for butter, and taking appropriate doses of folic acid supplement (see page 175).

*Eat E-rich foods.* In new large long-term studies, diets high in vitamin E–rich foods were found to reduce cognitive decline. This means we can "go nuts" for our brains, or perhaps we should consider taking supplements (see below).

*Drink wine in moderation.* Studies in Holland, Denmark, and the homeland of red wine, Bordeaux, found that moderate wine drinkers (especially those who imbibe red wine) were less likely to develop dementia as they got older. The antioxidant properties of flavonoids may limit free radical formation and inflammation—and also make platelets less sticky, so blood clots don't clog small vessels. (If you don't like wine, you may get similar benefits from drinking purple grape juice.)

*Exercise regularly.* This will help improve your glucose tolerance. Glucose intolerance with insulin overproduction has been linked to poor memory. Workouts also help lower cholesterol levels, and hence protect the blood vessels in your brain from fatty obstruction.

*Consider estrogen replacement.* Evidence has accumulated that initial postmenopause use of ERT can reduce our risk for AD. The conclusion of a 2002 international position paper reviewing evidence of estrogen's health effects: After weighing the various risks and benefits, women at high risk for AD due to genetics or family history may wish to consider ERT.

I spent a lot of time discussing the controversial Women's Health Initiative study. As I write this chapter, results were published in the *Journal of the American Medical Association* on the WHI Memory Study (WHIMS) showing that Prempro use after the age of 65 was correlated with a twofold *increase* in the development of dementia. Of 2,229 women assigned to taking this form of HRT, 40 developed dementia during four years of follow-up, compared with 21 among the 2,303 women taking a placebo.

It's possible that the progestin in Prempro counteracted any positive effect from estrogen, or that in order for estrogen to "protect" the brain it needs to be given at the onset of estrogen loss, not fifteen years later when the vascular system may be more susceptible to small clots, and the dementia may be due to tiny strokes.

The WHI study is also assessing the effect of Premarin-only on memory. It may show that estrogen by itself is a brain-positive therapy, as we'd been led to expect from the studies that found it reduces amyloid accumulation, enhances neurotransmitter release and action, and protects against oxidative damage. Right now, I would *not* advise women who have never been on HRT to start it at 65 to attain future protection. Those at risk might want to use it when they first become menopausal, especially if they have had a hysterectomy and don't need to take progestin. For a woman whose uterus is intact, I would prescribe another form of progesterone (see page 56), then reevaluate whether to continue after a few years. We don't know if the WHI study applies to all forms of estrogen. The patch may be less likely to cause clotting and vessel problems that could compromise the brain.

## What can be done about Alzheimer's disease

*Pharmaceuticals.* Four drugs are currently approved by the FDA to help control symptoms of AD but not to treat the underlying causes: Aricept (donepezil), Cognex (tacrine), Exelon (rivastigmine), and Reminyl (galantamine). They all affect the neurotransmitter acetylcholine. Unfortunately, they seem to produce only a mild, temporary memory boost. Studies are under way to see if starting these drugs at the earliest possible stage (pre-AD) could increase their benefit. A few experts call them "smart drugs," but so far this appellation seems like wishful thinking. They are expensive, can cause gastrointestinal side effects, and should not be prescribed unless AD is clinically presumed or diagnosed.

Another medication, *memantine,* works on glutamate, a neurotransmitter released in response to trauma, seizure, stroke, or other brain injury. A certain amount is needed for learning and memory; too much allows excess calcium to flow into the brain cells, which harms or even kills them. Memantine helps "normalize relations" between glutamate and brain cells, and seems to slow memory decline at later stages of AD. In combination with an acetylcholine-affecting drug, it may actually improve memory and thinking ability. Memantine has been used for over a decade in Germany (under the name Axura). It's approved by the European Union (where it's called Ebixa) to treat advanced Alzheimer's, and is now under review by the FDA.

*Supplements.* Taking 2,000 IU of vitamin E daily seems to slow the pace of decline in people with AD. But there is concern that too much E can have unwanted side effects, including suppression of the immune response needed to fight off infections, an increased tendency to bleed, and bone loss. (If you want to use E as an Alzheimer's preventive, don't go beyond 800 IU a day from food and supplements unless you discuss it with your doctor.)

There is no good evidence that ginkgo or other herbs will prevent or cure AD. For healthy older adults, ginkgo has been found to be no better than a placebo in enhancing memory. However, ginkgo extract has been approved in Germany to treat symptoms of Alzheimer's disease (at a dose of 240 mg a day). A U.S. study found that persons with mild to moderate AD who took 120 mg a day of ginkgo extract showed a slight improvement in cognitive functioning, and their caregivers saw a small improvement in mood and social behavior. Their doctors, however, saw no improvements in the ginkgo group. And remember, the quality and contents of herbal supplements vary tremendously.

**What's on the horizon**

Cholesterol-lowering statins and antihypertensive medications might reduce AD risk; I hope to see some confirming statistics in the next few years. (If you need to be on these meds for other reasons, they may be contributing to your future brain health.) There has been intriguing evidence that anti-inflammatory drugs, including aspirin, attack and dissolve plaques, and perhaps prevent new ones. Some studies have found lower rates of AD among frequent users of over-the-counter ibuprofen and aspirin. But a recent study of individuals with mild to moderate AD who took a prescription COX-2 inhibitor (rofecoxib) or naproxen found no improvement after a year of use, compared with a placebo.

## Alison's Story

Alison is a successful television writer with a wonderful sense of humor. She went through early menopause as a result of chemotherapy, which together with surgery and radiation successfully treated a breast cancer she developed in her early forties. Ten years later, we chatted as I did her annual exam. When I mentioned that I was writing the memory section of

## Treatable Memory Robbers

A number of medical conditions can affect memory, including diabetes, high cholesterol, hypertension, thyroid or endocrine disorders, infections, and depression. A very common culprit is the "silent" stroke, a small brain injury, caused by a blocked or ruptured blood vessel, causing no obvious symptoms. If your memory suddenly worsens (especially if you have high blood pressure), a silent stroke may have occurred—and is not so silent anymore.

A sensory problem such as gradual hearing loss can feel like forgetfulness. Stress and fatigue affect attention and recall. Antihistamines, painkillers, and drugs that treat hypertension, anxiety, or depression can fog your mind. If you start a new medication and suddenly can't remember if or when you took it, or just seem to be losing your focus, consult your doctor. These effects may wear off, or you may have to change the dose or switch to a different drug.

this book, she laughed and said, "Do you want to know what short-term memory loss can do? One day, I prepared some salad to take to work and put it in a plastic container. When I went to unlock the door of my car, I put the container on the roof. Not only did I forget about it as I got into the car, turned on the ignition, and started to back up . . . but when it fell on the hood, I exclaimed, 'What the hell is that?' "

Alison has learned to cope, but admits that she sometimes has to reread a scene she wrote the previous day in order to continue writing it. "But then it seems new, and I get the pleasure of being surprised that it's so good!"

Her sense of humor, and her ability to laugh at little memory lapses and concentrate on what her mind can do (she's a terrific writer), have made her short-term memory problems incidental rather than fundamental to her career and life.

## Keeping Your Brain Young

### Brain push-ups

Working it has definitely been shown to help prevent losing it. A recent study of 801 nuns, priests, and monks over 65 found that those who kept their minds active, took on new challenges, and inquired about new subjects (keeping up with the news, playing cards, doing puzzles, or visiting museums) were less likely to develop Alzheimer's disease four or five years later. The difference was extreme: The top 10 percent who were mentally busy were nearly 50 percent less likely to develop Alzheimer's disease than the least inquisitive 10 percent. Using their minds helped protect their working memory, speed of perception, and recall of recent events. Interestingly, years of education or amount of physical exercise did not make a difference in their AD risk.

This doesn't mean you should wait until you're 65 to begin your memory exercise. Researchers at Case Western Reserve University found that the risk for developing AD was three to four times lower in individuals who were intellectually active in their forties and fifties than in those who were not.

A mental workout doesn't require pounding music or trainers screaming at you (although listening to music—I suggest Mozart—does temporarily help organize thinking). It consists of a mental challenge, and is honed by practice. One interesting study found that mentally repeating a new skill, such as visualizing a finger exercise for the piano, stimulated the brain's motor center as much as physically playing the piano.

An experiment with 2,800 adults aged 65 to 94 found that training in memorization strategies, reasoning skills (using patterns to organize information), and speed-of-processing skills (tricks for locating information quickly even while distracted) could not only prevent decline but actually boost performance.

Find ways to keep your brain challenged. Register for a class, be it cooking or philosophy. Take up an instrument or a new sport. Have a young relative or friend teach you a computer game. Prepare for a trip abroad by learning the basics of a new language.

**Memory strategies**
The brains of people with exceptionally good memories are essentially no different from anyone else's. These "memory geeks" have learned and practiced recall techniques. For example, when remembering long lists of numbers, they imagine the numbers in different colors. Or they visualize a structure for the list of numbers: mentally "planting" them in distinct places along a well-known road, inside an imaginary room or city, or in a file cabinet. Imagery lets them draw on memory resources in more parts of their brains (particularly the hippocampus, associated with our ability to visualize in three dimensions). So think and sync in color and space.

If you have "I'm distracted and can't remember" moments, learn to compensate: Put important items (purse, keys, cell phone) in the same place every day. Keep a notebook handy to jot down to-dos and reminders, or track your tasks using a small tape recorder or your cell phone (the menu often has a brief recording device), PDA, or computer. You'll be using a new technical skill to boot. Before you set out to do something (look up a phone number, find the tape measure, or drive to a particular destination), take a second to mentally review your goal. We all need to remember where we're going, what we're doing, and even why we're doing it.

Remember the classic "Thirty days hath September, April, June, and November"? Did you or your children learn multiplication tables from the "Multiplication Rock" musical cartoons? Rhymes, songs, and acronyms are great for recall; I use them to remember medical terms, conditions, and patients. (Rest assured, however . . . I don't sing out loud or read poetry as I do pelvic exams or offer advice!) Here are some of my "help, there's so much to remember" tricks:

- When cramming for medical school exams, I used this mnemonic for the names of the twelve cranial nerves: On Old Olympus's Towering Top, A Finn And German Viewed Some Hops. The first letter of each word stands for the name of the nerve: Olfactory, Optic, Oculomotor, Trochlear, Trigeminal . . . since you don't need to memorize them, I won't list them all.
- ASCUS (Atypical Squamous Cells of Unknown Significance) signifies that the Pap smear is not quite normal. Rather than remembering the full term, I mentally recite what the cells are saying: "Ask us to catch us."
- HDL lipids start with an H, so ideally they should be *h*igh, and LDL lipids, *l*ow.
- The researchers who conduct large studies concoct acronyms so doctors can remember what they're about, such as HERS (Heart and Estrogen/Progestin Replacement Study) and MrFIT (Multiple Risk Factor Intervention Trial).

To remember phone and bank card numbers, connect them with a date, a measure, your childhood address, whatever confers delightful or distressing meaning. If the access code is 1821, think of the old and current legal drinking ages. I connect 45 with 58, the age I think I am versus my chronologic age.

Forgetting names can be particularly embarrassing. When meeting a new acquaintance, repeat her name to yourself a few times, make a comment about it, and use it in conversation (e.g., introduce her to someone else). Try associating the name with another word or image. If the name is unremarkable, take note of any striking features (such as her haircut or color, a pointed chin, a high voice, or freckles) and try to link the feature, or a pattern of features, to the person's name or profession, or to another person you know with a similar name.

Play with the names: Alexandra is overweight—which rhymes with Alexander the Great. Robin seems "flighty," and Shirley has hair that's curly (or seems surly). Once you make these kinds of silly connections, they're likely to stick.


## Getting Your Well-Earned Rest

For most of us, a good night's sleep means eight hours—although some women function well on six, and others need nine or ten to feel rested. But there's more to sleep than adding up hours; to feel fully refreshed, we need to spend quality time in each stage of sleep.

There are two basic types of sleep: REM (rapid eye movement, also known as our dreaming sleep) and non-REM (NREM) sleep. We cycle between NREM and REM every hour and a half during the night. NREM sleep actually consists of four separate stages, in which we go from "transition sleep" to "true sleep" to stages three and four, "slow-wave sleep." The latter is our deepest and perhaps most important sleep.

A lot happens in our bodies and brains while we're getting our Zs. The brain reduces adenosine levels, which build up as we expend energy during the day. Slow-wave sleep most efficiently reduces levels of adenosine, so any medication that suppresses this phase can leave you feeling tired despite a full night of what you thought was appropriate rest.

During slow-wave sleep, we also secrete growth hormone, restore our immune system, give our cardiac and pulmonary systems a breather (as our heart rate, breathing rate, and blood pressure decrease), lower our metabolic rate and body temperature, and generally allow all our systems to undergo recalibration and repair. If you are awakened during this maintenance phase, you may feel confused and groggy.

During REM sleep, as we dream (and have rapid eye movements— darting eyes behind closed lids) mental activity picks up, and heart rate, breathing, and blood pressure increase to "awake" levels. This is when it's easiest to wake up without feeling "out of it." The right mix of REM and non-REM sleep is important not only to how we feel the next day but to how our bodies function during the days, weeks, and even years to come.

## A woman's sleep is never done . . .

Most women aged 30 to 60 get less than seven hours of sleep on week-nights. Remember the phrase "Sleep is the sex of the nineties"? This continues to be true for most of us in the twenty-first century. It's a wondrous luxury that we can't afford as we hold down jobs, take care of our families, and multitask into the wee hours of the morning—or get up at those hours. This type of sleep deprivation (estimated to affect at least 40 percent of us) not only impairs our mental abilities but also leads to insulin resistance and elevated stress hormone levels—which go on to cause heart disease, diabetes, depression, and memory loss. It also makes us crave the wrong foods (sugar and caffeine), appear haggard, and both look and feel old.

Lack of proper rest not only harms our health, it can also hurt others; the National Highway Traffic Safety Administration estimates that fatigue plays a role in over 100,000 car accidents each year.

Setting aside time for sleep is clearly a health priority. If you can't put in the eight hours during the week, allow yourself an extra hour or two on the weekends to make up the sleep deficit. Short twenty-minute naps during the day help, but if they are more than thirty minutes you may end up changing your circadian rhythm (see below) and feel dazed instead of refreshed.

## Factors that contribute to poor sleep

*Changes in circadian rhythm.* Our sleep cycles are regulated by a cluster of nerve cells in the hypothalamus called the *suprachiasmatic nuclei*. This inner clock tells us when we're tired, when to go to sleep, and when to wake up. It responds to light/dark cycles by sending signals to other parts of the brain, including the pineal gland. As darkness falls, the pineal gland secretes more of the hormone melatonin, which causes drowsiness.

While teenagers' clocks work best with "late to bed and late to rise," the opposite is true as we get older: Melatonin spurts occur earlier, and we get less slow-wave sleep during the night. "Early bird" dinner specials are as much due to biology as to tight budgets; we're more likely to get hungry early, want to fall asleep before the ten o'clock news, and wake to darkness at 4:00 A.M. While this schedule is perfect for *Today* show staff, others may find it to be inconvenient.

You are particularly vulnerable if you work night shifts, where your work schedule and brain-rest schedule are not in sync. The same lack of brain-body synchronicity occurs when you cross several time zones and develop jet lag.

*Caffeine, alcohol, and cigarettes.* As I noted in chapter 4, many foods and drinks contain hidden caffeine. The half-life of caffeine is 7.5 hours, which means that afternoon pick-me-up coffee can disrupt your sleep cycle hours later. And while a glass of wine can make you drowsy, it causes midnight wakefulness. Cigarettes also stimulate, and that last smoke of the day may turn your night into a sleepless one.

*Sleep apnea.* We women joke about men's snoring, but the sleep-disturbing truth is that after menopause we are just as likely as men to suffer from this disorder. An estimated one in four women over age 65 suffers from *sleep apnea:* repeated pauses in breathing, followed by gasps and brief awakenings. Daytime tiredness and loud nighttime snoring (ask your significant other, or your neighbors) may be signs of apnea. Most sufferers don't receive the appropriate medical diagnosis—which can be fatal: Apnea is associated with an increased risk of high blood pressure, heart disease, stroke, and driving accidents.

*Limb movements. Periodic limb movement disorder* is surprisingly common as we get older. These "night moves" include repeated jerking and kicking, and trigger frequent waking. A similar disorder called *restless legs syndrome* causes tickling, aching, and jerking while sleeping.

*Night sweats.* About three-quarters of women will suffer from hot flashes during the first three to five years of menopause. The flashes may cause you to wake up, soaked in sweat—or you may not be aware of having them, but feel exhausted during the day because they interrupted your sleep pattern.

*Diseases and medications.* A number of illnesses, such as arthritis, osteoporosis, and heart disease, can interfere with sleep. Medications, such as those for asthma, often contain stimulants. Some antidepressants (including SSRIs; see page 380) and all the drugs used for attention-deficit disorder may cause insomnia. If you've started a new medication and find yourself unable to doze off or maintain restful sleep, consult with your doctor. Taking the drug in the morning, or changing the dose, may solve this side effect.

### Getting more and better Zs

*Exercise.* We need to get physical in order to sleep. A study published in the *Journal of the American Medical Association (JAMA)* looked at the effects of exercise on sleep among healthy (but tired) adults over 50. After four months of four exercise sessions per week—brisk walking and low-impact aerobics—they fell asleep in half the time, slept an average of an hour longer per night, and felt more rested in the morning. (A control group showed little change.) Don't expect a day of exercise to equate with a good night's sleep. In this study, it took more than two months of exercise for sleep to improve, so be patient and stick with it. And don't exercise just before bedtime; it raises the endorphins that make you more alert. Not what you need as your head hits the pillow.

*Light exposure.* Light exposure affects melatonin secretion. Especially during winter, it's easy to spend your day in less-than-bright environments. If you don't like an early-to-bed schedule, try getting some sun in the afternoon. (You can also ask your doctor about bright-light therapy.) If you work a night shift, you'll get better daytime Zs with lots of bright-light exposure at work, and low light in the morning before sleep.

Keep your room dark when you sleep. If nature's call wakes you during the night, keep the lights as dim as possible. Turning on a bright light may cancel your melatonin output, so your brain thinks it's time to get up.

*Bed equals sleep.* There are only two things you should do in bed: have sex and sleep. Reading or watching TV are no-nos if you have problems falling asleep. (You may find that upsetting newscasts or late-evening violent dramas make attainment of those Zs even more difficult.) If you can't fall asleep after fifteen or twenty minutes, get up and leave the bedroom. Play solitaire, have some warm milk or herbal tea and crackers (all of which can enhance relaxing neurotransmitters), read something dull . . . and go back to bed when you feel sleepy.

*A consistent schedule.* Keeping regular sleep and wake hours will help your circadian rhythms stay on track. Even if you just had a night of tossing and turning, get out of bed at the customary hour; over time, this will train your brain for better sleep. A prebed routine, such as a warm bath or restful book (read in a chair, not in your bed), may also help.

*Calm your mind.* Try to create a quiet and secure sleep environment. (Some women feel safer knowing a flashlight and phone are close by.) Don't lie there obsessing about being awake; worrying makes matters worse. Put soothing images before your mind's eye: calming ocean waves, black velvet, or soft green moss. A *JAMA* study of insomniacs over 55 found that making these kinds of changes in bedtime behavior, schedules, and thinking (known as *cognitive behavior therapy*) helped most of them achieve better sleep.

*Medical options.* If poor sleep seriously affects your daily functioning so that you can't concentrate, stay awake while driving, or, as often warned on medication bottles, safely operate heavy machinery, consult your doctor. Even if you somehow get through the day but sleep problems leave you depressed, anxious, or panicky for more than a couple of weeks, you should seek help. Start with your primary care physician, or go online and check with organizations such as the American Academy of Sleep Medicine (www.aasmnet.org), the National Sleep Foundation (www.sleepfoundation. org), or the National Institutes of Health (www.nhlbi.nih.gov/health/public/sleep) for referrals to sleep specialists and sleep clinics.

Some causes of insomnia have well-established medical treatments. Hormone replacement therapy does wonders for insomnia caused by night sweats (see chapter 2). Natural progesterone can induce sleepiness in doses of 200 mg. So if you have made a decision to take estrogen and need some form of progestin to protect your uterine lining, one pill may medicate two issues. For apnea, treatment can be as simple as a mouthpiece to correct jaw position and open the airway. The most effective therapy is usually CPAP (continuous positive airway pressure), a small pump that pushes extra air into the airway as you breathe. Weight loss can also make a huge difference in how the air travels down to your lungs.

In cases where the uvula, that fleshy projection in the upper palate, has enlarged and obstructs airflow, surgical reduction may allow sleep without the use of a nighttime air pump. Leg movement disorders can be treated with medications that increase dopamine levels. These include Mirapex and Klonopin. *Treating depression or anxiety* (see page 378) *with appropriate medications should also improve sleep.* One more drug, modafinil (Provigil), has been used to treat excessive daytime sleepiness in patients diagnosed with *narcolepsy*. The FDA has approved its use for patients with sleep apnea and for shift workers who suffer from fatigue and an inability to adjust their sleep patterns. Doctors also prescribe Provigil "off label" to treat severe fatigue associated with psychiatric disorders, chronic pain medication, and fibromyalgia. (The armed forces are testing it on soldiers who are sleep deprived.) Provigil can cause nausea, dizziness, nervousness, and headache. Long-term lack of sleep affects our physical and mental well-being. There is no assurance that this pill that can "pick you up now" won't let your health down later.

## What about sleeping pills?

I, like most physicians, am frequently asked to prescribe sleeping pills or hypnotics. Before doing so, I try to assess and treat the underlying cause of the sleeplessness. Depending on the circumstances, I may prescribe medication for short-term use.

Sleep medications fall into two categories—short-acting and long-acting—which work on different receptors in the brain. The *short-acting hypnotics,* Sonata (zaleplon) and Ambien (zolpidem), don't suppress deep sleep or REM sleep, and so have minimal effects on your next-day activities, nor do they seem to be addictive like the longer-acting medications (see below).

Sonata works almost immediately and wears off quickly (in one to two hours), making it ideal for those times when you wake up at four in the morning and can't go back to sleep. Ambien has a longer activity of two to three hours. This may be a good choice if you have problems falling asleep but once "there" can sleep until morning. For those of us who travel and suffer from jet lag, these short-acting medications can help us get to sleep in a new time zone.

Among the long-acting sleeping pills, called *benzodiazepines,* the brands most often prescribed include Halcion (triazolam), Restoril (temazepam), Dalmane (flurazepam), and Doral (quazepam). These literally calm your nerves, slowing central nervous system activity. This "brain calm" can provide temporary help with falling asleep and, depending on the pill and dose, last from several hours to more than twenty-four hours. They suppress deep and REM sleep, which can lead to next-day attention, memory, and thinking deficits. They can also cause lightheadedness and impair coordination, increasing the risk of accidents or falls.

Regular use of the benzodiazepines leads to tolerance, so that after a few weeks of nightly use they may no longer work. They can be addictive, causing rebound insomnia or a psychological need to continue or increase their use. Remember, they slow down the nervous system—and so does alcohol. Combining these can cause serious side effects and even death. I prescribe benzodiazepines for my patients who have sleep disturbances due to illness, sudden severe stress, or loss of a loved one, but I usually limit these prescriptions to thirty days.

If sleep problems are related to depression, some antidepressant medications can help (see page 378).

*Supplements.* Researchers have refuted the idea that we secrete less melatonin with age; it's the timing of the secretion that can change. Can taking melatonin supplements improve sleep? Perhaps. Small studies have found that low-dose melatonin supplements (under 1 mg) can help individuals who can't fall asleep in accord with their work or life schedule (delayed sleep phase syndrome), and recalibrate the sleep cycle for those with jet lag. But almost as many studies show contrary results: Melatonin supplements actually interfere with sleep quality. Since we have no way of knowing what's actually in the tablets, and long-term safety of this supplement is unknown, I don't encourage regular use. This is not a "sleep well to stay young" product. Bright-light therapy is a safer option for getting sleep schedules back on track.

*OTC sleep aids (antihistamines).* Histamine is an arousal chemical in the brain, so suppressing it makes you sleepy. Most over-the-counter sleep aids contain diphenhydramine (Sominex, Nytol) or doxylamine (Unisom), which are antihistamines. These pills are popular, but they can leave you groggy the next day. Moreover, they stop working if you take them every night. The best way to use them is for sleep emergencies (two or three nights in a row) to help get you back on a normal sleep schedule. The good news is they are not addictive. But OTC does not mean side effect free; these can give you dry mouth, drowsiness, constipation, or blurred vision. Rotating an antihistamine and a prescription sleeping pill may be reasonable, but do so only for a limited time and with your doctor's approval.

## Emotional Well-Being for "Long-Being"

### Coping with depression

You find yourself staring out the window, unable to concentrate on your work. Nothing is fun anymore. The present is bleak, and the future seems pointless.

### Beth's story

Beth had an eating disorder in her teens. She was briefly hospitalized and then treated as an outpatient for a number of years. Now, at 40, she was a disciplined eater who maintained a low but healthy weight and exercised faithfully. Beth married in her late thirties and decided, together with her husband, not to have children. She took enormous pride in her work as a television producer, and loved to cook (organic, of course), read, and travel. She had tried various birth control pills in the past but would always discontinue them after just a few weeks because she thought they made her gain weight or feel moody.

Beth came to see me complaining that over the past few months, she'd suffered from "terrible PMS all the time." She was sure I could fix it with the right brew of hormones. But her symptoms were not "just" PMS. She collapsed in bed when she came home from work, didn't want to get up in the morning, and cried at the slightest stress. Even offhand remarks from colleagues upset her. She didn't want to have sex, didn't want to read, and didn't want to discuss how she felt with her husband—in short, "didn't want" described her feelings about life. These symptoms were constant, although they intensified a week or two before her period. Beth was suffering from depression.

She joined the one-quarter to one-third of women who will experience at least one episode of clinical depression during their lives. ("Clinical" means it's a medically diagnosable and treatable condition.) According to the National Institute of Mental Health, each year 12.4 million women suffer from this disorder. It most frequently occurs between the ages of 18 and 45—and women are twice as likely to become depressed as men.

Beth was already at risk, and indeed may have been depressed in the past as she dealt with her eating disorder (the two often go together; in medical parlance, they are co-morbidities). I referred her to a psychiatrist. While he didn't think Beth needed to be hospitalized, he started her on aggressive antidepressant therapy, carefully monitoring her responses and progress. When I saw Beth three months later, she felt much better and was planning a trip to Europe with her husband.

We all feel rotten at times, often for very good and obvious reasons, such as the loss of a loved one, the breakup of a marriage, job stress, or financial woes. How can you tell if what you're feeling merits the medical label of major depression—a treatable, biological condition? There are clusters of symptoms, which often include unexplained fatigue, insomnia, anger, irritability, and sadness. The activities and events that used to bring you pleasure become "nothing." And nothing seems to comfort you. It becomes difficult to concentrate, think clearly, or perform tasks that normally were effortless. At its worst, the hopeless feelings can lead to thoughts of suicide or even suicide attempts.

Compared with men, depressed women are more likely to have symp-

## Is This Really Depression?

If you have at least three of these symptoms for more than a couple of weeks, see your doctor.

- Persistent sad, anxious, or "empty" mood
- Loss of interest or pleasure in activities, including sex
- Restlessness, irritability, or excessive crying
- Feelings of guilt, worthlessness, helplessness, hopelessness, pessimism
- Sleeping too much or too little; early-morning awakening
- Loss of appetite and/or weight—or overeating and weight gain
- Decreased energy, fatigue, feeling "slowed down"
- Thoughts of death or suicide, or suicide attempts

(Source: National Institute of Mental Health.)

toms related to food (weight gain or eating disorders) and sleep (problems falling asleep, or sleeping too much), and are more likely to feel anxious. Depression will often coexist with panic attacks, posttraumatic stress disorder, or obsessive-compulsive disorder.

Whenever we give the term "major" to a medical condition, there's usually a minor form; in this case, it's called *dysthymia*. If you manage to drag yourself through your daily routine but feel tired and don't seem to enjoy life adequately, and you've felt this way for a long time (say, a couple of years), you may have dysthymia. Another form of depression can cycle with manic periods of "high" or irritable moods, incessant talking, racing thoughts, and irrational overconfidence. This condition was once called manic-depression; the correct medical term is *bipolar disorder*. It is most frequently diagnosed in women in their late teens or twenties. Collectively, all these illnesses are classified as *mood disorders*.

### Factors that contribute to depression

*Genes.* We are all vulnerable to depression, but it often runs in families. If a parent or sibling has been diagnosed as depressed, your own risk increases two to four times.

*Hormones.* Our hormonal ups and downs affect serotonin levels and also change the sensitivity of receptors in our brains to this feel-good substance. When our estrogen levels peak, just before and during ovulation, we may feel our best; when they bottom out, just before our periods, we may feel our worst. This is premenstrual depression.

An abrupt decline in estrogen (together with progesterone) can also trigger postpartum depression. At no other time in our lives do our hormones plummet so drastically as when we give birth to a baby and expel the placenta—which produced huge quantities of estrogen and progesterone. Most of us get the "baby blues," but 8 to 10 percent of us will become clinically depressed. And what happens to our emotions after having a baby can foreshadow future neurotransmitter response and vulnerability. Women with postpartum depression are at greater risk for future depression; in fact, many have already had previous, undiagnosed episodes. And half of women who have one episode of clinical depression (whatever the cause) will experience another.

Gradual loss of hormones (as with natural menopause) usually does not cause a clinical mood disorder. The incidence of depression does not rise after menopause. But if you're already vulnerable and have a history of previous episodes, the onset of menopause can trigger a recurrence.

*Physical illness.* Serious illness and chronic pain frequently cause depression, due in part to stress, isolation, and loss of fulfilling social roles. Pain also reduces our coping skills and overwhelms our brains with the "wrong" neurotransmitters. Antidepressant therapy has become an important addition to chronic pain therapy.

*Social roles and pressures.* Girls are reared to please others, a source of unreasonable pressure from the get-go. We may be told not to display our ambition or assertiveness, even though we need these to advance in life. Most of us need to earn a living, and would prefer to do this through a fulfilling career—which requires education and dedication. This dichotomy adds to our mental disharmony. Then, too, we are the gender expected to nurture our mates, children, and aging parents.

*Experiencing violence and abuse.* At least one-third of women have been sexually abused in their past—and 25 to 50 percent are currently sexually or physically abused by a partner. A history of abuse, and the attendant feelings of self-blame, helplessness, and isolation, are strongly linked to depression.

*Stresses and losses.* About 48 percent of women have unintended pregnancies, and 10 percent experience infertility. One-third of widows have symptoms of major depression a month after their spouse's death; a year later, half of these women will not have recovered. Grief is, of course, natural and not a sign of disease, but prolonged and severe grieving can plunge some women into a clinical depression that warrants medical treatment.

I'm overwhelmed by this list. It's amazing that any of us get by without experiencing clinical depression. As a gender, we're phenomenally resilient.

## Depressed mood depresses your health and longevity

Depression can also lead to health problems that can become fatal. Women and men over 65 who are depressed have a higher risk of death, regardless of social or economic factors, or other health problems. A government survey of over five thousand women showed that those who were depressed were 73 percent more likely to develop heart disease. Depression changes exercise and eating habits, and also chronically elevates levels of stress hormones known to induce cholesterol plaque and inflammatory changes in blood vessels.

Chronic elevation of stress hormones (adrenaline and cortisol) may also be the reason that depressed women are more likely to develop osteoporosis. If they drink because they are depressed (or are depressed because they drink), the combination of osteoporosis and inebriation is likely to break their bones. Older women with depression have a 40 percent higher risk of nonvertebral fractures.

## What can be done?

Unfortunately, there is no simple medical test for depression (or recovery from it). Without treatment, an episode of depression will continue for an average of nine months. Toughing it out is not necessary; 80 percent of women will feel and function significantly better with treatment. Before you start a course of treatment, your doctor should check to make sure that what you're experiencing is not due to a physical illness or a medication side effect—which can sometimes mimic depression.

*Psychotherapy.* Modern psychotherapy rarely involves a Freudian approach of "lie here for years and tell me about your childhood and desire to have been born a man." Discredited theories and bad movies have unfortunately distorted our sense of what can be accomplished by talking to a trained mental health professional. The approach that's most frequently used today is called *cognitive-behavior therapy.* Along with relief of symptoms, the goal of therapy is to help you regain a sense of control and hope. The therapist works with you to determine what problems and situations might contribute to your depression, and helps you find ways to solve or improve them. You might examine past behavior patterns and relationships to see what worked well or failed miserably, and set goals for making gradual changes. A good therapist can also help you understand how distorted thinking may perpetuate depression (see box, opposite).

This process works! Studies using PET scans show that talk therapy can actually create brain changes similar to those induced by medications. Sixty percent of women with mild or moderate depression get better by talking it out and altering self-destructive thoughts and behavior.

During the first few sessions, you and the therapist should be able to settle on goals for the treatment, and estimate how long it will take to get there. Modern psychotherapy does not last for years; typically it takes six to twenty weekly visits to get the depression under control. You may be dismayed to find, however, that your health insurance will only pay for a few sessions. (A few states require that major depression be covered to the same extent as other biological illnesses. This is known as mental health parity, and is a hot political issue.)

Psychotherapy can take longer to work than pharmacological therapy, so to speed recovery and reduce the odds of a recurrence, doctors often recommend a combination of psychotherapy and medication, especially if the depression is considered more than mild. The right therapist can be a clinical social worker, psychologist, or psychiatrist. (Often the first two will have you consult with a psychiatrist, or your primary care physician, if medication is indicated.) Make sure this person is licensed by the state. A trusting therapeutic relationship is important to recovery. If you just don't "click" with the therapist after a few sessions, don't give up; get a referral to someone who's more compatible.

*Medications.* Stigmas and wrong conceptions about psychiatric medications abound. Many women feel guilty that they are "popping a pill" to improve their moods. It's important to know that antidepressants correct imbalances of the neurotransmitters in your brain; they are not "uppers" and won't work if you are not depressed.

Antidepressants don't give immediate relief. Most doctors will start you out at a low dose and gradually increase it; this helps minimize side effects. Once you reach the recommended and research-supported therapeutic level, it still takes time before you notice an improvement in your symptoms. If you've been on a full dose for six to eight weeks and it's not working, or if side effects are persistent and bothersome, talk to your doctor about switching medications. (Generally, only physicians can prescribe antidepressants. In a few states, psychologists and nurse-practitioners with additional specialized training may do so.)

## A Point of View for Mental Health

The way you interpret and explain everyday events can reinforce depression and low self-esteem—or help lift you out of that negative groove. Researchers have found that with consistent effort, you can actually change your "explanatory style" and become happier and more optimistic. Here are some examples of unhealthy thinking patterns:

1. You see setbacks or problems as permanent instead of temporary: "I'll never be able to lose weight!" versus "I need to get some help and a plan that I can follow so I can lose weight." "My husband is always yelling at me" versus "My husband is in a bad mood; he must have had a rough day."

2. You see problems as general, rather than specific to a person or situation: "I always seem to get stuck with bad bosses" versus "I have a personality clash with this supervisor." "Men always leave me" versus "It just didn't work out with this guy."

3. You view bad things that happen as based on internal causes ("I've got no talent for math") and good things on external causes ("I got this job because no truly experienced or talented people applied"). Optimists think the opposite. Bad things usually have outside causes, and good things come from internal ones under your control: "I've gotten good at writing proposals" instead of "I got lucky with that one."

4. You engage in all-or-nothing thinking; it has to be perfect or you think you're no good: "I really lost it with my daughter today. I'm just a lousy parent" instead of "I let my stress get to both of us. I'll do better tomorrow."

5. You discount praise and brood over criticisms: "When they said my outfit was flattering, they meant I normally look fat" versus "Wow—this really makes me look good!" (My personal variation on this: "You're complimenting this dinner; were all the others awful?" Since I rarely cook, this may be true.)

6. You tend to expect the worst: "I just know everyone will fight on that long car trip." You don't consider all the trips that went well, or try to figure out what made them work so you can repeat it.

*(continued)*

7. You take things personally, and assume responsibility for events outside your control: "It's my fault my daughter (or husband, or anyone else I feel responsible for, including the dog) had a bad day, or that I can't cheer her (him, it) up." If a friend passes you on the street without saying hello, is it more likely that you somehow made her angry and she's ignoring you on purpose—or that she was hurrying or deep in thought and just didn't see you?

Unfortunately, pharmacologic knowledge does not always translate into certainty as to which pill is likely to help which person, so it's very common to have to try more than one medication before you and your doctor find the right one. In the future, a brain scan may indicate whether the medication is effective, even before you feel a difference, or medications may be matched to your particular genetic makeup. Today, the right choice often comes down to a balance between effectiveness and side effects. Each medication has different side effects; ask your doctor what symptoms to watch for, and read the patient information sheet that comes with your pills.

Ultimately, all antidepressant drugs affect serotonin levels. SSRIs (selective serotonin uptake inhibitors) are often the preferred first-line treatment. Brands include Celexa (citalopram), Lexapro (escitalopram oxalate), Luvox (fluvoxamine), Paxil (paroxetine), Prozac (fluoxetine), and Zoloft (sertraline). Don't assume that none of them will work if one doesn't—or that if it worked for a friend or relative, it will for you. (Patients often tell me how well a friend is doing on a particular drug, so they want to try it.) The drugs also vary in the speed in which they become effective, and the length of time (*half-life*) that it takes for them to leave your system; among the SSRIs, Prozac has the longest half-life. Some of the SSRI drugs are starting to lose patent protection; fluoxetine is now available as a generic. (To counter this, the makers of Prozac have developed a once-weekly version, and gained FDA approval for a "new" indication, PMS, which allows them to market Prozac as Sarafem.)

SSRIs can dampen sexual desire. If you lose interest in sex after you start this medication, tell your doctor. Other antidepressants such as Wellbutrin (available as generic bupropion), Effexor (venlafaxine), Serzone (nefazodone), or Desyrel (trazodone) may be less likely to cause sexual side effects. And remember, it's not always the med that's the culprit; when we're depressed, few of us feel like having sex.

Two other classes of antidepressants, tricyclics and MAO inhibitors, are less expensive, but can have more side effects—and so tend to be reserved for those who "fail" with the newer drugs. The tricyclics (named for the three carbon rings in their chemical structure) affect a range of neurotransmitters, including serotonin, norepinephrine, and dopamine. Brands include Elavil, Anafranil, Norpramin, Tofranil, and Sinequan. Elavil is often prescribed to block the neurotransmission of pain stimuli in patients with chronic pain and fibromyalgia. While tricyclics can be very effective, common side effects include dry mouth, blurred vision, dizziness, drowsiness, or tremors.

MAO inhibitors have nothing to do with the former Chinese ruler. MAO stands for *monoamine oxidase,* a brain enzyme that breaks down neurotransmitters, including serotonin and norepinephrine. Drugs in this class, which include Nardil, Parnate, and Marplan, block the action of MAO and cause a rise in these brain chemicals. These drugs unfortunately interact with many other commonly prescribed drugs, so make sure all your doctors and your pharmacist know that you are taking a MAO inhibitor. You should also avoid aged or fermented foods, which means cheese and beer are out. (In fact, it's prudent to avoid alcoholic beverages and mood-altering drugs while taking any antidepressant, unless okayed by your doctor.)

Any antidepressant can affect sleep. Prozac, Zoloft, and Wellbutrin tend to be the most energizing, and Luvox, Anafranil, Desyrel, and Serzone the most sedating. You may have to try more than one until you get the desired effect, such as better sleep or less fatigue.

Antidepressant medications are not like antibiotics—to be taken briefly for a cure and then stopped. Provided their side effects are manageable (and in most cases these should decrease with time), doctors advise that you continue the medication for six to twelve months after a bout of clinical depression. Many experts feel that if you've had more than one episode, staying on medication is the best way to prevent recurrences. So far, most of the newer medications seem safe for long-term use.

If you have a serious physical illness, don't assume you can't take antidepressants. Since an accompanying depression can make physical illness worse, antidepressants could be lifesavers, especially if you have heart disease. A 2002 study found that sertraline (Zoloft) was safe to use even in patients with unstable cardiac disease.

Finally, we have to consider our uniquely female hormonal status.

Although the postmenopause decrease in estrogen is associated with a decrease in serotonin levels, episodes of clinical depression are no higher, and indeed may be lower, in postmenopausal women than younger women. But some psychiatrists believe a minimum threshold of estrogen is important to facilitate antidepressant medications, and often ERT (or, if needed, HRT) boosts the effect of the medication and depression relief after menopause.

Women who take birth control pills may feel that their underlying depression is either not improved or becomes worse. Switching to a pill with higher estrogen versus progestin activity (such as OvCon) or a pill that contains a progestin more like natural ovary-produced progesterone (such as Yasmin) may help.

### Alternative therapies

*St.-John's-wort.* This is often used in European countries (old and new) to treat mild depression. The National Institute for Complementary and Alternative Medicine is conducting several trials to see whether it is indeed effective, for whom, how long, and at what dose. A 2002 study published in *JAMA* found no benefit for moderately severe depression. Herbal treatments can be risky, due to unregulated, nonstandardized contents, as well as interactions with other medications. If you want to try St.-John's-wort (or if you're already on it), be sure to discuss this with your doctor. (See chapter 5.)

*Regular exercise.* It doesn't have to be sweat therapy. Just walking can improve depression, especially when used to boost other forms of treatment. Studies have shown that it also helps prevent relapse.

*Bright-light therapy.* This is used for a very specific form of depression called seasonal affective disorder (SAD). Those whose brain chemicals are light challenged don't respond as well to antidepressants as those with nonseasonal depression. Daily doses of very bright fluorescent light (twelve times brighter than ordinary room light) helps block melatonin release and alter serotonin levels. While you don't need a prescription to get a light box, you should consult a doctor to help you determine when to use it (morning or night) and for how long. Most women with SAD will feel better after "lighting up" (this is the only time I will use this expression in a positive fashion!) for just half an hour daily. Recent research suggests that light therapy might also benefit women with other forms of depression.

## Coping with chronic stress

Our bodies have evolved a number of useful ways to cope with stress: When we need to elude dangerous beasts (or careening cars) or prepare for a big hunt (or exam), our adrenal glands secrete stress hormones (adrenaline and cortisol). Increased heart rate, blood pressure, and respiration rush extra oxygen to our muscles, and our immune system is put on high alert. Strong emotions fix the memory in our minds, helping us recall, judge, and in the future avoid similar dangers. Our less urgent functions, such as digestion and reproduction, are temporarily diminished or halted (this is not a desirable way to lose weight or prevent pregnancy, but in extreme conditions our bodies have more important things to do).

When honking horns, looming deadlines, and other modern pressures create a chronic state of stress, our bodies' stress management methods start to hurt instead of help. We become irritable, and may resort to bingeing on high-carb and high-fat snacks, or drinking too much. Over time, we become more prone to colds and other infections. Chronically elevated cortisol levels encourage fat to lodge around our waists (as noted in chapter 4); this puts our hearts at risk. Brain cells in the hippocampus can actually shrink, contributing to memory problems.

How can you stop this harmful cycle? If you're gritting your teeth and holding on by your fingernails until your next relaxing vacation, stop. Just as you can't make up for missed sleep with a weekend bed-rest binge, research shows it's much healthier to reduce day-to-day stress than to alternate long periods of frazzle with oases of rest.

## A few ways to interrupt the stress cycle

- Squeeze a series of five- or ten-minute walks into your daily schedule. As noted in chapter 3, this can also prevent weight gain and add years to your life.
- Pay attention to posture and muscle tension. Are your shoulders hunched as you sit at your desk? Is your brow tense and furrowed? Most of us have areas where we tend to hold tension. Find yours and consciously relax (or stretch) those tight spots throughout the day.
- Breathe deeply. Before you rush to your next appointment, sit down, place a hand on your belly, and feel it rise and fall as you breathe. (When tense, we tend to breathe shallowly.) You can turn this into a mini-meditation by mentally repeating a calming word or phrase. It doesn't

have to be a foreign-sounding mantra; try the words "relax, relax." I use "ease off, ease off."

- Take a mental vacation. Picture a relaxing place, perhaps a peaceful beach with gently rolling waves; imagine yourself strolling along, feeling the warm sand between your toes. Or lose yourself for a while in a humorous novel, a sitcom, or an enlightening or mood-lightening movie.

## Recipe for a longer life: what the research shows

*Accentuate the positive.* The evidence is piling up: A positive attitude and optimistic outlook are linked with longer life, and a chronically hostile, negative attitude may shorten it. A study of 255 doctors found that those physicians whose personality tests showed high hostility levels were far more likely to have died twenty-five years later on—mostly due to heart disease—than those who were easygoing. (I use this stat as affirmation of my need to be nice to patients, friends, and family.)

Although I don't want to sound like one of those "think good, feel good, be good" gurus, thoughts and feelings do affect your physical health. Basic emotions (anger, fear, happiness, sadness, disgust) as well as complex emotional states (anxiety) affect your autonomic nervous system, which runs your body without your conscious control, keeping your heart beating, glands secreting, vessels contracting, and so on. Over time, too much time spent in negative emotional states—or trying to suppress your emotions rather than expressing them—takes its toll on these functions. On the happier side, optimism about the future, and explaining life with the "glass half full" approach, seem to counterbalance the damage done by negative emotions.

Consider this unusual study of autobiographies written by 180 nuns before taking their vows. The number of positive words these novitiates used to describe their lives (gratitude, happiness, hope, contentment, amusement, love, interest) versus the negative ones (anger, contempt, disgust, fear, sadness, shame, disinterest) predicted their death rates six decades later. The least positive nuns were 2.5 times more likely to have died than the most positive ones.

*A healthy attitude toward aging.* Your attitude toward getting older can make a difference in whether you get there, and in what condition. In one survey, 660 people over 50 were questioned about their attitudes toward aging ("I am as happy now as I was when I was younger" versus "Things keep getting worse as I get older" and "As you get older, you are less useful"). Decades later, those who gave optimistic answers were found to have lived, on average, 7.5 years longer than those who bemoaned their age.

It's fascinating to note that when older adults (in their sixties to eighties) are exposed subliminally to awful words representing negative stereotypes about aging (*confused, decrepit, dependent, incompetent, diseased,* and *senile*), their confidence about and performance on simple tests (such as counting backward) are diminished. These diminishing words also trigger a cardiovascular stress response, including changes in blood pressure and heart rate. Although it takes longer, exposure to positive words (*sage, accomplished, advise, insightful, astute,* and *creative*) has been found to have a protective effect and can speed recovery from stress.

*The right kind of work.* A demanding high-pressure job can be stressful, but won't necessarily shorten your life, as long as you feel you can exert some control over what you do and the conditions in which you do it—and you develop an emotional link with your colleagues. What does hurt is lack of inclusion in decision making, no determination of workflow or conditions, and lack of social support on the job.

*A little help from my friends . . .* Whether you live alone or with others, having strong ties to relatives and friends promotes mental and physical well-being. Isolation is counterproductive to brain health. Get out there and communicate, socialize, and make emotional connections.

My recipe for keeping the female brain healthy and young: Exercise it to keep it in shape, rest it when it's fatigued, heal it when its neurotransmitters and electrical impulses are improperly discharged, and calm it when stresses abuse it. And don't forget it!

# Epilogue: My "120"

There is a Hebrew blessing that is added to every birthday solicitation, *"Ad meyah ve esrime"*: "[May you live] until 120." Scientists who have probed the molecular basis of human aging and mortality concur. This, they say, is the utmost limit of our cellular viability. Do I have the audacity to think I can reach this age? No, but why not use this number to overachieve and help make sure I reach the more modest goal of staying healthy and active and looking young in the present and upcoming decades.

The question that is posed by many of my patients after I've discussed their symptoms and test results, reviewed the relevant studies, and advised them about their care, is "What do you do?" Like most women, I have done the good, the bad, and the lazy. So in this final chapter, I'll continue the women's stories I've told in this book but, this time, the woman is me.

I'm a baby-boomer "starter," born at the end of World War II in 1945. I went to college in the sixties, raised a family in the seventies and eighties, and stood back in wonderment as I passed the half-century mark in the nineties. How old do I feel? Forty-five.

This chapter is not meant to be a prolonged autobiography, so I'll follow (and rename) the chapter headings of this book to share some personal life events—education, marriage, child bearing, child raising, divorce, remarriage, having a medical practice, and the psychosocial adjustments—that have fashioned my "120" pursuit.

## WHEN IT COMES
## TO REPRODUCTION

As I was the oldest daughter, my adrenarche (when adrenal hormones pour forth, causing blemishes, axillary and pubic hair growth, and body odor) was greeted with parental horror and frequent visits to the dermatologist's office for acne treatments. In an attempt to "burn that pimple away," I had multiple sessions of sunlamp therapy. I now blame some of my wrinkles on this dermatological travesty. But the oily olive-colored skin that was the despair of my teen years may have helped prevent a more pronounced photoaging in my forties and fifties.

I trained arduously at a professional ballet school and as a result had less than the average teenager's subcutaneous fat and breast development. I consumed the healthy diet of the time: whole milk, lots of "wholesome" meat and butter, as well as frozen vegetables cooked until the green was out of them. My parents thought they were guarding my nutrition and my weight by prohibiting sugar, baked goods, pasta, and pancakes (and for this I am grateful). By the time I reached the age of 16, it was clear I was not genetically blessed with a "body by Balanchine"—the short torso, long legs, straight arch, and foot structure (my second toe is longer than the first; not good for pointe shoes)—that would get me into the New York City corps de ballet. Nor, quite frankly, did I have the talent.

At Barnard, I discovered the wonder of education and the joy of doughnuts, two A.M. meatball submarines, and coffee. I tried to smoke but could not inhale without feeling I had aspirated burning charcoal. During a junior year abroad in Israel, I met my future husband, a law student just back from his paratrooper unit duties. It was awe at first sight . . . I started taking the Pill. The dose was five times greater than that currently prescribed, providing me with a preview of future morning sickness.

During the first years of marriage, I abstained from all unnecessary physical exertion with the reluctant exception of housecleaning (Israeli men don't clean). I had begun medical school; cooking was time-consuming and our hours were irregular, so we ate "whatever" until Friday-night family dinners, when my mother-in-law prepared a Jewish feast. During the week I filled up on dairy products—leban (a kind of yogurt) and cheese—and gobbled loaves of wonderful fresh white bread.

After the Six-Day War, like so many wives whose husbands survive armed conflict, I tried to get pregnant. Nothing happened the first three months and, at the age of 23, I sought immediate action to cure my infertility. A wise gynecologist suggested I postpone therapy (at least that kind) and let a few more months go by. They did, and I conceived and went on to have severe nausea, vomiting, and a bout of pneumonia that required hospitalization. I have since been most empathetic to women with pregnancy-related nausea. Days before I was due to deliver, I waddled into my pathology final wearing a tight maternity dress and holding up my belly. The three male professors administering the oral exam showed great concern (they were not obstetricians) and rushed through the most rudimentary of questions. I got an A but, three days later, had a more difficult time during the labor of my eight-pound daughter, who was finally delivered with forceps. I breast-fed, but since I had to return to classes, did so for only six weeks.

Medical school, followed by internship and residency, was not overly conducive to hands-on motherhood and family life. I have since apologized to my daughter who, despite this, developed into a beautiful, talented, and intelligent young woman.

I went back on the Pill. In my second year of residency, after assisting a "meticulous" (slow) surgeon in a seven-hour procedure, I developed leg pain, which was diagnosed by my chief resident as a deep thrombophlebitis. His exact words were: "Damn it, Reichman, you probably have a clot." In retrospect, I wonder if it wasn't just a leg cramp. Today, the diagnosis would have been verified with vascular ultrasound. I briefly started taking anticoagulant therapy and sadly bade the Pill farewell.

Several years later, I became pregnant with my second daughter. I was now one of the doctors in charge of an obstetrics and gynecology department and taught at the University of Tel Aviv Medical School. This time nausea was not a problem and I felt that pregnancy at 33 was no big deal until I performed an ultrasound on myself at twelve weeks and discovered that, in addition to an enlarged uterus and a viable pregnancy, there was a large solid mass that appeared to be an ovarian tumor. While the doctor in me weighed the possible diagnoses, procedures, and prognoses, the woman in me panicked. I returned to the University of Chicago where I had trained, and underwent exploratory abdominal surgery. I was still giving orders about the incision, retractors, and a course of action for every contingency when the anesthesiologist mercifully put me under. Fortunately, the tumor was a benign fibroid that could be removed. I continued the pregnancy at bed rest, taking medications to stop contractions, and delivered my healthy second daughter at term.

I had been taught to separate myself from patients' fears in order to dispassionately wield my instruments. Having had this surgery, I now knew what that fear was like and found that although I could still be "the objective surgeon" during a procedure, objectivity was more difficult before or after. Compassion and postoperative care are as important to a patient's healing and recovery as are informed consent and technical know-how.

## TO TAKE OR NOT TO TAKE
## HORMONES? I TOOK

I awoke at two in the morning drenched in perspiration. Did I eat something weird; was it the wine I had with dinner? The next evening I ate carefully and abstained from alcohol, yet once again the late-night soaking occurred. It was May and a lovely sixty degrees outside, but needing an instant remedy, I turned on the air conditioner. Thankfully, the white sales were on, so the next day I sallied forth to the mall where I saved 50 percent on a lightweight comforter. My husband protested, "What's this skimpy thing we're sleeping under?" Only then did I stop and consider: "Could this, dare this, be hormonal?"

I was 46 years old. The answer lay not in the comforter; my future comfort lay in hormonal comprehension. The estrogen dip before my period had irritated my "older" inner thermostat, which then directed my body to cool down through vessel dilation and profuse water evaporation. Once my period was over, my estrogen level rose and my thermostat quieted down, allowing me to sleep dryly, encased in my down cocoon. Perimenopause had become personal.

I had been using a copper IUD for contraception, and at the same time I experienced night sweats, my periods were becoming heavy and prolonged. I asked a colleague to remove the IUD and perform a pelvic ultrasound. I had several small fibroids in the outer uterine wall. Remembering a previous (and tentative) diagnosis of a blood clot in my leg, I ran coagulation blood tests, which were normal. Deciding that the clot had been misdiagnosed and/or was due to immobility, I started low-dose birth control pills in order to redirect the estrogen highs and lows of peri-menopause. The Pill provided me with hormonal stability during the next six years. I would take the active pill two, sometimes three months at a time, going off only when it was convenient to get my period. I had no hot flashes, night sweats, or menstrual cramps. My red-blood count soared, as my periods become infrequent and light (I had always been slightly ane-mic), and my skin was clear. Moreover, I seemed to be wrinkling less than many of my same-aged friends and patients. Was this genetic or due to consistent estrogen levels, which helped maintain my skin's collagen con-tent? I suspect both were involved. The small fibroids didn't grow, possi-bly as a result of the constant opposition of the progestin to the estrogen in the Pill. I was also protecting myself from future ovarian and endome-trial cancer.

At the age of 52, I figured that the time had come to ascertain my menopausal status. In order to see whether my ovaries had run out of fol-licles, I stopped the Pill and tested my FSH and estrogen levels. The for-mer was high and the latter low. I was there, and during the month that I was off the Pill, I had ample clinical evidence of severely diminished es-trogen: night sweats, frequent nighttime awakening, and hot flashes. The perspiration that accumulated on my forehead as I performed surgery was not due to undue physical labor. My requests that the nurse wipe my brow and that the room temperature be lowered to sixty degrees greatly amused the barely-out-of-puberty residents. I also found I was searching for heretofore easily remembered words, names, and numbers; this was what patients meant when they said their brain was in a fog! I started hor-mone replacement therapy (a transdermal estrogen patch and a daily dose of oral progesterone) expecting to feel different, perhaps develop bloat-ing, breast tenderness, or breakthrough bleeding. None of these side ef-fects occurred. The hot flashes and night sweats disappeared, and I felt like my previous self. By now I was wondering what all the fuss about HRT was about! I started with a dose of 0.075 mg and, after a few months, I tried lowering it to 0.05 mg. One day, as I sat on the *Today* show set with Katie Couric, I found myself groping for words. I went back to the higher dose, and blood tests show this provides me with the estrogen equivalent of what my ovaries would produce in the first week of the re-productive cycle (60 to 80 picograms).

Have I second-guessed my decision to go on HRT? Sometimes . . .

The second most traumatic physical event in my life occurred three years later, when it was discovered that I had precancerous cells in my breasts.

My mother had undergone a radical mastectomy for breast cancer at the age of 46 (and is doing well more than thirty years later). I knew this raised my own breast cancer risk, but I tried to placate my genetic fears by concentrating on our physical differences. I was small-breasted, had been athletic during puberty, and outwardly resembled my father, so genes be damned! My yearly mammograms were declared clear. During the last test the mammographer who followed me and so many of my patients suggested we do an ultrasound, "just to make sure" everything was okay. It wasn't. The ultrasound showed an area of questionable density. A few days later a colleague excised the pinpointed (literally) tissue under local anesthesia. The pathologist, also a friend, looked at the tissue and declared it most probably benign. Two days later she called me crying (a sobbing pathologist is not reassuring). Further testing had revealed atypical ductal hyperplasia, and these abnormal cells were ominously creeping throughout the specimen.

When I look back at the ensuing weeks, all I remember is an eerie calmness, a sense of relief that I could and would finally deal with my deeply suppressed concern about breast cancer. Years before, I had diagnosed breast cancer in a patient and friend in her early forties. Her mother also had breast cancer at an early age. Despite aggressive therapy she died several years later. At that time I talked to an oncologist about having a prophylactic mastectomy.

My previous query about prophylactic mastectomy didn't seem so crazy now. I made the rounds—oncologists, surgeons, plastic surgeons, and geneticists. I underwent BRCA-gene testing (I was negative). I knew I could opt to go on Tamoxifen and that, statistically, this would give me up to an 86 percent chance of remaining cancer-free. But I, the surgeon, preferred a surgical solution that would reduce my odds of breast cancer even further. A bilateral mastectomy would allow me to get rid of abnormal tissue (and make sure there was nothing worse) in both breasts so that I could get on with my life. How bad could it be; it wasn't abdominal surgery (so speaketh a surgeon who performs only abdominal and vaginal surgery). On the plus side, I would get implants that could fill a B-cup bra! The surgeons and I agreed that I would recover quickly and could go back to work two weeks after surgery. I should have known better; surgeons nearly always minimize recovery time. The procedure took six hours, and it took six days before I could use my arms to feed myself.

There were times when the pain, which felt as if a spiked bra was hammered into my chest wall, was so bad that I cried through the night. But recover I did, and two weeks later, I was able to get through the day with just a Vicodin or two. Despite the exhaustion, which I tried to ignore, I went back to work and my nurses (who were the only ones who knew I had the surgery) kept my patient-load light.

The discomfort on one side continued and, a few months later, I had a second procedure to free up scar tissue around the implant. I later had the expanders (implants that are slowly filled with saline) removed and replaced by permanent silicone implants. The pain subsided, and I reveled in my ability to lie on my stomach at night or during an occasional massage. It took months to find a bra that fit, was comfortable, and looked right. I still don't gaze in the mirror when I step out of the bath, and I'm not completely comfortable with my upper body. I will, on occasion, go braless if I'm wearing a loose-fitting shirt.

Would I do this again? Probably—pain is something we forget. Otherwise, how would we go through childbirth more than once? Now that I know that the atypical cells are not there, I don't have cancer, and with great probability won't in the future, I'm tremendously relieved. This doesn't mean that I suggest that my patients or other women who have similar histories and biopsy reports follow the surgical course I chose. Each of us has to assess our risk and understand all of our options. I just don't want to hide what I did beneath my white coat.

In light of all of this, do I regret taking hormones? I don't think that they (or my prior use of birth control pills) instigated the precancerous changes. Most of the research suggests that if HRT does anything, it may be through stimulation of growth of cells that already are cancerous, but that it doesn't cause normal cells to become malignant. I never blamed HRT, and now that I have had the surgery, I don't want to stop the therapy. This is a quality-of-life decision. I feel good, look good (although recent photos with inadequate lighting cause some concern), and I sleep. (I recently tried to lower the dose of my patch and awoke repeatedly with sweats.) My cholesterol levels and C-reactive protein are fine. Sex doesn't hurt (on the contrary, it feels great!). I tried the testosterone drops I discuss in chapter 2 but, after I sprouted pimples, stopped. My libido isn't low enough to warrant acne.

I am probably among the 15 to 20 percent of women who continue to have menopausal symptoms for fifteen years or more. Antidepressants may diminish some of these symptoms, but they have side effects, and the few times I tried an SSRI (after divorce and family illness), I experienced adverse effects. Right now, transdermal estrogen works for me and helps me want to continue in my personal quest of 120.

## ROCK AROUND THE CLOCK? NO, BUT I WORK OUT

Once I gave up my ballet workouts, I have to admit to becoming a bottom-heavy nerd who proclaimed, "I don't have time for that stuff," as I sat through my education.

I didn't reverse my sedentary habits until the age of 37, after I had moved to Los Angeles and went through a divorce that freed up many of my evenings. I tried everything—step classes, jazzercise, spinning, and high-impact aerobics (the latter at the Jane Fonda Workout Studio, where I found it difficult to follow the routine while trying to pull down the "required" thonglike leotard). I started running and felt exhilarated, but one day I tripped, fell in the street, and just lay there while cars with staring strangers sped past. Aside from the indignity, I had multiple contusions on my legs, some of which left scars. I ceased running. I then dated a neurosurgeon who taught me to ski, mostly by taking me to the top of a mountain and telling me to follow him down. I joined a gym, hired a trainer, and had to pay him whether or not I showed up, so I did.

I'm proud to report I have finally achieved exercise independence. For the past ten years, I've kept going without trainers. I walk at a four-miles-an-hour pace on my treadmill for thirty minutes, three times a week; I lift dumbbells (7 and 10 pounds) and do exercises with leg weights for an additional fifteen minutes. I try to get to a local gym once or twice a week where I use the elliptical runner, followed by thirty minutes of pushing, shoving, and pulling on weight machines. We have a house in Ojai, a small town nestled in the mountains near L.A. On the weekends I get to go there, I love to hike, bike, or just walk. I'm convinced that exercise, together with eight hours of sleep, is my most reliable way to look, feel, and remain young. Before I sound like a born-again athlete, let me hasten to add that, like most of my friends and patients, I use excuses to desist: I think I'm getting sick, I am sick, I worked a fourteen-hour day and deserve to rest, it's a secular holiday, a religious holiday. . . .

A funny thing happened on the way to completing this book. I stopped exercising for nearly three months (after I wrote the exercise chapter). I had to meet publishing deadlines, got a cold, traveled to Ethiopia, and got another cold. But now as I write this last chapter, I am "excused out" and have to face my clock. I'm back in my routine. My muscles are a bit sore, but that seems inconsequential compared with my sharpened focus, energy, improved sleep, and assuaged guilt. As I pedal out of my driveway on my way to the bike path, I feel less daunted by what I can and will do as I get closer to that 120.

## NOSHING ALL THE WAY

Contrary to the suspicion of many of my patients who ask my nurse, "Does she starve herself?" I don't. I eat frequently, noshing throughout the day. I don't eat junk food, rarely have a calorie-dense dessert, and stop eating when I get that "I'm stuffed and can't move" feeling. I don't practice combining, separating, or eating before six P.M., nor do I drink designer water to fill my stomach and appease my appetite. I'm not a vegetarian—it just wouldn't fit into my lifestyle, as I grab food between patients, before surgery, while traveling, or in restaurants. I did give up red meat fourteen years ago, after the Nurses' Study showed a correlation between red meat consumption and colon cancer. I promptly lost eight pounds. I have had no desire to go back to any kind of beef, lamb, or pork, although I used to make an awesome steak au poivre and miss demonstrating my cooking skills with this dish. What I do eat is an "L.A. meets Mediterranean" diet.

On a typical weekday, I'll have:

**Breakfast (a meal I never miss)**
- A two-egg omelet with low-fat cheese, mushrooms, or tomatoes; or
- A combination of one whole egg and one egg white fried in a nonstick pan sprayed with olive oil
- Two pieces of whole-grain toast, "buttered" with Smart Balance nonhydrogenated spread
- 4 to 6 ounces of calcium-enriched orange juice

**Two to three hours post-breakfast**
- A cappuccino with nonfat milk from the coffee shop near my office
- One-half low-fat or oatmeal muffin (I immediately share or throw the other half away so as not to consume the entire 400-

calorie entity), or a banana with a cup of nonfat yogurt sweet-
ened with a sugar substitute

## Lunch
- A salad with chicken, tuna, or nuts mixed with vinaigrette dressing; or
- A homemade sandwich of whole wheat bread with nonpro-
cessed turkey or tuna in water, garnished with nonfat mayon-
naise or mustard, tomato, and/or avocado slices; or
- Leftovers from dinner

## Two to three hours post-lunch ("low" time)
- A cappuccino with nonfat milk (the local coffee shop loves me!)
- Nuts or a cup of nonfat yogurt (if I don't have this in the morn-
ing); or
- One-half whole wheat pita with hummus

## Dinner (after 7:30)
- Salad containing tofu, soybeans, goat cheese, and walnuts with
vinaigrette dressing
- Grilled or roasted chicken (white meat) or fish (salmon, sea bass,
or trout); or
- Roast turkey (breast)
- Steamed vegetables (usually broccoli, cauliflower, and carrots)
- Brown rice, pasta, or couscous
- Mixed fresh fruit

## Two to three hours post-dinner
- One-half cup nonfat frozen yogurt or low-fat ice cream

## Beverages
- Water or iced tea with meals or when I'm thirsty
- Occasionally, one glass of white wine (red wine gives me a
headache)

I realize my "daily bread" may sound boring, but in all honesty, this
represents my Monday-to-Friday schedule when I don't go out and don't
travel. I also make sure I "cheat" once a day with a piece or two of dark
chocolate or a goodie that my staff or patients bring to the office. At

restaurants, I try to order the simple, less sauce-laden food items and either share an entrée or take some home for lunch the next day. I'm always willing to try a spoonful of a companion's dessert; I have a deep-seated belief that what I don't order shouldn't count. I appreciate good cooking and, when presented with gourmet delights, delight in tasting. The greatest pleasure is in those first few mouthfuls, after which the joy of ingestion becomes palpably diminished. Why continue to the point of feeling bloated and uncomfortable? I no longer suffer remorse about what I don't put on my plate or leave uneaten.

## A VITAMIN OR TWO A DAY

I have yet to discover a vitamin or herb that either bears the label "until 120" or reputably claims that it will get me to that goal. But I want to play it long, safe, and without regret, so I'm not relying solely on my nutrition to safeguard my health and longevity. I don't grow my own food nor can I ascertain what nutrients and chemicals have left or entered the soil whence it sprouted or was fed. Moreover, my sustenance was transported, stored, chilled, and cooked. Hence, I take the following daily supplements:

- 1 multivitamin with iron
- 400 units vitamin E
- Calcium (citrate) with vitamin D, 600 mg in the morning and 600 mg at night (if I haven't had enough yogurt or milk products)

I will take echinacea capsules if I think I'm getting a cold, but stop once I feel better. Beguiled by ads, I have tried evening primrose and dong quai for PMS (I thought I felt better as I swallowed six capsules a day, but didn't feel worse when I stopped). I took St.-John's-wort and SAMe for mild depression (they seemed to make no difference; I then read that the latter product didn't contain the levels purported to work in clinical trials, at which point I knew that I was not better). To sharpen my mind, I took ginkgo biloba, but stopped when studies showed that it probably would not. I don't think I became more cerebrally challenged without this herb and don't want to risk bleeding by mixing it with low-dose aspirin.

## PHYSICIAN, HEAL THYSELF

Like most medical students, I "developed" some of the diseases I studied (myocarditis, lymphoma, a cerebral aneurysm). I survived all of these diagnoses and, once I graduated, stopped personalizing signs, symptoms, and syndromes. Over the next decade I did my best to disdainfully ignore my health, until I was pregnant with my second child and had surgery. Despite this call to vulnerability I remained a slow convert to health-consciousness and had most of my age-appropriate exams (mammograms, Pap smears, and colonoscopy) in order to achieve a doctor-patient authority—"If I could do it, so should you"—as well as physiological superiority: My tests wouldn't dare be abnormal. It was somewhat humbling when, in my early fifties, a bone-density test showed I had osteopenia in my hips. I increased my previous haphazard calcium supplementation and developed a taste for plain nonfat yogurt. I also started hormone replacement therapy.

I now take my health tests more seriously. My most personal disease prevention and detection for a longer life was the breast ultrasound that led to the diagnosis of my precancer. I currently order ultrasounds (in addition to yearly mammograms) on my patients at the drop of a hat or, more precisely, the mention of dense lumpy breasts. I check my blood tests (cholesterol, liver, kidney function, thyroid, C-reactive protein, and blood count) every two years. Last time a heart disease lipid marker (lipoprotein-a) was elevated. Nothing other than high doses of niacin and perhaps estrogen is known to lower this. I considered whether I should start statin therapy to medicate away heart attack risk. I had a CT scan, which demonstrated the absence of any calcified plaque on my coronary arteries. After consulting a well-known cardiologist (who I happened to meet in the hospital parking lot), I decided to simply continue eating right, recheck my blood, and take low-dose aspirin.

Will I get scanned from head to toe with CT scans or MRI on a regular basis, "just in case"? No, not until the literature can convince me that this will improve and prolong my life. I will get the basic tests I've outlined in chapter 6—not to set an example, but to set the criteria for my health in the years to come.

## "LIGHT FROM BELOW, SHOOT
## FROM ABOVE": LOOKING GOOD

My husband, the director, told me years ago (when I didn't have to worry about it) that my facial lines would disappear on camera if light was beamed from below and the camera was held high. When we took the cover shot for this book, my talented and agile photographer stood on a ladder! As I scrutinize my face, chin, and neck to apply makeup, I consider everything I wrote in chapter 7. I've had facials and bought expensive cleansers, masks, and rejuvenating and moisturizing creams sold at spas and department stores. I've queried dermatologists and plastic surgeons about skin care secrets. I've read dermatologic articles and books. In the end, I've settled on the fairly basic skin care I've outlined in the chapter "Looking Young from the Outside In." I start by blocking the sun's rays. Before I leave my bathroom in the morning, I apply over-the-counter Cetaphil moisturizer with Parsol (SPF 15). When I apply makeup, I use a nonoil base with additional SPF protection. I go to a higher 45 waterproof block for outdoors in strong sunlight. I wear a hat, long-sleeved shirt, and pants to hike or bike, and seek shade whenever possible. I wash my face at night with Cetaphil cleanser and then dab 0.5 percent Retin-A or Tazorac 0.1 percent gel under my eyes or on my cheeks where I have some pigmented (dare I say "age") spots. I then apply a 0.5 percent compounded estriol cream to my face and neck. Once a week I use 10 to 15 percent glycolic acid before I start this evening routine.

Prior to going on camera for the *Today* show, I'll apply some Preparation H gel under my eyes, which tend to get puffy from the L.A.–New York commute and jet lag. When I notice that my skin seems excessively dry, and fine lines become crevices, I use a smidgen of cream from my keep-as-long-as-possible $90 jar of Crème de la Mer. Eight years ago, I asked a prominent Beverly Hills dermatologist to inject collagen in the nasolabial folds near my mouth. A few days later, one of my kids asked me why I looked good. But as the collagen filler gradually wore off, I didn't think I looked worse and didn't repeat the injections. Five years ago, I had fine capillaries around my nose buzzed with a laser. That's all I've done to my face . . . so far.

I see many patients who have had fillers, lasers, peels, or plastic surgery and look fantastic. I go home and pull at my face, neck, and abdomen to see how I might look if I had similar procedures. But then a patient shows up looking stretched and so unnatural that I vow to leave those areas untouched. For now I'll just continue my simple face-saving routine accompanied by exercise, sleep, and good nutrition. Having had breast reconstructive surgery, I'm not eager to undergo any other procedures. One day, however, when those footlights and high-held cameras don't suffice, I might consider more invasive medical or surgical options.

## MINDING TIME

I used to think that an occasional memory lapse was due to either over-stuffing my brain with information or "under-hormoning" my cerebral synapses with estrogen. I continue to cling to these theories, but am also cognizant of the fact that I'm over 50 and the passage of time might have affected the memory centers in my brain. The FDA has recently defined certain types of mild memory loss in over-50-year-olds as *age-associated memory impairment* (AAMI—one more acronym to remember!).

The studies correlating initial and continued education and brain stimulation with a decreased risk of Alzheimer's are, however, encouraging. I'm trying hard to activate my neurotransmitters, as well as exercise and renew my neuronal connections. I peruse the *New York Times* and the *Los Angeles Times* each morning (arguably some of the articles are not going to work), as well as three weekly newsmagazines. I attempt to get through the very thorough articles in *The New Yorker*. A character in the play *Collected Stories* remarked that "life is too short for *The New Yorker*"—but not if it will make my brain live longer. I look forward to the weekly and monthly medical journals that inexorably advance across my desk. If my brain can make sense of the complex linguistics used by the experts and absorb their reports, it will, I hope, remain fit. This should let my patients continue to pick my brain (just one brain pun).

"Start *new* activities, get a hobby," exhort the experts. My "new" has been the acquisition of sufficient computer skills to enable me to use e-mail and access websites for news, general information, and medical searches. I regret that my parents discouraged my acquisition of typing skills when I was a teen, lest I get a job rather than an advanced degree. I'm still a slow typist, but my two (sometimes four) fingers are reconditioning circuits in my motor cortex. I'm still working on developing a hobby—I envy my friends who collect, paint, master bridge, or play golf. Shopping probably doesn't count.

The association between optimism and longevity has given me some cause for concern. I come from a long line of appropriately depressed Eastern European Jews who had to deal with pogroms and the Holocaust, followed by the need to succeed as new immigrants in this country. So far I see little evidence of genetic optimism. I placate my moroseness with the belief that surgeons should possess obsessive-compulsive tendencies, and good clinicians have to consider "what can go wrong" in the best of circumstances. When these personality traits manifest toward family, friends, and co-workers, they can, unfortunately, create problems—some of which I've tried to work out by talking to them and to therapists. Am I "cured"? Have I become the positive person who will get to be a centenarian? I have the next forty-two years in which to try . . .

The last but not least important factors that have been shown to influence our longevity clock are spiritual belief and commitment. I'm certain, within the "soul" center of my brain, that when we concentrate our efforts on a selfless goal, we promote the production of the neurotransmitters that help overcome brain wear and tear and prevent the apathy of decrepitude.

As I finished the previous chapters in this book, I, to put it nonmedically, entered a funk. I hated letting go of this yearlong project and felt a loss of control as I relegated the manuscript to the editors and publisher. I worried whether I had run out of things to say, facts to report, or concepts to pitch for my next *Today* show segments. I was worn out by the L.A.–N.Y. commute; the Middle East was still in turmoil; my older daughter moved back to live in Israel; my younger daughter was between jobs; and my husband was busy . . .

Just as I was wallowing in situational pity, I was asked to accompany the CEO of Save the Children on a trip to Ethiopia in order to survey the organization's emergency response to the severe famine in that country. Upon my return I was asked if what I saw on the trip had made me depressed. The answer was a resounding "No." I felt renewed and even elated by the commitment of the many aid and government workers and the projects I witnessed. They were making a "small" difference by saving the life of a starving child and a large one by helping a country overcome huge social, economic, and health problems. The trip reinforced my personal commitment, optimism, and sense of wonderful fortune. I, and those I teach, treat, and love, have the resources to acquire the knowledge, access the health care, and make the behavioral changes that will slow our clocks down. We can make pretty-darn-good better as we head toward "120."

# For More Information

If you'd like to know more about the health issues I've covered in this book, here are some places to start. (This is by no means an exhaustive list!) I've tried to include sources that won't go out of date and will provide the most up-to-date information.

## GENERAL HEALTH TOPICS

- The Agency for Healthcare Research and Quality, a scientific research agency of the federal government, offers reviews of the latest women's health research at www.ahrq.gov/research/womenix.htm.
- The U.S. Department of Health and Human Services also has a women's health information site, www.4woman.gov with research summaries and fact sheets on a range of conditions.
- The Federal Trade Commission (FTC) has a consumer website (www.ftc.gov/bcp/menu-health.htm) with practical information on all kinds of health issues, from sun-protective clothing to weight-loss fraud.
- The National Institutes of Health (NIH) site (www.nih.gov) is brimming with free information on every aspect of health, including the latest news.

- The National Women's Health Resource Center (www.healthywomen.org) is a nonprofit clearinghouse for information and resources, offering research updates and an extensive library of books and other materials to view and/or purchase.

## REPRODUCTIVE ISSUES

- Resolve: The National Infertility Association (www.resolve.org) has information on diagnosing and treating conditions that cause infertility, alternatives such as assisted reproductive technologies and adoption, and coping with the emotions and stress that can accompany fertility problems.
- The American Society for Reproductive Medicine (www.asrm.org) has patient information related to fertility and menopause, including help with selecting an IVF/GIFT program.

## HORMONAL ISSUES

- The North American Menopause Society website (www.menopause.org) offers a summary of hormone replacement research, as well as other useful articles.
- While the American College of Obstetricians and Gynecologists site (www. acog.org) is geared primarily to physicians, it offers authoritative special reports and treatment recommendations for women's medical concerns.

## EXERCISE

- You can download the entire contents of the Surgeon General's Report on Physical Activity and Health or "just the fact sheets" on women and exercise at www.cdc.gov/nccdphp/sgr/women.htm.
- The Physician and Sportsmedicine Online (www.physsportsmed.com) is a medical journal site that also features practical "personal health" articles on fitness, nutrition, and ways to exercise if you have health problems.

## DIET AND WEIGHT

- The National Library of Medicine's Medline Plus website (www.nlm.nih. gov/medlineplus/weightlossdieting.html) offers links to a wealth of consumer information from the National Institutes of Health, medical associations, university and hospital websites, and more—along with the latest popular news coverage on food and weight.

## DIETARY SUPPLEMENTS

- The NIH Office of Dietary Supplements has fact sheets and safety information. See www.dietary-supplements.info.nih.gov.
- The National Center for Complementary and Alternative Medicine (www.nccam.nih.gov) has general and specific supplement information, safety alerts, and searchable results from clinical trials.

## DISEASE PREVENTION AND DETECTION

- The Nurses' Health Study website (www.channing.harvard.edu/nhs) has abstracts of dozens of study publications, as well as newsletters that sum up the findings.
- The Arthritis Foundation website (www.arthritis.org) answers questions about arthritis, provides links to useful products and services, and connects people who are coping with arthritis.
- The American Cancer Society site (www.cancer.org) lets you search for specific information on cancer types and on ways to cope with the disease (from making treatment decisions to building a support network).
- Katie Couric cofounded the National Colorectal Cancer Research Alliance; visit their site (www.nccra.org) for news, links, resources—and motivation to schedule that screening test.
- Whether you're a cancer survivor, looking for a clinical trial to join, or want to cut your cancer risk, the Women's Cancer Network (www.wcn.org)—a site jointly developed by the Gynecologic Cancer Foundation and Cancer-Source—has something for you. You'll find a plethora of factual articles, personal stories, and useful links.
- The American Diabetes Association (www.diabetes.org) offers facts, recipes, community resources, and its own monthly magazine.

- The American Heart Association site (www.americanheart.org) gives the latest on diseases, conditions, treatments, and prevention. Some of the health-promotion programs are specifically for women.
- The American Lung Association (www.lungusa.org) features research and advocacy on lung diseases and—especially important—support for conquering your cigarette addiction.
- The National Osteoporosis Foundation's easy-to-type site (www.nof.org) informs both patients and professionals about risk factors, prevention, medications, and exercise.

## LOOKING YOUNG

- AgingSkinNet (no explanation needed!) is sponsored by the American Academy of Dermatology (www.skincarephysicians.com).
- The American Society for Aesthetic and Plastic Surgery site (www.surgery.org) includes descriptions of cosmetic surgery procedures.
- The Food and Drug Administration's website has information on cosmetics, creams, and hair products, including research findings and safety alerts. See www.cfsan.fda.gov/~dms/cos-prd.html.

## YOUNG AND HEALTHY IN MIND

- The Nun Study has its own site (www.mc.uky.edu/nunnet) with updates on aging with grace and preventing Alzheimer's disease.
- The National Institute of Mental Health has user-friendly fact sheets, reports, and brochures on mental illnesses at www.nimh.nih.gov/publicat.
- The Alzheimer's Association site (www.alz.org) promotes research and advocacy. It also links to many resources for people diagnosed with AD and their families and friends.
- The National Sleep Association site (www.sleepfoundation.org) is a hub for information on sleep disorders, and includes a special section for women.

## LIVING LONGER

- The AARP (formerly the American Association of Retired Persons) aims to cover all aspects of well-being for people over 50, including health information and advocacy (www.aarp.org/health).

- The National Institute on Aging site (www.nia.nih.gov) offers many free publications on health topics, and a searchable "resource directory" for organizations that serve older adults.
- The International Longevity Center–USA, an affiliate of Mount Sinai School of Medicine, has links to the latest publications on aging and related health topics, at www.ilcusa.org.

# Index

# BOOKS BY JUDITH REICHMAN, M.D.

### I'M NOT IN THE MOOD
#### What Every Woman Should Know About Improving Her Libido
ISBN 0-688-17225-3 (paperback)

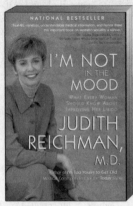

The "hormone of desire," testosterone, acts on the brain to stimulate sexual interest, sensitivity to sexual stimulation, and orgasmic ability in both sexes. Dr. Reichman reveals the effectiveness of small doses of testosterone in reviving sexual desire and pleasure for women.

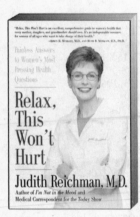

### RELAX, THIS WON'T HURT
#### Painless Answers to Women's Most Pressing Health Questions
ISBN 0-06-095932-0 (paperback)

This book is the ultimate answer for any woman who's ever wished she could spend unlimited time quizzing her doctor during a routine office visit. What's the ideal contraceptive for me? How can I make sure I don't have cancer? What can I do about cramps and PMS? What should I do if I have problems getting pregnant? And much more.

### SLOW YOUR CLOCK DOWN
#### A Woman's Complete Guide to a Younger, Healthier You
ISBN 0-06-052728-5 (paperback)

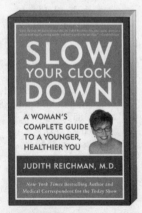

Written especially for women in their forties and fifties, *Slow Your Clock Down* shows them how to extend the minutes and hours of their bodies' internal and external clocks. While the aging process is inevitable, Dr. Judith Reichman argues that we can offset the effects of genetics by living better and healthier.

---

**Don't miss the next book by your favorite author.**
**Sign up for AuthorTracker by visiting *www.AuthorTracker.com*.**

**Available wherever books are sold, or call 1-800-331-3761 to order.**